The European health report 2009
Health and health systems

The World Health Organization was established in 1948 as the specialized agency of the United Nations serving as the directing and coordinating authority for international health matters and public health. One of WHO's constitutional functions is to provide objective and reliable information and advice in the field of human health. It fulfils this responsibility in part through its publications programmes, seeking to help countries make policies that benefit public health and address their most pressing public health concerns.

The WHO Regional Office for Europe is one of six regional offices throughout the world, each with its own programme geared to the particular health problems of the countries it serves. The European Region embraces some 880 million people living in an area stretching from the Arctic Ocean in the north and the Mediterranean Sea in the south and from the Atlantic Ocean in the west to the Pacific Ocean in the east. The European programme of WHO supports all countries in the Region in developing and sustaining their own health policies, systems and programmes; preventing and overcoming threats to health; preparing for future health challenges; and advocating and implementing public health activities.

To ensure the widest possible availability of authoritative information and guidance on health matters, WHO secures broad international distribution of its publications and encourages their translation and adaptation. By helping to promote and protect health and prevent and control disease, WHO's books contribute to achieving the Organization's principal objective – the attainment by all people of the highest possible level of health.

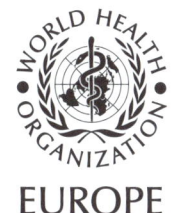

The European health report 2009

Health and health systems

WHO Library Cataloguing in Publication Data

The European health report 2009 : health and health systems.

1. Health status 2. Health status indicators 3. Mortality – statistics 4. Morbidity – statistics 5. Delivery of health care – organization and administration 6. Regional health planning 7. Health policy 8. Europe

ISBN 978 92 890 1415 1 (print) NLM Classification: WA 900
ISBN 978 92 890 1416 8 (ebook)

ISBN 978 92 890 1415 1

> Address requests about publications of the WHO Regional Office for Europe to:
>
> > Publications
> > WHO Regional Office for Europe
> > Scherfigsvej 8
> > DK-2100 Copenhagen Ø, Denmark
>
> Alternatively, complete an online request form for documentation, health information, or for permission to quote or translate, on the Regional Office web site (http://www.euro.who.int/pubrequest).

© **World Health Organization 2009**
All rights reserved. The Regional Office for Europe of the World Health Organization welcomes requests for permission to reproduce or translate its publications, in part or in full.

The designations employed and the presentation of the material in this publication do not imply the expression of any opinion whatsoever on the part of the World Health Organization concerning the legal status of any country, territory, city or area or of its authorities, or concerning the delimitation of its frontiers or boundaries. Dotted lines on maps represent approximate border lines for which there may not yet be full agreement.

The mention of specific companies or of certain manufacturers' products does not imply that they are endorsed or recommended by the World Health Organization in preference to others of a similar nature that are not mentioned. Errors and omissions excepted, the names of proprietary products are distinguished by initial capital letters.

All reasonable precautions have been taken by the World Health Organization to verify the information contained in this publication. However, the published material is being distributed without warranty of any kind, either express or implied. The responsibility for the interpretation and use of the material lies with the reader. In no event shall the World Health Organization be liable for damages arising from its use. The views expressed by authors, editors, or expert groups do not necessarily represent the decisions or the stated policy of the World Health Organization.

Contents

Contributors vii
Abbreviations.. viii
   Technical terms viii
   Country groups... viii
Foreword ix

Part 1. Introduction... 1
   Aims of the report 3
   Structure of the report 4
   References 5

Part 2. Health in the European Region 7
   Key health status indicators: averages and trends 8
      Life expectancy 8
      Mortality 13
      Burden of disease... 26
      Challenges for the future 30
   Factors influencing health 31
      Environment and health... 31
      Lifestyle and behaviour 39
      Social determinants of health.. 44
   Current and future challenges 50
      Changing demographics in the European Region 51
      Mitigating the burden of communicable diseases 56
      Continuing rise of chronic diseases.. 63
      Rising health care costs 70
   Health systems' role in improving population health 73
      Improving health outcomes 74
      Increasing coverage and financial protection 81
      Reducing inequity in health and access to health care 88
      Contributing to health and societal well-being 93
   References 96

Part 3. Strengthening health systems 113
   Investing in health systems 114
      Delivering integrated and cost-effective services 114
      Investing in human and capital resources 118
   Reinvigorating primary care in Europe for people-centred services................ 121
      Putting people first: the meaning of people-centred care 121
      Diversity of primary care in the WHO European Region............................ 122
      Achieving people-centred care in the WHO European Region 122
      Overcoming challenges to people-centred care: European examples........ 126
   Sustaining performance through health financing policy................................. 128
      Reallocating public funds to health despite tighter fiscal constraints 128

Strategic purchasing of health care: resources allocated to providers linked with
performance information or population needs 133
Conclusion 136
Exercising stewardship for healthy public policies 136
Stewardship and health systems 137
Examples of stewardship for healthy public policies in practice................................. 138
Health in all policies: instruments and challenges 139
Conclusion 141
Assessing health system performance for accountability 141
Accountability for better health outcomes and health system stewardship 142
Assessing health system performance in European countries 143
International trends, key challenges and the way forward 146
References 147

Part 4. Annex 157
Table 1. Population of the WHO European Region, 2007 (or latest available year)
and 2020 (projected) 158
Table 2. Basic socioeconomic indicators in the WHO European Region,
2007 or latest available year 159
Table 3. Improving health outcomes in the WHO European Region 160
Table 4. Factors influencing health – environment, lifestyle and behaviour –
in the WHO European Region, 2007 or latest available year 161
Table 5. Health system financing, immunization and Stop TB Strategy
in the WHO European Region 162
Table 6. Human resources for health in the WHO European Region,
2007 or latest available year 163
Table 7. Health service delivery in the WHO European Region,
2007 or latest available year 164
Definitions of the indicators included in the tables 165

Contributors

The European health report 2009 was produced under the overall direction of Enis Barış, Director, Division of Country Health Systems at the WHO Regional Office for Europe, and staff of the Health Intelligence Services unit: Enrique Loyola, Anatoliy Nosikov and Govin Permanand. The contributors (listed below in alphabetical order) were, except where otherwise indicated, staff of the Regional Office at the time that the report was prepared.

The writers and principal contributors were: Sara Allin (University of Toronto, Canada), Enis Barış, Jill Farrington (University of Leeds, United Kingdom), Ann-Lise Guisset, Matthew Jowett, Theadora Koller, Joseph Kutzin, Jeffrey Lazarus, Julia Lear, Enrique Loyola, Francesco Mitis, Anatoliy Nosikov, Martina Pellny, Govin Permanand, Michaela Schiøtz (University of Copenhagen, Denmark), Mike Sedgley, Sarah Simpson and Jeremy Veillard.

Other contributions came from: Roberta Andraghetti, Franklin Apfel (World Health Communication Associates, United Kingdom), Andrea Bertola, Chris Brown, Cristina Comunian, Mikhail Ejov, Tamás Evetovits, Josep Figueras, Bernhard Gibis (Kassenärztliche Bundesvereinigung (KBV), Germany), Michala Hegermann-Lindencrone, Sonja Kahlmeier, Michal Krzyzanowski, Suszy Lessof, Rebecca Martin, Martin McKee (London School of Hygiene and Tropical Medicine, United Kingdom), Lars Møller, Ole Norgaard, Francesca Racioppi, Annemarie Rinder Stengaard, Marc Suhrcke (University of East Anglia, United Kingdom), Srdan Matic, Brenda Van den Bergh, Martin van den Boom, Trudy Wijnhoven, Isabel Yordi and Erio Ziglio.

The WHO Regional Director for Europe, Marc Danzon, and the Deputy Regional Director, Nata Menabde, contributed suggestions, comments and criticism. Other support in preparation of the report was provided by Grace Magnusson, Hanne Wessel-Tolvig and Kate Willows Frantzen.

We at the WHO Regional Office for Europe would like to extend a special note of appreciation to Anatoliy Nosikov not only for his work on this report and several of its predecessors but also for his 20 years of service to the Organization. We wish him well in his retirement.

Abbreviations

Technical terms

BMI	body mass index (weight in kg divided by height in m^2)
DALYs	disability-adjusted life-years
DOTS	WHO-recommended strategy for tuberculosis control
ECDC	European Centre for Disease Prevention and Control
GP	general practitioner
GDP	gross domestic product
MCV1	first dose of measles-containing vaccine
MDGs	Millennium Development Goals
MDR-TB	multidrug-resistant tuberculosis
NHS	National Health Service (United Kingdom)
OECD	Organisation for Economic Co-operation and Development
PPP	purchasing power parity
SDR	age-standardized death rate
TB	tuberculosis
THE PEP	Transport, Health and Environment Pan-European Programme
UNECE	United Nations Economic Commission for Europe

Country groups

CARK	central Asian republics and Kazakhstan: Kyrgyzstan, Tajikistan, Turkmenistan, Uzbekistan and Kazakhstan
CIS	Commonwealth of Independent States, comprising Armenia, Azerbaijan, Belarus, Georgia, Kazakhstan, Kyrgyzstan, the Republic of Moldova, the Russian Federation, Tajikistan, Turkmenistan, Ukraine and Uzbekistan when the data were collected
EU	European Union
EU15	15 countries in the EU before 1 May 2004
EU12	12 countries joining the EU since 1 May 2004
Eur-A	27 countries with very low child and adult mortality: Andorra, Austria, Belgium, Croatia, Cyprus, the Czech Republic, Denmark, Finland, France, Germany, Greece, Iceland, Ireland, Israel, Italy, Luxembourg, Malta, Monaco, the Netherlands, Norway, Portugal, San Marino, Slovenia, Spain, Sweden, Switzerland and the United Kingdom
Eur-B	17 countries with low child and adult mortality: Albania, Armenia, Azerbaijan, Bosnia and Herzegovina, Bulgaria, Georgia, Kyrgyzstan, Montenegro, Poland, Romania, Serbia, Slovakia, Tajikistan, the former Yugoslav Republic of Macedonia, Turkey, Turkmenistan and Uzbekistan
Eur-C	9 countries with low child but high adult mortality: Belarus, Estonia, Hungary, Kazakhstan, Latvia, Lithuania, Republic of Moldova, the Russian Federation and Ukraine

Foreword

Investing in health and health systems is especially important during times of crisis. The WHO Regional Office for Europe has worked with Member States to improve health system performance for several years. Now, more than ever, health systems must meet increased demand and expectations in the face of global challenges and crises. Some experts emphasize the "four Fs": the fuel, food, flu and financial crises. Nevertheless, additional trends affect health, such as climate change and populations' longer life expectancy. Meanwhile, the cost of pharmaceuticals and health care technologies continues to rise. All these factors affect the long-term financial sustainability of health systems.

To address these issues, governments and policy-makers must have access to information that is current, accurate, comparable and digestible. Policy-makers across the WHO European Region are working to improve the collection, analysis and reporting of health indicators and information. The fragmentation of measurement and monitoring systems often frustrates policy-making at different levels of government and health systems. The Regional Office supports health ministries and governments in making use of better information on public health and health system performance to steer effective reforms in a complex environment.

The European health report 2009 *is designed to provide Member States with essential public health information. The Regional Office's main objective continues to be to support countries in choosing the best possible investments in health based on current knowledge, and we hope that the report will thus encourage them to use the best available evidence when designing policies to ensure universal access to high-quality care despite today's challenges. In this regard, we further hope that the report will be a resource not only for health ministries but also for our partners, inside and outside government, working to promote health. Indeed, as Jonas Gahr Støre, Norway's Minister of Foreign Affairs, stated at a meeting in Oslo in April 2009 on health in times of global economic crisis: "at the end, we are all, in one way or another, ministers of human health".*

Marc Danzon
WHO Regional Director for Europe

Part 1.
Introduction

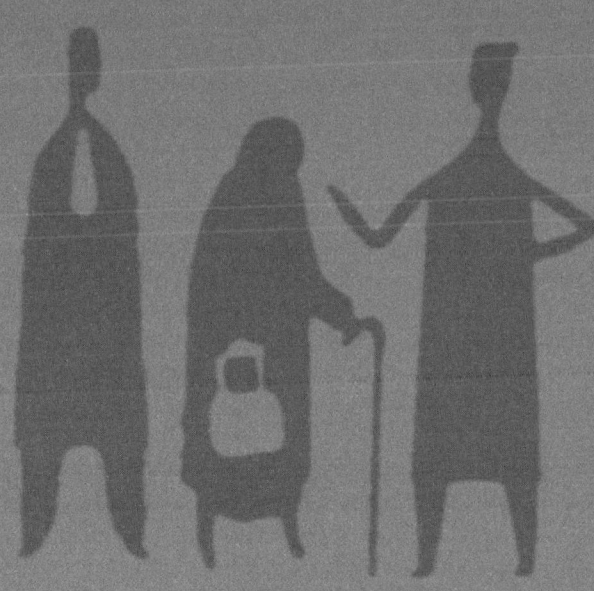

The WHO European Region includes 53 Member States and nearly 900 million people living in diverse cultural, economic, social and political circumstances. Although the Region has the highest average score on the Human Development Index of any WHO region, significant inequity remains within and between countries or population groups, especially in health; inequity in health is the avoidable and unjust systematic differences in health status between groups in a given society (1). How well do Member States in the Region fulfil their aim of promoting health and reducing inequity, given the demographic, epidemiological, technological, environmental, socioeconomic and fiscal challenges that they face?

The European health report 2009 reviews and assesses public health indicators and trends during the past four years. Since 2005, European governments have taken a health systems approach towards combating ill health, promoting healthy lifestyles and reducing inequality in health. This report reflects the fact that the European Region is experiencing great change, internally through reforms of health systems and externally due to global crises, causing great uncertainty in both health systems and outcomes. Although several global trends affect health, the global economic recession and the new pandemic (H1N1) 2009 influenza are the most acute.

First, the severe economic crisis will have many implications and long-term consequences: economic growth seems unlikely to recover soon, and debt may constrain public finances for years to come. Slowing economic activity and rapidly rising unemployment seriously threaten or already affect the living conditions of millions of individuals and families in the European Region and the revenue base of health and social protection schemes. Experience from previous economic recessions suggests the vital importance of ensuring a high degree of solidarity and social security, maintaining public expenditure and basic health services and scaling up disease prevention and health promotion activities.

On 1–2 April 2009, the WHO Regional Office for Europe, in cooperation with the Norwegian Ministry of Health and Care Services and the Norwegian Directorate for Health, held a high-level meeting called Health in times of global economic crisis: implications for the WHO European Region (2). The participants agreed that all economic recovery packages must explicitly include health-related action. Health systems are not merely an important part of social protection networks but also an intelligent actor in the economy, as the Tallinn Charter: Health Systems for Health and Wealth (3) emphasizes. The WHO Regional Office for Europe has to exercise strong leadership in aligning the agendas of stakeholders in joint collaboration.

The second challenge is the pandemic (H1N1) 2009 influenza. The emergence of the pandemic virus was first detected in late April 2009; as of 20 November 2009, over 206 countries and overseas territories or communities have reported laboratory-confirmed cases of pandemic (H1N1) 2009 influenza, including over 6770 deaths. As many countries have stopped counting individual cases, particularly of milder illness, the case count is likely to be significantly lower than the actual number of cases. WHO declared a pandemic in June 2009, reflecting the geographical spread and reach of the virus, not its severity.

This is a new influenza A(H1N1) virus that has never before circulated among humans and is not related to previous or current human seasonal influenza viruses. It appears primarily to affect people aged 25–45 years or under 15 years, while most seasonal influenza predominantly affects older people. Most cases seem to be mild and self-limited and do not require admission to hospital. Nevertheless, many Member States are experiencing significant strains on their health care delivery systems as they face sharp increases in demand for services. International experience of the pandemic (H1N1) 2009, especially in the southern hemisphere, has shown that poor clinical outcomes are associated with delays in seeking health care and limited access to supportive care. In addition, the virus has shown its ability to cause rapidly progressive, overwhelming lung disease, which is very difficult to treat. WHO recommends prioritizing the prompt use of antivirals to treat individuals at risk of severe or fatal disease associated with pandemic (H1N1) 2009 virus infection.

By late November 2009, countries throughout the European Region reported high or very high intensity of influenza transmission, especially in children up to the age of 15 years, with 652 deaths since April 2009. Vaccination campaigns had started in 17 countries and 8 countries were eligible to receive vaccine donated to WHO.

The influenza pandemic confirms, once again, that ill health has no borders. It is testing the 2005 International Health Regulations *(4)* for the first time in a public health emergency affecting multiple countries and is providing important lessons on the importance of preparing people and institutions for such emergencies. Key features of the response have included real-time exchange of information and a multistakeholder approach. Many countries affected so far have stressed the importance of universal access to health care and the need for strong primary health care.

Health systems are vital at all stages of the response to the pandemic: detecting and confirming cases, providing care, treatment and advice to the people affected and coordinating with other sectors to maximize impact. WHO has worked closely with countries in the European Region to support the capacity of their health systems, activating their pandemic preparedness plans and strengthening their response capacity. Investment in health systems is proving essential in responding to this and other threats and in saving lives.

Aims of the report

This report summarizes facts and public health trends in the European Region and discusses the strengthening of health systems in each of their functions: service delivery, resource generation, financing and stewardship. The Annex provides some of the data used in the analysis and conclusions on the current and future health challenges in the European Region. The evidence presented includes:

- the burden of disease from specified conditions;
- how strongly specific risk factors affect specific diseases and conditions;
- selected public health interventions that can clearly improve health if the contextual factors for successful implementation are considered; and
- the role of health systems in addressing the myriad health issues in the Region.

In 2008, health ministers of the countries in the European Region adopted the Tallinn Charter *(3,5)*. It highlights the importance of health systems in producing health and wealth, provides guidance and a value-based strategic framework for strengthening health systems in the Region, offers a platform for regional and national policy dialogue and urges political commitment and action from all Member States. Two recent follow-up meetings have discussed implementation of the Tallinn Charter. In February 2009, Member States agreed to work with WHO to develop a framework for health system performance assessment and a platform to share and learn from their experiences *(6)*. In April 2009, the participants at the high-level meeting, Health in times of global economic crisis, made 12 recommendations to minimize the negative health effects and to strengthen the performance of health systems during the severe economic recession *(2)*. These recommendations emphasize a commitment to the principles of the Tallinn Charter and the importance of health ministries' leadership in ensuring that health issues are high on the economic and social agendas and that governments recognize that every minister is a health minister.

Structure of the report

Part 2 of the report describes current health trends, factors influencing health, present and future challenges and health systems' role in contributing to improved population health in the European Region. Although health status indicators such as mortality continue to improve in the Region, subregions and groups within countries still have dramatic differences in health closely linked to demographic or economic transition or degrees of social disadvantage. Examples of widening gaps include the alarming spread of multidrug-resistant tuberculosis (TB) and environmental health problems due to air pollution in urban industrial centres and the combustion of solid fuel in homes. Intersectoral action and multifaceted strategies should ensure a focus on disadvantaged groups to minimize these disparities.

Trends pose present and future challenges to health policy-makers. Low fertility levels, increasing ageing and immigration could place additional demographic pressure on health and welfare systems. Emerging and re-emerging epidemic infections place additional burdens on the capacity of public health to prevent, detect and respond to the spread of communicable diseases. Modern lifestyles and behaviour are leading to growth in chronic diseases and conditions such as obesity, hypertension and diabetes. Average health care expenditure in the European Region rose from 7.4% of gross domestic product (GDP) in 1998 to 7.7% in 2005. Rising incomes may also raise individuals' expectations for newer and more expensive health technologies.

Health systems must be dynamic and flexible enough to anticipate or respond to these health trends, as well as emergent external factors such as the severe economic recession or the outbreak of a new influenza virus. Health systems have the essential role of improving health outcomes by delivering health care and by providing intersectoral leadership and coordination. Within the European Region, health ministries are committed to ensuring that everyone can use the services they need without becoming impoverished by out-of-pocket health expenditure. Significant progress has also been made towards identifying action to address socially determined inequity in health and to derive principles on good practices and criteria for assessing projects designed to reduce inequality in access to health care. Policy-makers setting priorities for health care expenditure could also consider that increased spending on effective health care contributes substantially to a more productive economy and to improving health and well-being. Strengthening health systems based on sound evidence of cost–effectiveness and performance assessment provides the potential to improve health, increase wealth and enhance societal well-being.

Part 3 of the report further demonstrates that governments in the European Region have undertaken a process of wide-ranging reform to improve health systems' performance within all four functions: service delivery, resource generation, financing and stewardship. One area of special attention has been the renewed commitment to modernize primary health care as a coordinated, integrated, people-centred and comprehensive service. The reform process is conveying a clear message that health-financing policy should focus on policy objectives and not on implementing specific mechanisms. Financing policy should aim to sustain good health system performance, orienting the system in accordance with the underlying values of equity, solidarity and participation while managing resources in a fiscally responsible manner.

Member States in the Region differ widely in the availability and quality of data, accountability structures and processes, citizens' participation and the transparency and maturity of their culture of performance measurement and continuous quality improvement. The Regional Office supports health ministries and governments in using better performance information to steer complex reforms in environments with growing financial constraints and rising expectations.

Focusing on health systems can improve health outcomes now and in the future. It is hoped that this report will encourage the successful implementation of effective health system reforms and policies that will improve health systems' performance in providing efficient, patient-centred, high-quality health care.

References

1. Equity [web site]. Geneva, World Health Organization, 2009 (http://www.who.int/healthsystems/topics/equity/en, accessed 28 June 2009).
2. *Health in times of global economic crisis: implications for the WHO European Region, Oslo, Norway, 1–2 April 2009. Meeting report.* Copenhagen, WHO Regional Office for Europe, 2009 (http://www.euro.who.int/document/HSM/Oslo_report.pdf, accessed 28 June 2009).
3. *The Tallinn Charter: Health Systems for Health and Wealth.* Copenhagen, WHO Regional Office for Europe, 2008 (http://www.euro.who.int/document/e91438.pdf, accessed 28 June 2009).
4. *International Health Regulations (2005)*, 2nd ed. Geneva, World Health Organization, 2005 (http://www.who.int/ihr/9789241596664, accessed 28 June 2009).
5. *WHO European Ministerial Conference on Health Systems: "Health Systems, Health and Wealth", Tallinn, Estonia, 25–27 June 2008. Report.* Copenhagen, WHO Regional Office for Europe, 2009 (http://www.euro.who.int/InformationSources/Publications/Catalogue/20090122_1, accessed 28 June 2009).
6. *First Regional Follow-up Meeting on the Tallinn Charter: Health Systems for Health and Wealth, Copenhagen, Denmark, 5–6 February 2009.* Copenhagen, WHO Regional Office for Europe, 2009 (http://www.euro.who.int/healthsystems/20090128_1, accessed 28 June 2009).

Part 2.
Health in the European Region

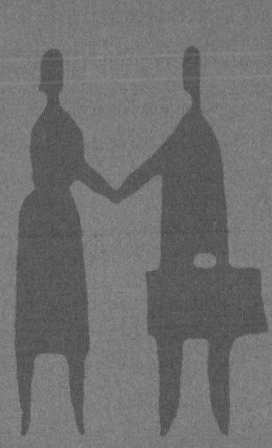

Key health status indicators: averages and trends

The health status of the population in the WHO European Region has improved in the past decades, as indicated by longer life expectancy at birth. Nevertheless, important and growing inequality in longevity is associated with gender and social and economic factors. Gains in life expectancy have been attributed to overall decreasing mortality, mainly from declining communicable diseases in early childhood and delays in premature death among adults due to improved health care *(1)*. In addition, changes in lifestyles and behaviour have led to further changes in the patterns of mortality and the burden of disease, with chronic noncommunicable conditions, injuries and violence affecting health more strongly.

Groups of European countries vary substantially. The Commonwealth of Independent States (CIS), including the central Asian republics and Kazakhstan (CARK), in general have higher mortality and disease rates, which have been linked to demographic, social and economic transitions. The 15 countries in the European Union (EU) before 1 May 2004 (EU15) and the 12 countries joining the EU since 1 May 2004 (EU12) in general have lower mortality and disease rates. As health systems require further delineation of country situations and needs, to adjust and respond accordingly, this section describes mortality and the burden of disease and their recent trends in the Region. While Part 2 of this report discusses patterns and trends for groups of countries, information on many of the topics covered is available for each country in the Region in seven tables in the Annex. The Annex also contains definitions of some of the technical terms used.

Life expectancy

Life expectancy roughly but comprehensively measures overall population health, as it summarizes, in a standardized format, current information on the health situation of all age and sex groups of populations. As such, it reliably indicates overall health performance in a society at a specific time *(2)*. This broad indicator reflects societies' performance in improving health and not solely the performance of health systems. This distinction is key, as it links to public health's greatest idea: that human health and disease embody the successes and failures of society as a whole *(3)*.

The highest life expectancy at birth in the European Region was 82.0 years in Switzerland (2006) and the lowest, 66.4 years in Kazakhstan (2007). Life expectancy for the Region as a whole increased from 73.1 years in 1990 to 75.6 years in 2006 (Table 2.1).

Life expectancy has increased steadily and considerably in the EU countries (Fig. 2.1). Remarkably, the averages for EU15 and EU12 countries have both improved by 5% from already high levels. This reflects a consistent reduction in mortality rates at all ages, due to such factors as higher living standards and educational levels, healthier lifestyles and improved access to and quality of health services.

Unfortunately, the CIS countries have not been able quickly to recover from the rising mortality in the early 1990s. The average life expectancy for these countries deteriorated sharply between 1991 and 1994 and then recovered only partly. Since the late 1990s, the CIS average has essentially stagnated.

Table 2.1. Life expectancy at birth (years) by country group, WHO European Region, 1990 and 2006

Country group	1990	2006	Index in 2006 (%) (1990 = 100%)
European Region	73.1	75.6	103
EU15	76.5	80.3	105
EU12	70.8	74.3	105
CIS	69.7	67.9	97
CARK	69.1	69.1[a]	100

[a] Data for 2005.
Source: European Health for All database (4).

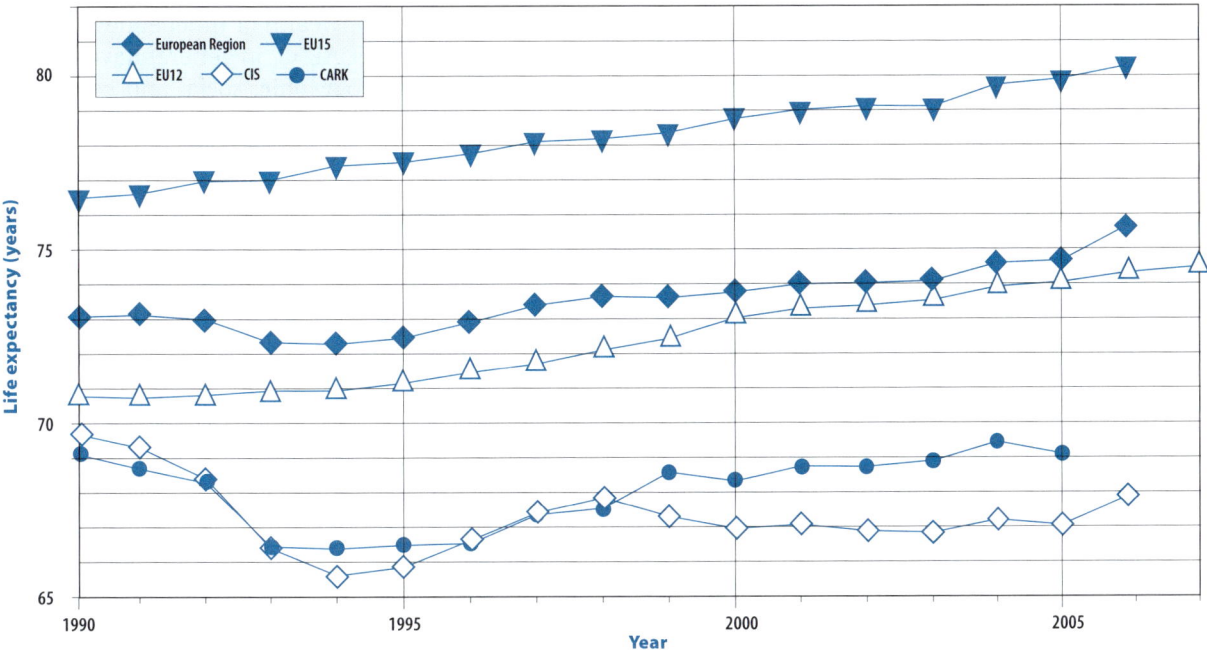

Fig. 2.1. Life expectancy at birth by country group, WHO European Region, 1990–2007

Source: European Health for All database (4).

The Russian Federation's large population strongly influences average life expectancy in the CIS. Many researchers have focused on the unfavourable trends in the country, finding clear associations between life expectancy and socioeconomic trends. For example, the increases in mortality in 1991–1994 and in 1998–2003 paralleled the critical socioeconomic situation in those periods, and the relative declines in mortality in 1994–1998 and 2003–2006 were associated with relative economic improvement (5). Moreover, excessive alcohol intake by much of the population caused much of the premature mortality, particularly among men, although many alcohol-related deaths were wrongly attributed to diseases of the circulatory system (see below) (5).

Nevertheless, several CIS countries (such as Armenia, Azerbaijan, Tajikistan and Uzbekistan) have performed relatively well and been able to improve life expectancy slightly from their 1990 levels (Fig. 2.2). This indicates that, despite converging trends in the past, more recent national policies have made a difference. Comparative analysis is needed to identify the specific

Fig. 2.2. Life expectancy at birth (three-year moving averages), selected CIS countries, 1990–2005

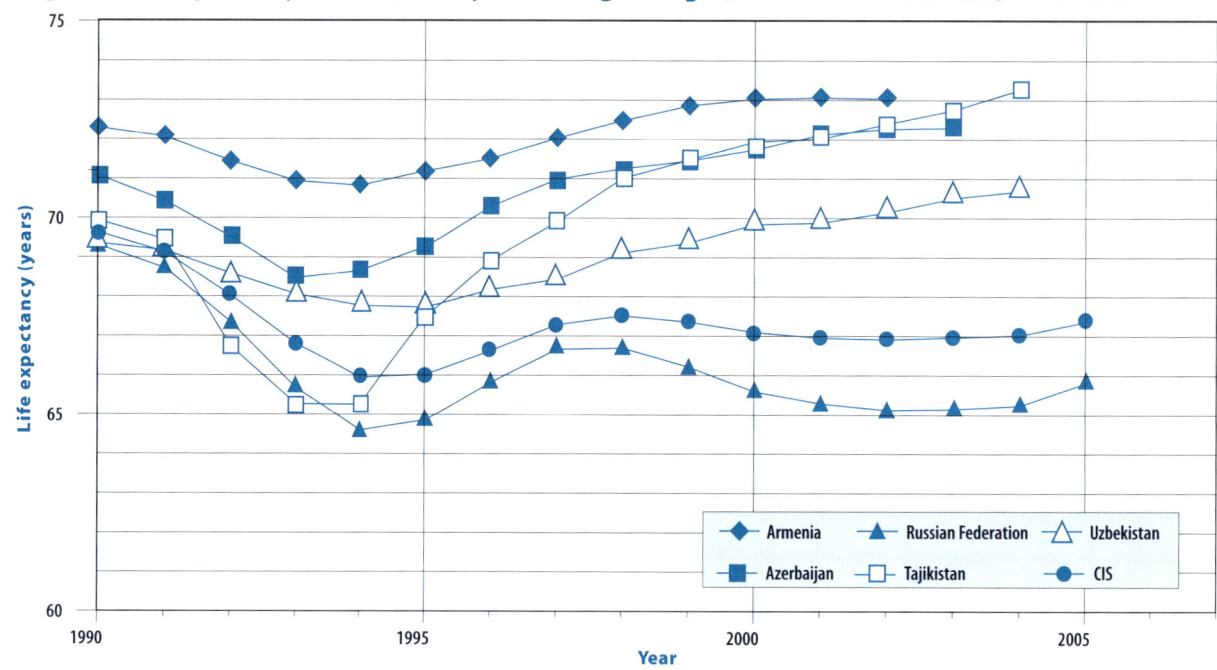

Source: European Health for All database (4).

policies that have played a role in these countries, but research evidence from a broad range of other countries suggests that the policies affecting the socioeconomic circumstances in which people live and work usually have more influence than policies related solely to health care.

The increasing trends in life expectancy in the European Region are similar for people younger and older than 65 years. The reduction or loss of life expectancy from death before 65 years of age is a very useful measure of premature mortality. Table 2.2 shows that, except for CIS countries, the years of life lost to this cause are decreasing in the Region.

Table 2.2. Years of life expectancy lost as the result of death before 65 years of age, WHO European Region, 1990 and 2006

Country group	1990	2006	Index in 2006 (%) (1990 = 100%)
European Region	7.8	6.7	86
EU15	5.6	4.2	75
EU12	8.7	6.9	79
CIS	10.3	11.3	110
CARK	11.5	10.0[a]	87

[a] Data for 2005.
Source: European Health for All database (4).

Estimating the relative contributions of the numerous health-related and other, mainly socioeconomic factors that might affect the variation in life expectancy over time and across countries is difficult. In general, higher national income is associated with higher life expectancy at birth. Expenditure on health services is also important in improving health. Countries with similar levels of income and health expenditure may differ substantially in life expectancy, however, and countries with similar life expectancy may vary considerably in income and health expenditure. Although this is observed globally, the relationships between GDP and health, GDP and total health expenditure, and total health expenditure and health are not necessarily deterministic or linear; some countries have better outcomes than others owing to many other factors, including the performance of their health systems.

For example, Denmark and Portugal have the same life expectancy, but Portugal has 60% of the income and 64% of the health expenditure per person (in international dollars adjusted for purchasing power) as Denmark (Table 2.3). Similarly, Georgia has the same life expectancy as Hungary, but 19% of the income and 24% of the health expenditure. Further, Croatia and Lithuania spend similar amounts on health and have similar GDP, but life expectancy differs by 5 years.

Table 2.3. Comparison of three pairs of countries on life expectancy, income and health expenditure, WHO European Region, 2007 or latest available year

Indicator	Denmark	Portugal	Hungary	Georgia	Croatia	Lithuania
Life expectancy at birth (years)	78.1	78.3	73.0	73.1	76.0	71.0
GDP per person (in US$ PPP[a])	33 973	20 410	17 887	3 365	13 042	14 494
Total health expenditure per person (in US$ PPP)	3 169	2 034	1 329	318	1 001	862

[a] PPP: purchasing power parity (see definition in Annex).
Source: European Health for All database (4).

The Commission on Social Determinants of Health highlights the fundamental but frequently ignored role of the social determinants of health (6,7). The principal driving force behind the differences observed is the differently graded relationships between socioeconomic status and health. This means that societies differ in the gradient, or slope, of the systematic decline in the health status of socioeconomic groups from the top down. The principle is, however, that the slope is not fixed; it changes continually owing to changes in socioeconomic structure, but still persists in all populations across time and space. For example, the political changes in about 1990 in some EU12 countries very clearly enabled them to align their previously stagnant life expectancy trends with the slope of the EU average (Fig. 2.3).

In general, the differential but modifiable effect of socioeconomic status on health influences equity in health. This results in inequity in health between countries and even more so within countries, which can be determined by comparing various indicators.

Gender inequity in health is the first choice of example. According to Marmot (8), "the differential status of men and women in almost every society is perhaps the most pervasive and entrenched inequity". The gender gap in life expectancy was 7.5 years for the European Region in 2006 (Table 2.4): 71.9 years among males and 79.4 years among females. This gender gap in country subgroups in the Region in recent decades has largely changed because of changes in the differences between men and women in risk-taking behaviour and the uptake of preventive and curative health services, which in turn have responded to socioeconomic shifts.

Inequality within countries is greater than that between countries for most factors. The magnitude of the inequality reported depends on the method used. One global study examining more than 9000 life tables (2) concluded that about 90% of the inequality in life expectancy is within countries. In the EU specifically, a comprehensive review of inequality in health (9) found considerable socioeconomic inequality in health. The populations studied differ markedly in the health conditions and determinants of health that are mainly responsible for the health gaps, which also strongly indicates that inequality in health can be reduced.

Fig. 2.3. Life expectancy at birth (three-year moving averages), selected EU12 countries versus the EU15 average, WHO European Region, 1970–2006

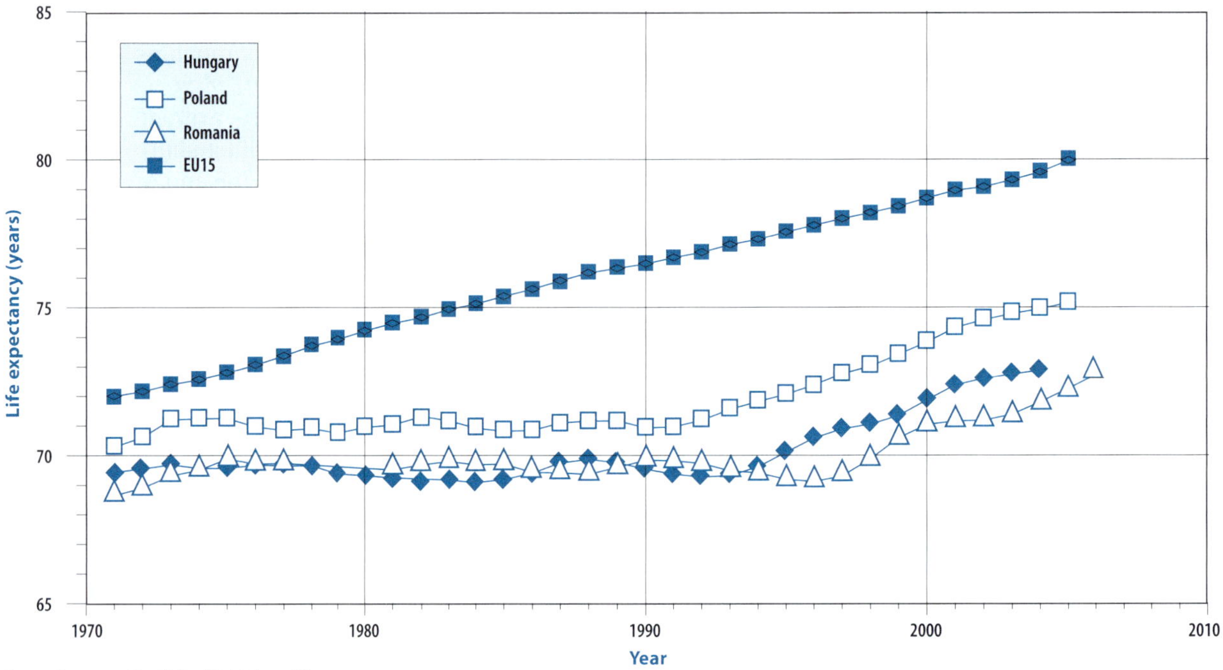

Source: European Health for All database (4).

Table 2.4. Differences in life expectancy at birth (years) among males and females by country group, WHO European Region, 1990 and 2006

Country group	1990	2006	Index in 2006 (%) (1990 = 100%)
European Region	8.0	7.5	94
EU15	6.8	5.7	84
EU12	8.2	8.1	99
CIS	9.6	10.9	114
CARK	7.6	7.1	93

Source: European Health for All database (4).

Life expectancy is not a good measure of health systems' performance. For example, a report on health trends in Norway by the Norwegian Directorate of Health (10) confirmed a conclusion made earlier: that "the increase in life expectancy appears to have been constant for the last 150 years". This constant rate of annual increase is 0.3 years and applies to industrialized countries. As health systems have not had the same effect over time, the constant rate suggests that demonstrating the effects of health system reforms on life expectancy is not easy. Although improved access to effective health care increasingly saves lives, directly linking changes in the mortality rates with the contributions of the health system in terms of disease prevention and therapeutic intervention is often difficult (see the section below on the role of health systems in improving population health). Life expectancy and mortality as currently determined are simply not sensitive enough to monitor how health system reform affects public health (see the section below on measures of avoidable mortality and disability-adjusted life-years).

Various indicators have been used to summarize overall health, such as life expectancy and the effects of disability and disease at different ages. Thus, healthy life expectancy at birth takes account of years lived in less than full health *(11)*. Healthy life expectancy in countries in the European Region varies similarly to life expectancy at birth, differing by as much as 21 years among males (range: 74–53) and 19 years among females (range: 76–57) in 2007 *(12)*. In addition, although women live an average of 7.5 years longer than men, the average difference in healthy life expectancy is only 5 years, meaning that women live a smaller share of their lives in good health or free of disability than men (Fig. 2.4). Thus, towards the end of life, women have accumulated a larger burden of ill health than men as a result of both longer longevity and multiple illnesses. In general, healthy life expectancy is nearly 20% lower in the CIS countries (median 58.0 and 61.5 years for males and females, respectively) than in the EU15. This inequality has been suggested to be associated with such socioeconomic factors as educational levels and health expenditure by the public sector (as a percentage of both GDP and total government expenditure) *(13)*. Health information systems therefore need to be improved by introducing, on a large scale, the available non-mortality-based indicators that can verify the specific and potentially invaluable contributions of health systems to overall population health. The expected rewards for the ever-increasing spending on health systems must be demonstrated to the public. This information is also crucial for managing health reforms responsibly. Efforts to strengthen health systems without good measurement and monitoring could unnecessarily waste capacity and resources. Improving information systems requires dedicated resources, but the damage that societies suffer from poor health monitoring and a lack of evaluation undoubtedly costs more in the long term.

The future challenges to health systems are often discussed in relation to the continuing increase in life expectancy and the resulting ageing of the population. Increasing life expectancy, in combination with stable or decreasing fertility rates, will increase the proportion of the population older than 65 years. The need for health care services increases as people age, and increases in the use and thus costs of health care are therefore often predicted. These predictions may, however, be overstated *(14)* and are addressed below.

Mortality

Mortality is a robust indicator of a population's health situation that is widely used in the European Region. In some parts of the Region, however, registries have poor coverage and quality, requiring that available figures be treated with a degree of caution. The overall mortality rate from all causes of death in the Region gradually declined during the past decade to reach an average age-standardized death rate (SDR) of 888.2 per 100 000 population in 2006. The rates vary significantly, increasing from the countries in the western part of the Region to the eastern countries (Fig. 2.5) *(15)*.

Since the mid-1990s, overall mortality in the European Region has followed two trends: decreasing in EU countries, with an SDR 20–25% lower in 2006, and stagnant or increasing in the CIS countries (including CARK), with an SDR nearly 10–15% higher (Table 2.5). In addition, males (SDR: 1177.9) have 75% higher mortality than females (SDR: 672.9) in the Region as a whole, but the excess is larger in the CIS countries (90%) than in the EU15 countries (61%). Mortality has increased substantially in the CIS countries with more than 10 million population, with SDRs increasing nearly 35% in Belarus, Kazakhstan, the Russian Federation and Ukraine between 1990 and 2006. Mortality decreased by more than 10%

Fig. 2.4. Estimated life expectancy at birth and healthy life expectancy among males and females, WHO European Region, 2007

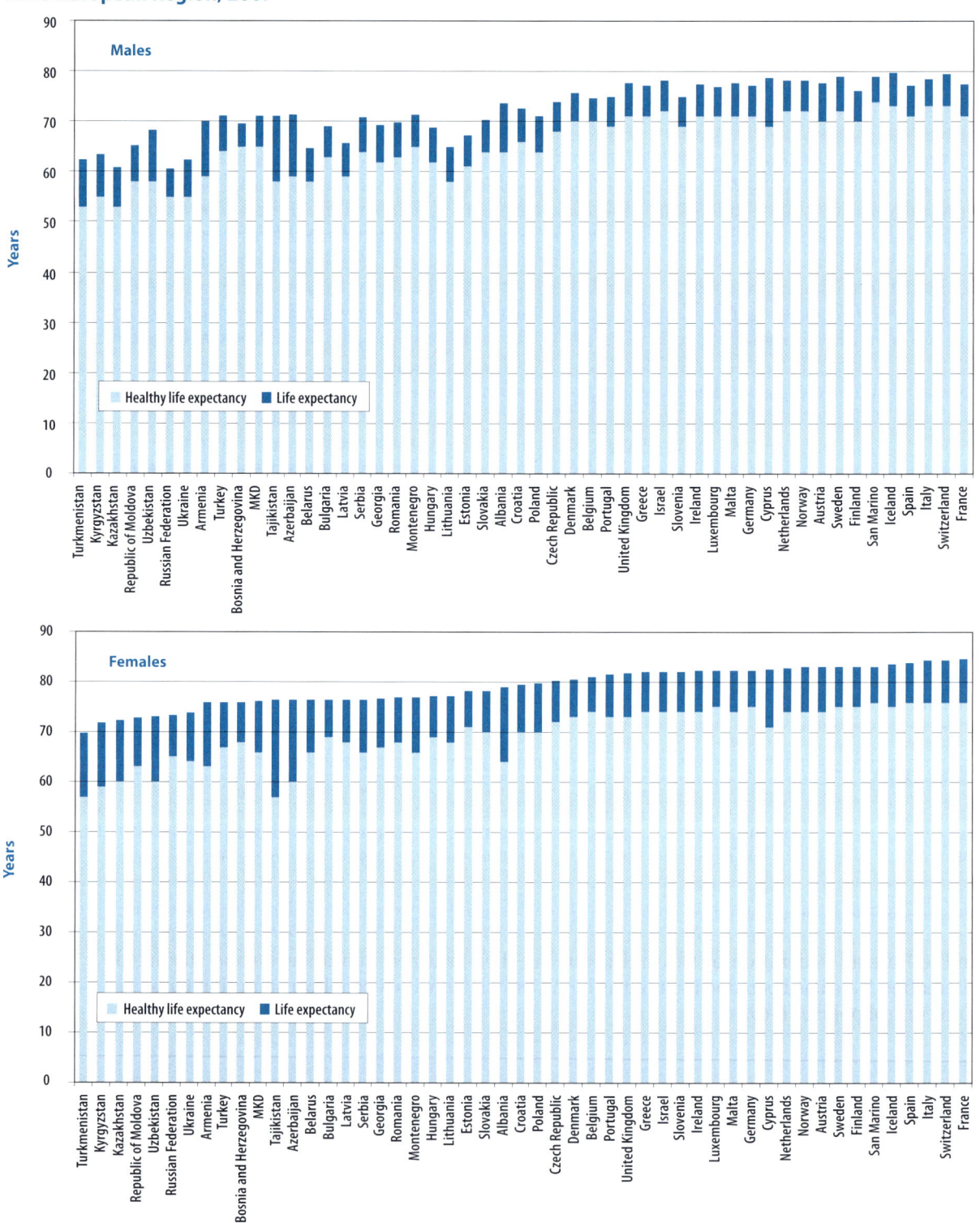

Note. MKD is the International Organization for Standardization (ISO) abbreviation for the former Yugoslav Republic of Macedonia.
Source: World health statistics 2009 (12).

Fig. 2.5. Mortality from all causes: SDRs per 100 000 population, WHO European Region, 2007 or latest available year

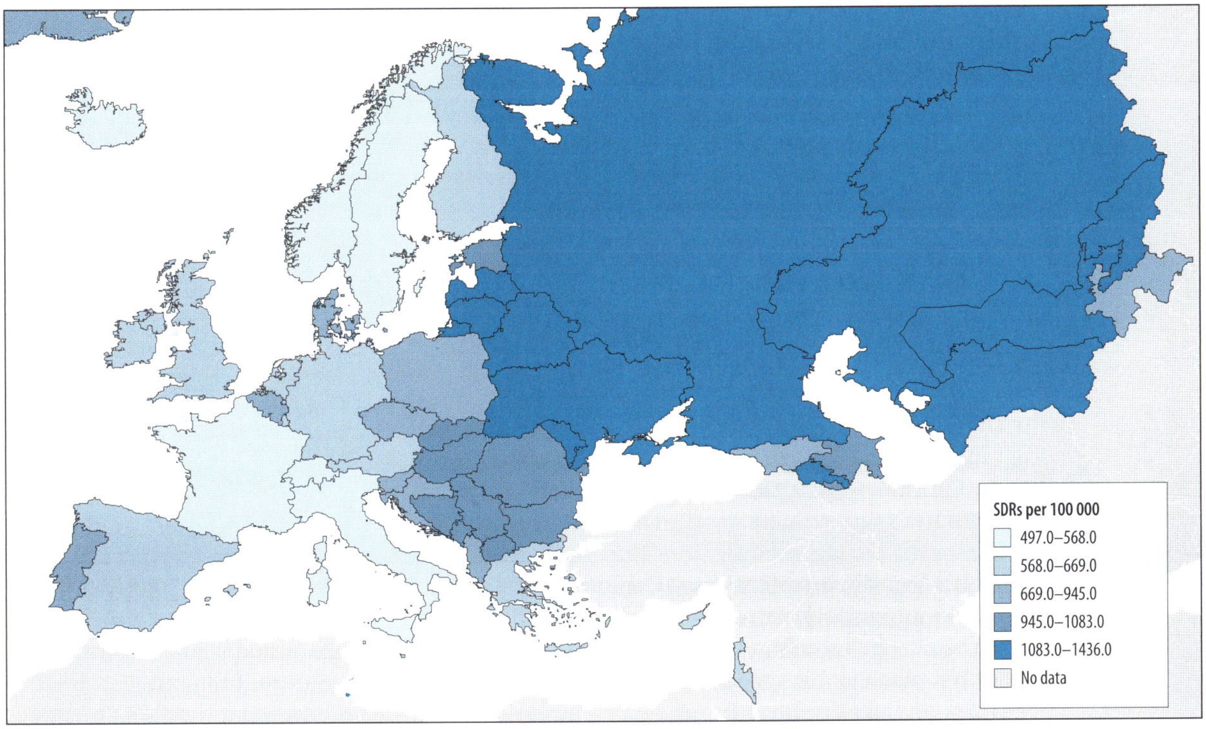

Source: European mortality database *(15)*.

Table 2.5. Mortality from all causes: population-weighted SDRs per 100 000 population by country group, WHO European Region, 1990–2006

Country group	1990	1995	2000	2005	2006	Index in 2006 (%) (1990 = 100%)
European Region	967.1	1038.3	964.2	926.1	888.2	92
EU15	780.4	722.1	658.2	599.9	580.7	74
EU12	1141.1	1124.9	1003.9	944.8	923.7	81
CIS	1154.4	1448.6	1375.8	1394.6	1326.6	115
CARK	1107.6	1366.7	1266.7	1240.0	NA	112[a]

Note. NA: not available.
[a] Figure for 2005.
Source: European mortality database *(15)*.

in the Russian Federation by the mid-1990s but then returned to peak levels and stagnated thereafter. This has been documented as being associated with alcohol consumption patterns and control policies *(16)*.

Age groups affected

Mortality rates in the European Region tend to increase with age, although patterns differ according to country group (Fig. 2.6). For example, CIS countries and CARK have higher mortality rates than the Region as a whole regardless of age, but the rates tend to converge at older ages. In addition, mortality rates among younger people in CARK are more than twice the rates for the Region as a whole, suggesting the impact of communicable diseases. In CIS countries, the mortality rates peak among the economically active population, which suggests associations with cardiovascular diseases, injuries and violence.

Fig. 2.6. Age-specific mortality: population-weighted SDRs per 100 000 population and rate ratios by country group, WHO European Region, 2007 or latest available data

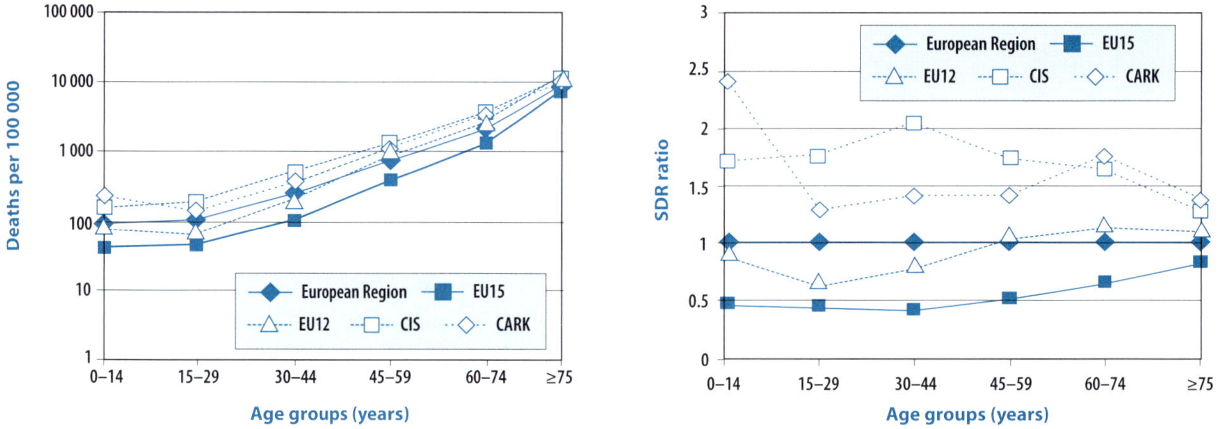

Source: European mortality database *(15)*.

Mortality rates by age group in the European Region have decreased overall, but not in all countries. Although mortality has decreased among children younger than 15 years in all groups of countries, the differences among adults are dramatic, with either slower decreases or increases in the 1990s, especially in CIS countries. The relative magnitude of rates still differs substantially by age group (Fig. 2.7). These differences show inequality in health, suggesting an association with lifestyles and access to health care among adult and older population groups.

Infant and maternal mortality

Infant mortality before 1 year of age indicates living conditions and access to health care. It has fallen by more than 50% since 1990 in the European Region. The rate for the Region in 2006 was 7.3 deaths per 1000 live births (Table 2.6). Although the declines have been similar across country groups, rates still differ greatly, varying from a low rate ratio, compared with the Region, of 0.54 in the EU15 countries to 2.43 in the CARK.

Maternal mortality indicates access to and the quality of health care. It declined to 12.9 deaths per 100 000 live births in the European Region in 2006, nearly 50% of the 1990 level (Table 2.7). The decline has been steepest in the EU12 (nearly 75%) and lowest in the EU15 (30%), even though the latter have 60% lower maternal mortality than the Region as a whole. In contrast, ratios in CIS countries (including the CARK) are twice as high, suggesting health care problems. Haemorrhage, abortion and toxaemia combined, which are mostly preventable, account for nearly 40% of maternal deaths in CIS countries and 30% in the CARK (data not shown), further substantiating this view.

The Millennium Development Goals (MDGs) are intended to break the cycle of poverty and ill health by establishing targets for countries to achieve by 2015, with a starting year of 1990 *(17)*. MDG 4 aims to reduce the mortality of children younger than 5 years by two thirds and MDG 5, to reduce the maternal mortality ratio by three quarters. This acknowledges that most of these deaths are preventable. Child mortality in the European Region is the lowest of any WHO region, and there is an overall trend towards achieving the MDG 4 target in the Region.

Fig. 2.7. Mortality from all causes: population-weighted SDRs per 100 000 population by age and country groups, WHO European Region, 1981–2006

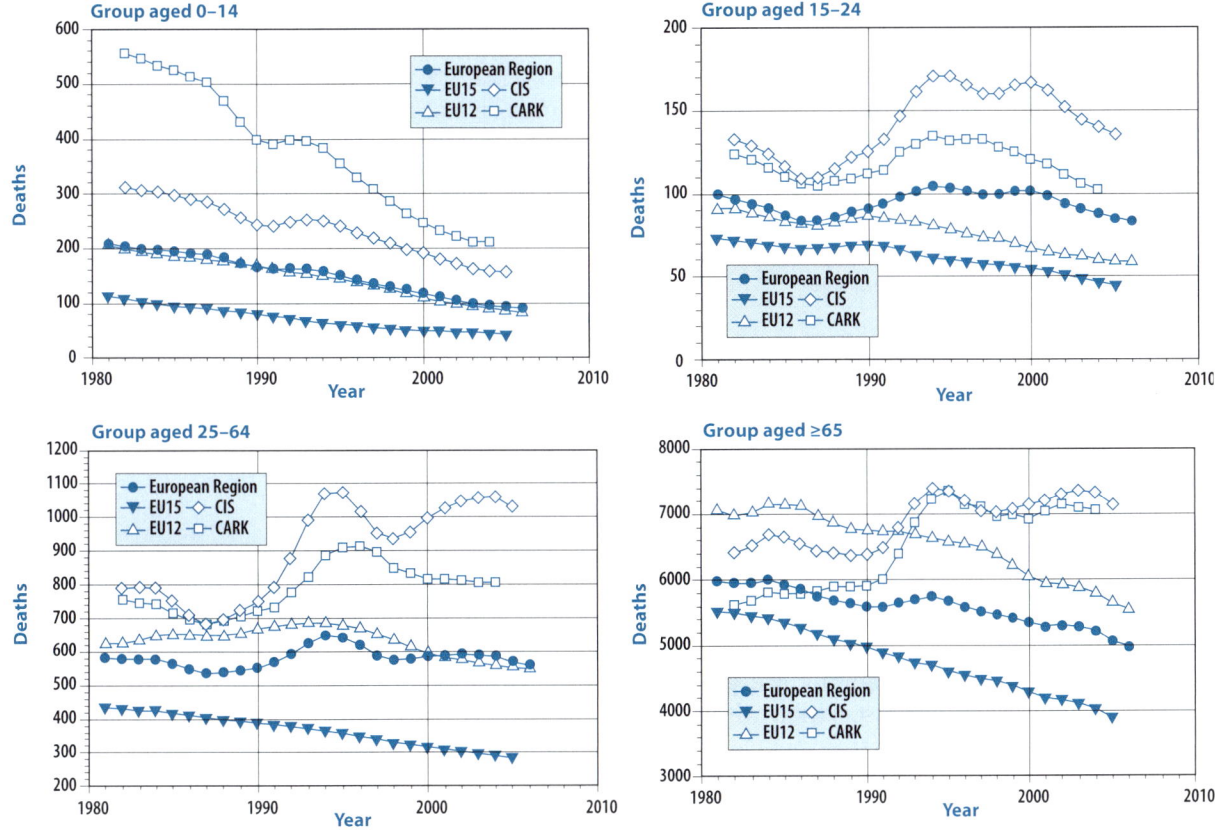

Source: European mortality database (15).

Table 2.6. Population-weighted infant mortality rates per 1000 live births by country group, WHO European Region, 1990–2006

Country group	1990	2006	Index in 2006 (%) (1990 = 100%)	Rate ratio (European Region = 1)
European Region	15.4	7.3	47	1.0
EU15	7.6	4.0	52	0.5
EU12	16.9	7.9	46	1.1
CIS	22.3	12.8	57	1.8
CARK	33.8	17.7	52[a]	2.4[a]

[a] Figure for 2005.
Source: European mortality database (15).

Table 2.7. Population-weighted maternal mortality rates per 100 000 live births by country group, WHO European Region, 1990–2006

Country group	1990	2000	2005	2006	Index in 2006 (%) (1990 = 100%)	Rate ratio (European Region = 1)
European Region	25.1	18.6	14.3	12.9	52	1.0
EU15	7.8	5.3	4.9	5.6	71	0.4
EU12	29.3	16.5	8.8	8.0	27	0.6
CIS	44.9	39.2	28.2	27.4	61	2.1
CARK	55.3	43.8	36.7	NA	67[a]	2.8[a]

Note. NA: not available.
[a] Figures for 2005.
Source: European mortality database (15).

Nevertheless, child mortality varies between and within countries. For example, it is declining more slowly in the CIS countries, and five of them are unlikely to reach the target. Three more may reach it only with additional effort.

The situation of maternal mortality and MDG 5 is more variable. Similar to child mortality, four CIS countries have higher rates and are not on track to reach the target, and four more may be able to attain it if they increase their efforts. Some EU countries that already have low mortality rates face their own difficulties, with four showing increases between 1990 and 2000. On the positive side, the maternal mortality ratio in Turkey fell by about 90%. In 1973, Turkey's ratio was more than 8 times the average of the countries in the Organisation for Economic Co-operation and Development (OECD), but it was down to about 2.5 times the OECD average by 2006, and is now estimated at 21.2 per 100 000 live births *(18)*. This progress is largely due to making maternal mortality a political priority, funding it accordingly, pursuing policies and providing services in a culturally sensitive manner. This includes establishing pre-delivery care homes for expectant mothers near a hospital and providing land and air transport free of charge for obstetrical emergency cases, greatly reducing the distance and time needed to access appropriate and high-quality specialized care.

Mortality by causes

Noncommunicable diseases produce the largest burden of mortality in the European Region (see the section below on current and future challenges), accounting for more than 85% of the 9 million estimated deaths between 2003 and 2007 in the Region *(19)*. Diseases of the circulatory system continue to be the main cause of death. They account for 48% of all deaths in the Region, ranging from 35% in the EU15 countries to 65% in the CIS countries, and are declining in most EU countries (Fig. 2.8).

Fig. 2.8. Proportional mortality from broad groups of causes of death by country groups, WHO European Region, 2006 or latest available year

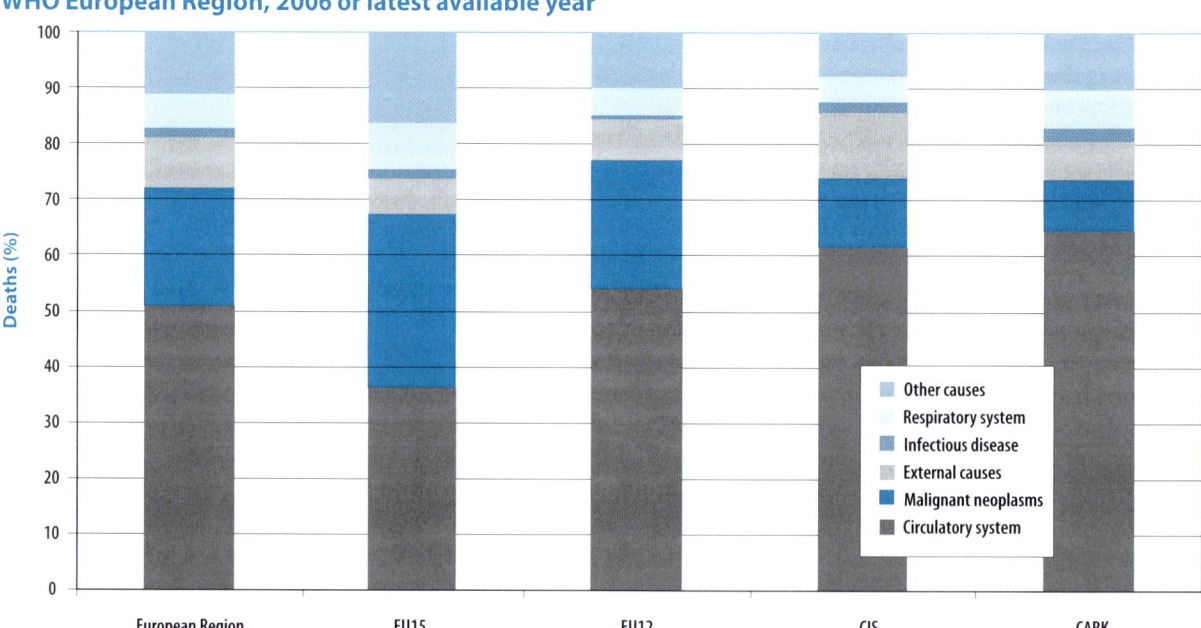

Source: European mortality database *(15)*.

Cancer (malignant neoplasms) is the second most important cause of death, accounting for more than 20% of total deaths in the Region, with figures ranging from 7% to 30% between countries. Cancer comprises a greater proportion of causes of death in the countries in the western part of the Region. External causes of injury and poisoning, and respiratory diseases are the two other major causes of death, accounting for 8% and 6% of deaths in the Region, respectively, although they occur more frequently in the CIS, CARK and EU12. These four groups of causes account for almost three quarters of all deaths. Infectious and parasitic diseases cause 16% of deaths globally but less than 2% in the European Region, although up to 8% in some countries in the eastern part of the Region.

Mortality profiles in the Region differ greatly by cause of death, age and sex. For example, external causes of injury and poisoning account for more than 70% of deaths among adolescents and young adults (especially men). Diseases of the circulatory system and cancer become leading causes as age increases (Fig. 2.9) *(20)*. In early childhood, diseases of the respiratory system and "other diseases" comprise the largest share (nearly 90% of deaths), affecting boys and girls similarly. Infectious and parasitic diseases have declined among young children, accounting for less than 5% of deaths, but are becoming increasingly important among adults.

Fig. 2.9. Mortality profiles by cause of death, age and sex, WHO European Region, 2007

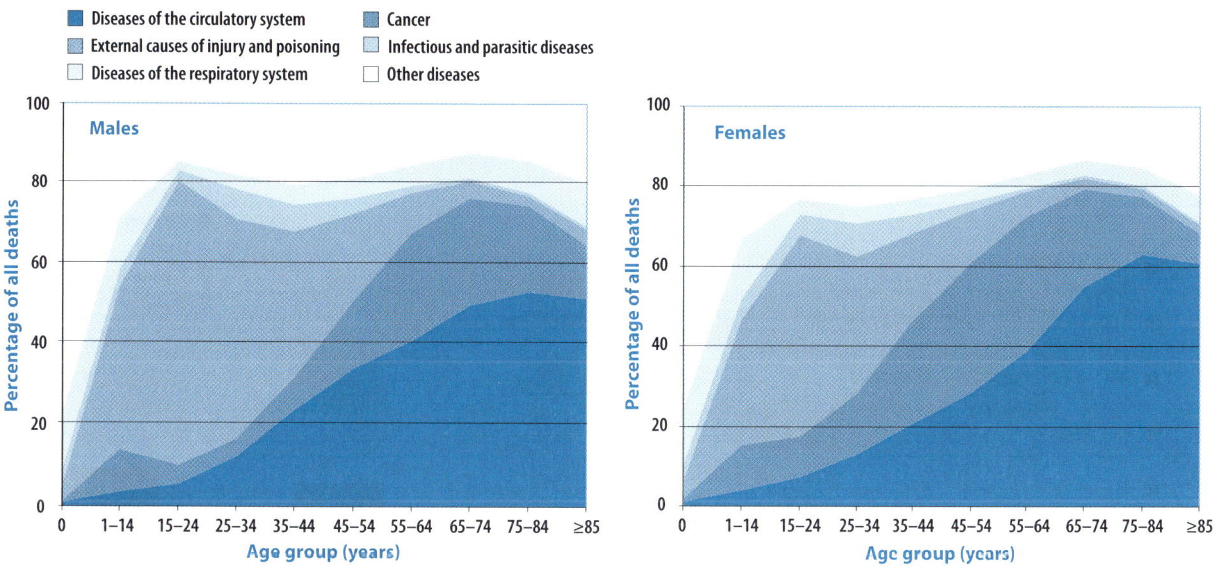

Source: Atlas of health in Europe (20).

Mortality from specific causes

The predominant causes of death in the European Region are chronic noncommunicable diseases, representing around 80% of all mortality. The SDR was 736.5 deaths per 100 000 population in 2006: almost 1% of the population in that year. This mortality has declined during the past two decades, reaching an overall reduction of 10% in 2006 (Table 2.8). In addition, the EU15 countries (26% decline) and EU12 countries (19% decline) have made strong progress. In contrast, mortality from this cause increased in the CIS countries (including the CARK) by 13% from 1990 to 2006. People in these countries have more than 40% excess risk of death compared with the European Region average.

Table 2.8. Population-weighted mortality rates from chronic noncommunicable diseases per 100 000 population by country group, WHO European Region, 1990–2006

Country group	1990	2006	Index in 2006 (%) (1990 = 100%)	Rate ratio (European Region = 1)
European Region	814.3	736.5	90	1.0
EU15	675.3	501.6	74	0.7
EU12	977.0	794.1	81	1.1
CIS	946.1	1071.9	113	1.5
CARK	930.0	1052.9	113	1.4

Source: European mortality database (15).

The mortality rate from diseases of the circulatory system closely resembles and shapes the time trends of overall mortality, including the differences between countries and country groups (Fig. 2.10). Diseases of the circulatory system cause nearly 50% of deaths in the Region, ranging from 35% to 65% among different country groups, with the overall mortality rate, 430 per 100 000 population. This rate is nearly 50% lower in the EU15 countries but almost twice as high in the CIS countries (including the CARK). In contrast, the mortality rate from cancer in the EU15 is similar to that of the European Region, but the proportion of deaths caused by cancer is 50% higher than that of the Region and twice as high as in the CIS and CARK, suggesting that the EU15 countries have improved the control of diseases of the circulatory system more than that of cancer.

Fig. 2.10. SDRs per 100 000 population by cause of death, WHO European Region, 2007 or latest available year

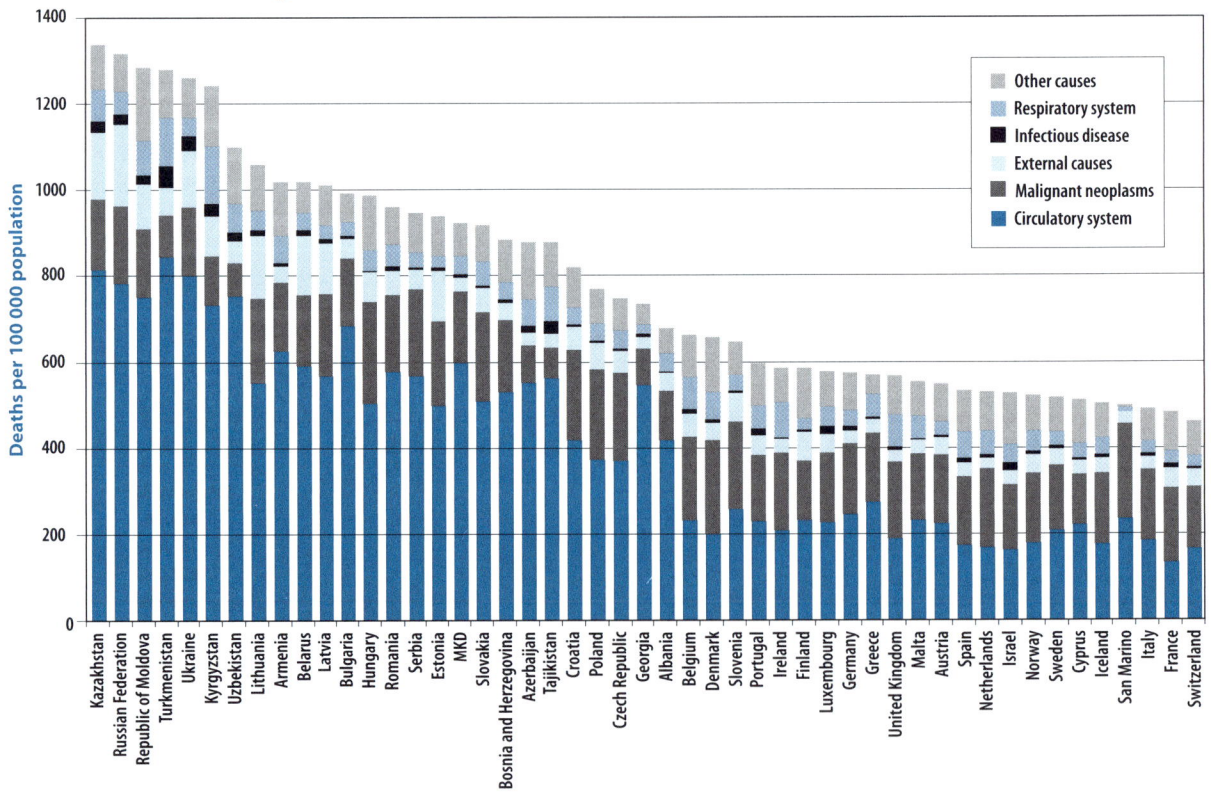

Note. MKD is the International Organization for Standardization (ISO) abbreviation for the former Yugoslav Republic of Macedonia.
Source: European mortality database (15).

The distribution of diseases of the circulatory system, mainly ischaemic heart and cerebrovascular diseases, varies considerably by age, sex and other factors. For example, the risk of dying from ischaemic heart disease increases with age and is almost 25 times higher among people 65 years or more than younger people (SDR: 1270.1 versus 55.8 per 100 000 population). Further, this risk is 90% higher among males than females (SDR: 274.0 versus 152.2 per 100 000 population). In addition, countries in south-western Europe have the lowest mortality rates from ischaemic heart disease (SDR: 21–71 per 100 000 population) *(21)*, and the risk is 5–7 times higher in the easternmost parts of the Region (Fig. 2.11). The trends for cerebrovascular disease are similar for age and increasing west-to-east gradient, but people 65 years and more have 31 times the excess risk of younger people (SDR: 803.3 versus 25.8 per 100 000 population). Males have only 30% higher mortality than females (SDR: 134.5 versus 106.0 per 100 000 population). The differences between the western and eastern parts of the Region have been suggested to result from interaction between key lifestyle factors (diet, smoking and physical activity) and psychosocial factors (stress), but other aspects, such as access to and the quality of health care, are thought to play a role *(11)*.

Fig. 2.11. Ischaemic heart disease: SDRs per 100 000 population by country, WHO European Region, 2007 or latest available year

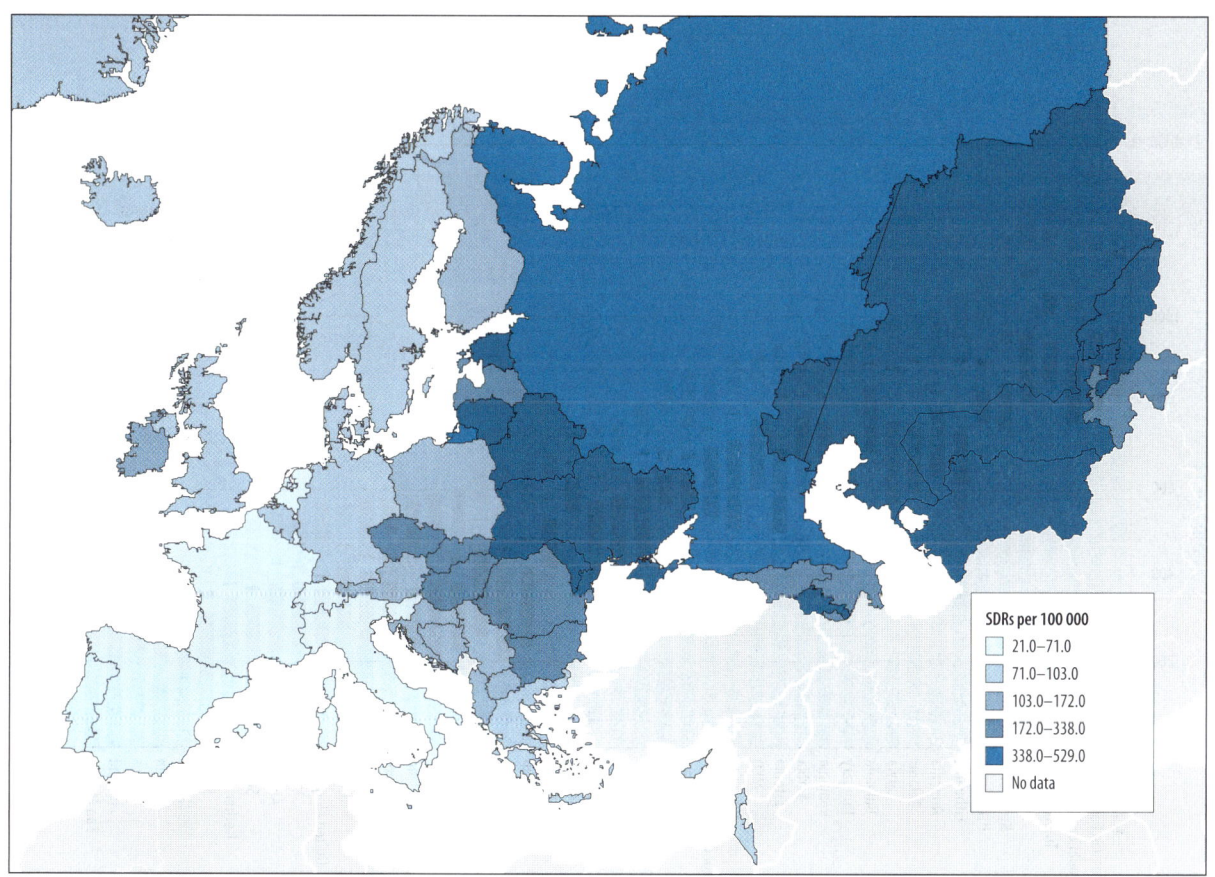

Source: European mortality database *(15)*.

Studies in the Russian Federation support this view, strongly associating changes in cardiovascular disease mortality in recent decades with high alcohol consumption and poisoning *(5)*. Additional research has further suggested that socioeconomic factors, such as mass privatization and the consequent unemployment that occurred in the Russian Federation and other countries in the post-Communist era, dramatically promoted rapid social and political changes. These, in turn, have aggravated the mortality situation, especially in the countries that already had lower life expectancy and incomes, thereby exacerbating existing inequality in income and health *(22,23)*. Studies indicate that high social capital – in the form of participation in social organizations – reduced these effects and further suggest that social policies may be useful in the future in reforming systems.

The overall SDR for cancer in the European Region was 168.1 per 100 000 population in about 2007, accounting for nearly 20% of all deaths. The mortality rate is more than 10 times higher among people aged 65 and more than among younger people (SDR: 912.0 versus 79.6 per 100 000 population) and 80% higher among males than females (SDR: 229.1 versus 127.0 per 100 000 population). Cancer of the trachea, bronchus and lung, colon, stomach, liver and prostate accounts for nearly 50% of mortality from cancer among men. Cancer of the breast, trachea, bronchus and lung, stomach, liver, colon, cervix uteri and ovary accounts for 60% of mortality from cancer among women. In contrast to cardiovascular diseases, cancer has the highest mortality rates in the EU12 countries (Fig. 2.12). This has been suggested to be the result of increasingly high smoking rates, especially among women *(1)*.

Fig. 2.12. Cancer: SDRs per 100 000 population by country, WHO European Region, 2007 or latest available year

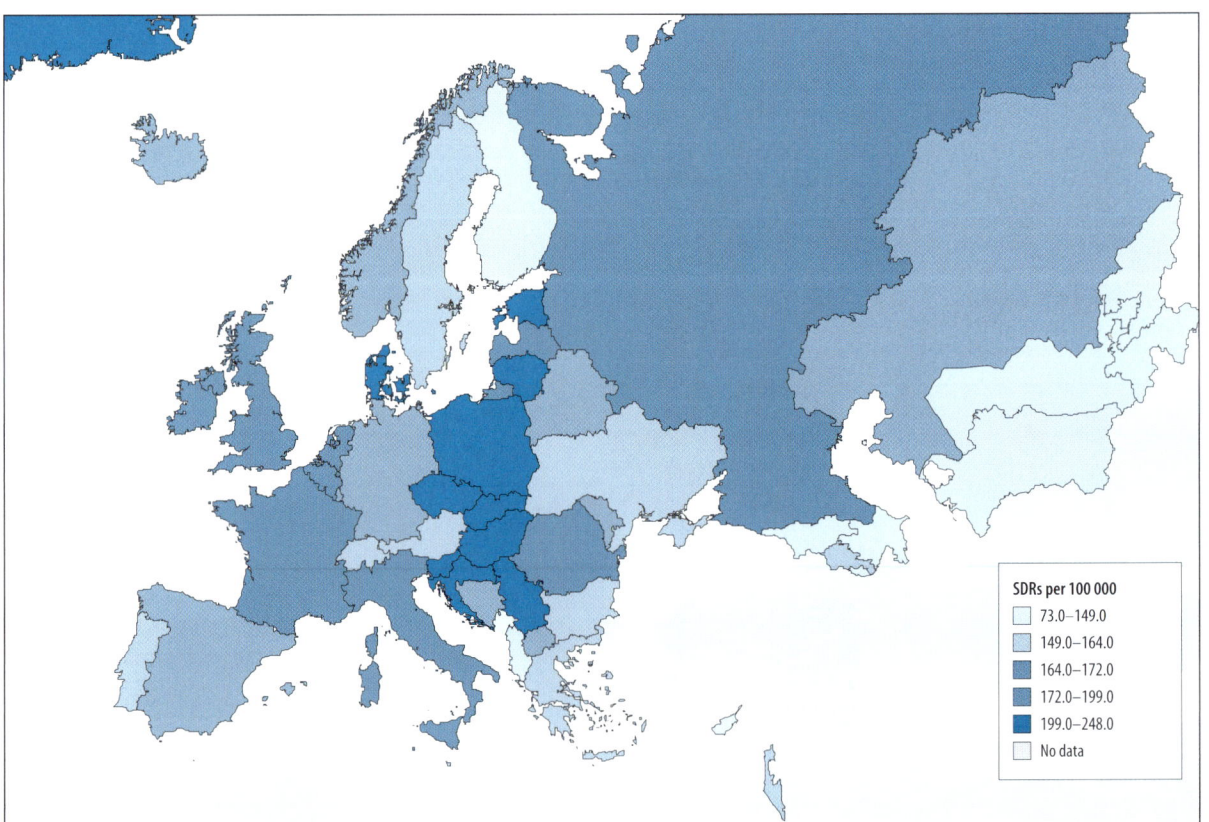

Source: European mortality database *(15)*.

External causes of death – particularly injuries from accidents (including falls), transport-related causes and violence, both self-inflicted and done to other people – result in considerable mortality in the Region. External causes account for 8% of all deaths. The overall SDR from this cause in the European Region was 71.8 per 100 000 population in 2007, declining more than 10% since 1990 (Table 2.9). People 65 years and older have the highest rate, almost twice the average (SDR: 135.3 per 100 000 population), but the age-related excess risk varies by specific cause. The excess risk for older people is 2 times higher for transport crashes (SDR: 12.7 per 100 000 population), suicide (SDR: 13.8 per 100 000 population) and homicide (SDR: 4.8 per 100 000 population) but 9 times higher for falls (SDR: 26.9 per 100 000 population). In addition, mortality from external causes is nearly four times higher among males than females (SDR: 124.9 versus 34.2 per 100 000 population). Similar to all-cause mortality, the geographical distribution tends to increase from west to east in the European Region, with CIS countries having 2–3 times higher risk overall and for specific causes. The differences for accidents, suicide and homicide have been attributed to various lifestyle and socioeconomic factors, including high alcohol intake, roads and vehicles in poor condition, and limited enforcement of the law *(1)*.

Table 2.9. Population-weighted SDRs per 100 000 population from external causes of death by country group, WHO European Region, 1990–2006

Country group	1990	2006	Index in 2006 (%) (1990 = 100%)
European Region	79.9	71.8	90
EU15	49.8	34.3	69
EU12	87.3	63.7	73
CIS	115.9	145.0	125
CARK	87.8	81.1[a]	92[a]

[a] Figures for 2005.
Source: European mortality database *(15)*.

Mortality from infectious and parasitic diseases decreased dramatically from the 1950s, reaching the lowest SDR for the European Region (10.1 per 100 000 population) in 1990 (Table 2.10). This progress resulted from improved overall living conditions and maternal and child health care, particularly improved access to water and sanitation, immunization and antibiotics, and better nutrition. Nevertheless, mortality increased by 40% in the mid-1990s and then stagnated, with an SDR of 14.5 per 100 000 population in 2006. TB, HIV and hepatitis are the main causes of this resurgence and stagnation. The increased mortality has affected mainly the EU15 and the CIS countries, whose rates are nearly 60% higher than in 1990. Even so, the 1990 and current levels in the CIS are almost three times those in the EU15.

Table 2.10. Population-weighted SDRs per 100 000 population from infectious and parasitic diseases by country group, WHO European Region, 1990–2006

Country group	1990	2006	Index in 2006 (%) (1990 = 100%)	Rate ratio (European Region = 1)
European Region	10.1	14.5	143	1.0
EU15	5.8	9.2	158	0.6
EU12	8.7	6.9	79	0.5
CIS	16.0	25.3	158	1.8
CARK	31.1	27.8	90	1.9

Source: European mortality database *(15)*.

Avoidable mortality

Avoidable mortality has been proposed to indicate the potential premature mortality that may be reduced by timely and effective intervention by the health system. This may include health promotion, primary prevention (to reduce exposure) or secondary prevention (to diagnose and treat disease). It may also include the participation of non-health sectors such as environment, transport and others (13,24,25). Accordingly, avoidable mortality can be further separated into amenable (treatable) and preventable. Amenable mortality is considered a better indicator of health care services and helps to indicate how much they contribute to health, either positively or negatively (see the section below on health systems' role in improving population health).

The SDRs for ischaemic heart disease and cerebrovascular disease were 186 and 113 per 100 000 population, respectively, in about 2007. Thus, the two causes account for more than 70% of cardiovascular mortality and nearly 35% of total mortality in the European Region. Mortality from ischaemic heart disease among people aged 0–64 years (SDR: 55.8 per 100 000 population) varies widely between countries, with the ratio between the highest and lowest SDR exceeding 13.5. The rates are 50–80% higher than the regional average in Azerbaijan, Georgia, Kyrgyzstan, Latvia, Lithuania, the Republic of Moldova and Uzbekistan and more than twice the regional average in Belarus, Kazakhstan, the Russian Federation, Turkmenistan and Ukraine. This situation has been attributed to a combination of preventable factors, such as high alcohol intake and binge drinking, stress and feeling lack of social support, all exacerbated by economic and social crises (21).

The highest SDR for cerebrovascular diseases among people aged 0–64 is 17 times the lowest. Mortality rates are 50–80% higher than the regional average (SDR: 24.1 per 100 000 population) in Azerbaijan, Belarus, Bulgaria, Georgia, Romania, the former Yugoslav Republic of Macedonia, Ukraine and Uzbekistan, and nearly twice as high in Kazakhstan, Kyrgyzstan, the Republic of Moldova and the Russian Federation. Recent studies have shown great variation in the prevalence of cerebrovascular diseases worldwide and higher rates in low-income countries, perhaps because of limited access to and quality of health care (26). In addition, the prevalent risk factors are poorly correlated with and fail to predict mortality from this cause. The differences are suggested to be due to higher case fatality and less aggressive treatment in low-income countries.

Deaths from cancer of the trachea, bronchus and lung have declined nearly 25% among people aged 25–64 years in the European Region (SDR: 29.3 per 100 000 population) since 1990. This decline is particularly steep in CIS countries (SDR: 27.7 per 100 000 population) and the CARK (SDR: 16.2 per 100 000 population), with rates falling by 40–50%. Lung cancer among women, however, has risen dramatically (by 40–50%) in EU countries (SDR: 18.2 per 100 000 population), particularly the EU12 (SDR: 17.8 per 100 000 population).

Mortality from colon cancer was once one of the main causes of death in the European Region, but has declined by 12% since 1990 among people aged 25–64 (SDR: 11.8 per 100 000 population). The decline has reached 15–25% in all country groups, except the EU12 countries (SDR: 14.6 per 100 000 population) where rates are stagnant. Nevertheless, the rate among men (SDR: 18.8 per 100 000 population) – but not women (SDR: 11.0 per 100 000 population) – in the EU12 countries increased by nearly 20%, suggesting that the stagnation mainly reflects dietary and lifestyle factors and, to a lesser extent, access to health care (1).

Mortality from breast cancer among women aged 25–64 years in the European Region (SDR: 24.4 per 100 000 population) has decreased by more than 15% since 1990, despite increasing by 10% in CIS countries (SDR: 26.2 per 100 000 population). The rates are twice as high among older women, and have increased by nearly 40% in the CIS countries, suggesting that the increases may be due to low quality of care (both diagnosis and treatment). Cervical cancer among women aged 25–64 years in the Region (SDR: 5.9 per 100 000 population) has declined 7% since 1990, but mortality remains high in the EU12 (SDR: 11.6 per 100 000 population) and CIS (SDR: 9.0 per 100 000 population), including the CARK (SDR: 8.3 per 100 000 population). The rates have increased solely in the CIS countries (20% since 1990), including the CARK (13% since 1990), largely because of a lack of prevention and control of sexually transmitted infections (mainly human papillomavirus) and limited access to diagnosis and health care *(1)*.

Diabetes is another important cause of amenable mortality; the SDR in the European Region was 12.7 per 100 000 population in 2006 (Table 2.11). Mortality rates differ significantly by age. They are 21 times higher among people aged 65 years and more than among younger people (SDR: 83.8 versus 3.9 per 100 000 population) and 15% higher among males than females (SDR: 13.6 versus 11.7 per 100 000 population). Trends from 1990 to 2006 varied geographically, with declines of 12–15% in EU countries and increases of 40–98% in CIS countries. The mortality rate among people aged 0–64 years is three times higher in the CARK (SDR: 12.1 per 100 000 population) than in the Region as a whole. The ratio of mortality to incidence (an approximation of case fatality) has been suggested as a good indicator of the performance of health systems *(27)*. The CARK and some other CIS countries (such as Belarus) have high mortality from diabetes at early ages. This may suggest that other causes related to limited access to and the quality of health care play a role, in addition to the changes in lifestyle factors that increase vulnerability to diabetes mortality.

Table 2.11. Population-weighted SDRs from diabetes per 100 000 population by country group, WHO European Region, 1990–2006

Country group	1990	2006	Index in 2006 (%) (1990 = 100%)
European Region	12.6	12.7	100
EU15	15.6	13.4	86
EU12	14.8	13.0	88
CIS	7.7	10.8	140
CARK	11.0	21.9[a]	199

[a] Figure for 2005.
Source: European mortality database *(15)*.

TB accounts for nearly 50% of the mortality from infectious and parasitic diseases among people aged 25–64 years in the European Region (SDR: 7.1 per 100 000 population). It is a main reason for increasing mortality from these diseases in the Region since 1990, especially in the CIS countries (SDR: 18.5 per 100 000 population), where the rate has more than doubled. Although mortality has declined recently, the situation is also critical in the CARK, with rates similar to those in the CIS as a whole. The mortality rate from TB increases with age in most country groups, except the CIS, where younger people have higher mortality. This suggests the effects of such factors as poor diet and alcohol intake, which are aggravated by poor socioeconomic conditions and coinfection with sexually transmitted infections, especially HIV.

Inequality in mortality

Mortality rates differ considerably by cause of death and age group in both country groups and individual countries. These patterns are reproduced within countries (Table 2.12). For example, geographical mortality rate ratios for subnational regions are relatively low (less than 1.5) for cancer and cardiovascular diseases but higher for infectious and parasitic diseases and external causes, suggesting the importance of environmental factors. In addition, subnational variations in some countries, mainly the Russian Federation and Uzbekistan, tend to be very high for all causes but particularly for external causes and infectious diseases. A notable exception is Ireland, where regional mortality rate ratios tend to be closer to 1, indicating a more even distribution of risk.

Table 2.12. Geographical and gender inequality in SDRs (per 100 000 population) for broad groups of causes of death in selected countries, WHO European Region, 2006 or latest available year

Country	Mortality from groups of causes of death											
	Diseases of the circulatory system			Neoplasms			External causes			Infectious and parasitic diseases		
	National value (SDR)	Regional highest-to-lowest mortality ratio	Male-to-female mortality ratio	National value (SDR)	Regional highest-to-lowest mortality ratio	Male-to-female mortality ratio	National value (SDR)	Regional highest-to-lowest mortality ratio	Male-to-female mortality ratio	National value (SDR)	Regional highest-to-lowest mortality ratio	Male-to-female mortality ratio
Austria	223.9	1.32	1.47	162.8	1.22	1.60	40.2	1.31	2.87	4.7	2.78	1.54
Bulgaria	685.4	1.26	1.50	157.4	1.23	1.81	45.0	1.23	3.69	7.2	2.34	2.29
Czech Republic	370.7	1.36	1.48	206.7	1.29	1.77	51.7	1.30	2.99	5.1	2.71	1.36
Finland	231.1	1.39	1.86	141.1	1.22	1.55	67.6	2.24	3.13	5.6	1.46	1.54
France	145.4	1.62	1.71	183.7	1.42	2.05	48.8	2.08	2.33	10.6	1.60	1.76
Hungary	502.4	1.27	1.60	248.2	1.10	1.92	80.0	1.36	3.17	4.1	1.91	2.42
Ireland	207.5	1.01	1.66	184.6	1.01	1.40	29.4	1.20	2.24	3.5	1.10	1.28
Netherlands	175.3	1.18	1.60	191.0	1.17	1.51	26.6	1.16	1.94	7.9	1.96	1.45
Russian Federation	807.0	3.24	1.69	190.7	2.45	2.06	224.1	15.27	4.40	24.3	9.76	5.04
Spain	173.5	1.59	1.50	169.3	1.19	2.25	32.9	1.59	2.98	12.1	4.31	1.98
United Kingdom	224.0	1.56	1.58	187.1	1.41	1.42	28.7	2.67	2.32	6.6	2.80	1.22
Uzbekistan	754.2	1.91	1.30	77.9	3.27	1.23	28.2	3.59	3.49	21.3	5.57	2.10
European Region	430.2	–	1.55	171.6	–	1.80	76.0	–	3.66	14.5	–	2.57

Source: European mortality database (15).

Mortality rates for men are consistently higher within countries and for all causes. Again, the disparity between men and women tends to be relatively less for cardiovascular diseases and closer to the European Region average (rate ratio < 1.6). For external causes of death, differences within countries are greater, and significantly exacerbated in the Russian Federation compared with other countries. In addition to the environmental factors linked to geography that may increase the risk of death, exposure to other lifestyle and behavioural factors associated with gender may further increase mortality risk among men. Nevertheless, these results should be interpreted cautiously since they represent only aggregated data and are thus open to ecological bias. Studies on inequality have reported similar results, with geographical gradients and smaller differences for cardiovascular diseases and cancer than for other causes of death that are consistent with these findings (28,29).

Burden of disease

WHO has proposed additional summary measures for the burden of disease, including disability-adjusted life-years (DALYs), to indicate both mortality and the effects of morbidity on population health (19). DALYs account for the years of life lost through premature death and the years of life lived in less than full health due to illness or disability.

The European Region represents nearly 14% of the world population but contributes 151.4 million DALYs lost, about 10% of the global burden, with an average 171 DALYs lost per 1000 population in 2004. The population in the low- and middle-income countries in the European Region[1] represents 54% of the regional total, but accounts for 67% of the regional DALYs, an average of 215 DALYs per 1000 population. The burden of disease in the Region is projected to decrease by 23% in 2030 if current trends in diseases and mortality continue. Projections for the low- and middle-income countries indicate an even larger reduction (31%) due to changes in age and cause-specific patterns.

Similar to mortality, the population aged 15–59 years has the largest burden of disease for all causes combined: 58% of DALYs lost in the Region, with 61% in its low- and middle-income countries (Fig. 2.13). In addition, males have 21% excess loss of DALYs compared with females in this age group, but this reverses after 60 years of age, with an excess of 42% among females, and the profiles are similar in the various country groups. Men aged 15–59 will still lose more DALYs in 2030 than older men: 58% of the total. In contrast, losses among women 60 years and older will predominate, accounting for 48% of the total for women. The increasing ageing of the population, especially among women, adds to the relevance of these figures (see the section below on changing demographic patterns in the Region). In low- and middle-income countries, the relative contribution of DALYs will increase slightly among middle-aged males and females as the contributions among children aged 0–14 years decline.

Fig. 2.13. Estimate (2004) and projection (2030) of the age and sex distribution of DALYs lost by country income level, WHO European Region

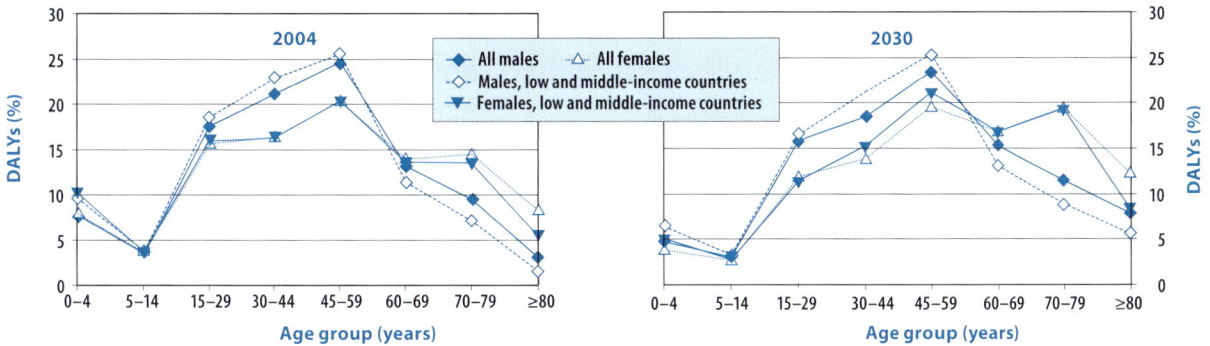

Source: The global burden of disease: 2004 update (19).

Causes of lost DALYs have been grouped into three broad categories: communicable, maternal, perinatal and nutritional conditions (Group I), noncommunicable diseases (Group II) and injuries (Group III), each with additional subgroups.[2] Worldwide, Group II conditions account for the largest share of the burden of disease, with 48% of lost DALYs, and Group I causes, an additional 40% (Table 2.13). In contrast, Group II conditions predominate in the European Region, with nearly 77% of all lost DALYs, followed by Group III with 13%.

---

[1] According to WHO (19), in 2004 this group of countries included: Albania, Armenia, Azerbaijan, Belarus, Bosnia and Herzegovina, Bulgaria, Croatia, Czech Republic, Estonia, Georgia, Hungary, Kazakhstan, Kyrgyzstan, Latvia, Lithuania, Poland, Republic of Moldova, Romania, Russian Federation, Serbia and Montenegro, Slovakia, Tajikistan, the former Yugoslav Republic of Macedonia, Turkey, Turkmenistan, Ukraine and Uzbekistan. Now, however, Montenegro and Serbia are separate countries.
[2] Disease subgroups involve the following categories: Group I – infectious and parasitic diseases, respiratory infections, maternal conditions, perinatal conditions and nutritional deficiencies; Group II – malignant neoplasms, other neoplasms, diabetes mellitus, nutritional and endocrine disorders, neuropsychiatric conditions, sense organ disorders, cardiovascular diseases, respiratory diseases, digestive diseases, diseases of the genitourinary system, skin diseases, musculoskeletal diseases, congenital abnormalities and oral diseases; and Group III – unintentional injuries and intentional injuries (19).

Table 2.13. DALYs lost according to broad groups of causes, WHO European Region and its low- and middle-income countries (LMIC), 2004

Cause	World[a] (DALYs)		European Region[b] (DALYs)		European Region, LMIC[c] (DALYs)		
	Number (thousands)	% of total	Number (thousands)	% of total	Number (thousands)	% of total	% of total for the Region
Total DALYs	1 523 259	100.0	151 461	100.0	102 130	100.0	67.4
I. Communicable diseases, maternal and perinatal conditions and nutritional deficiencies	603 993	39.7	15 391	10.2	13 094	12.8	85.1
Infectious and parasitic diseases	302 144	19.8	6 041	4.0	5 203	5.1	86.1
Respiratory infections	97 786	6.4	2 907	1.9	2 419	2.4	83.2
Maternal conditions	38 936	2.6	862	0.6	691	0.7	80.2
Perinatal conditions	126 423	8.3	3 687	2.4	3 173	3.1	86.0
Nutritional deficiencies	38 703	2.5	1 893	1.3	1 608	1.6	84.9
II. Noncommunicable conditions	731 652	48.0	116 097	76.7	72 613	71.1	62.5
Malignant neoplasms	77 812	5.1	17 086	11.3	8 813	8.6	51.6
Other neoplasms	1 953	0.1	283	0.2	103	0.1	36.5
Diabetes mellitus	19 705	1.3	2 660	1.8	1 349	1.3	50.7
Nutritional and endocrine disorders	10 446	0.7	1 266	0.8	549	0.5	43.3
Neuropsychiatric disorders	199 280	13.1	28 932	19.1	16 342	16.0	56.5
Sense organ disorders	86 883	5.7	8 429	5.6	4 608	4.5	54.7
Cardiovascular diseases	151 377	9.9	34 760	22.9	26 845	26.3	77.2
Respiratory diseases	59 039	3.9	5 910	3.9	2 992	2.9	50.6
Digestive diseases	42 498	2.8	6 945	4.6	4 755	4.7	68.5
Diseases of the genitourinary system	14 754	1.0	1 319	0.9	885	0.9	67.0
Skin diseases	3 879	0.3	331	0.2	242	0.2	73.1
Musculoskeletal diseases	30 869	2.0	5 435	3.6	3 263	3.2	60.0
Congenital abnormalities	25 280	1.7	1 845	1.2	1 298	1.3	70.4
Oral diseases	7 875	0.5	896	0.6	569	0.6	63.5
III. Injuries	187 614	12.3	19 973	13.2	16 424	16.1	82.2
Unintentional injuries	138 564	9.1	14 545	9.6	12 034	11.8	82.7
Intentional injuries	49 050	3.2	5 428	3.6	4 389	4.3	80.9

[a] Population (thousands): 6 436 826.
[b] Population (thousands): 883 311.
[c] Population (thousands): 476 019 (53.9% of the total for the Region).
Source: The global burden of disease: 2004 update (19).

The low- and middle-income countries in the Region account for 63% of the regional DALYs lost from Group II conditions but substantially more of DALYs lost from Group I (85%) and Group III (82%) conditions. In fact, these countries have the highest burden of Group III causes (injuries) (16%) of all WHO regions. The low- and middle-income countries differ slightly from the regional average in the distribution of the lost DALYs by cause subcategories. Neuropsychiatric conditions, which account for 3% of overall mortality in the European Region, comprise 19% of the lost DALYs, second only to cardiovascular diseases (23%). These two are also the leading causes of lost DALYs in the low- and middle-income countries in the Region. Moreover, malignant neoplasms, unintentional injuries and sense organ disorders are the next three leading causes of lost DALYs in the Region as a whole, versus unintentional injuries, malignant neoplasms and infectious and parasitic diseases in the low- and middle-income countries.

The share of Group II causes in the Region is projected to increase to 84% of all lost DALYs by 2030, mainly due to increases in neuropsychiatric conditions and malignant neoplasms, while cardiovascular diseases remain at the same level. The low- and middle-income countries in the Region are projected to follow a similar trend, with Group II causes increasing to 80% of the burden of disease and the contribution of Group III causes projected to decrease from 16% to 10%.

Twenty-five leading conditions account for more than 60% of DALYs lost in both the European Region as a whole and its low- and middle-income countries. Nearly two thirds of these conditions are in Group II, and some have non-fatal outcomes (Table 2.14). Ischaemic heart disease and cerebrovascular diseases are the leading causes of DALYs lost, together accounting for 17% of the burden in the Region and 20% in the low- and middle-income countries. Unipolar depressive disorder and alcohol use disorder are the main neuropsychiatric conditions, with a combined share of 9%.

Table 2.14. DALYs lost from 25 leading causes, WHO European Region and its low- and middle-income countries (LMIC), 2004

Cause	Region[a] (DALYs) Number	%	Cause	LMIC[b] (DALYs) Number	%
Total	151 461 416	100.00	Total	102 130	100.00
Ischaemic heart disease	16 825 931	11.11	Ischaemic heart disease	13 450	13.17
Cerebrovascular disease	9 531 199	6.29	Cerebrovascular disease	7 494	7.34
Unipolar depressive disorders	8 446 229	5.58	Unipolar depressive disorders	4 692	4.59
Other unintentional injuries	5 265 230	3.48	Other unintentional injuries	4 579	4.48
Alcohol use disorders	4 999 976	3.30	Alcohol use disorders	3 446	3.37
Hearing loss, adult onset	3 925 584	2.59	Road traffic accidents	2 660	2.60
Road traffic accidents	3 677 947	2.43	Cirrhosis of the liver	2 282	2.23
Trachea/bronchus/lung cancer	3 264 161	2.16	Self-inflicted	2 213	2.17
Osteoarthritis	3 140 275	2.07	Lower respiratory infections	2 194	2.15
Cirrhosis of the liver	3 098 534	2.05	Hearing loss, adult onset	2 099	2.05
Self-inflicted	3 092 210	2.04	Poisoning	2 036	1.99
Alzheimer and other dementia	3 071 924	2.03	Osteoarthritis	1 970	1.93
Chronic obstructive pulmonary disease	2 960 739	1.95	Violence	1 826	1.79
Diabetes mellitus	2 659 614	1.76	TB	1 695	1.66
Lower respiratory infections	2 617 929	1.73	Trachea/bronchus/lung cancer	1 637	1.60
Refractive errors	2 369 601	1.56	Chronic obstructive pulmonary disease	1 486	1.46
Poisoning	2 170 835	1.43	Falls	1 484	1.45
Falls	2 030 492	1.34	Diabetes mellitus	1 349	1.32
Violence	1 970 036	1.30	Congenital abnormalities	1 298	1.27
Colon and rectum cancer	1 894 627	1.25	Diarrhoeal diseases	1 279	1.25
Congenital abnormalities	1 844 624	1.22	Prematurity and low birth weight	1 269	1.24
Breast cancer	1 737 542	1.15	Refractive errors	1 179	1.15
TB	1 734 840	1.15	Inflammatory heart disease	1 168	1.14
Schizophrenia	1 612 050	1.06	Birth asphyxia and birth trauma	1 080	1.06
Bipolar affective disorder	1 555 355	1.03	Schizophrenia	1 040	1.02

[a] Population (thousands): 883 311.
[b] Population (thousands): 476 019.
Source: The global burden of disease: 2004 update (19).

Among adults aged 15–59 years, injuries account for 17% of the burden of disease in the European Region but more than 30% in its low- and middle-income countries (20). In contrast, women in this group are more affected by neuropsychiatric conditions, especially unipolar depressive disorders. In both the Region as a whole and in its low- and middle-income countries, most of the 10 leading conditions that account for more than 40% of DALYs lost have been related to such major risk factors as alcohol, smoking, road safety and other factors that may affect citizen safety (19). More specific analysis is required to further understand the main causes and vulnerable groups affected at the country level and to address them through adequate policies and interventions.

Finally, the DALYs lost to cardiovascular diseases, both ischaemic heart disease and cerebrovascular diseases, are projected to increase marginally by 2030, especially in low- and middle-income countries *(20)*. Malignant neoplasms will also increase in these countries, but remain at current levels in other parts of the Region. Meanwhile, injuries and communicable diseases are expected to decline in importance as causes of the burden of disease. Since people will live longer (see the section below on changing demographic patterns in the Region), the burden of disease has been projected to decline overall by 10% (and by 30% per person) from 2004 to 2030, mainly due to shifting disease patterns (especially associated with non-fatal disabling outcomes such as unipolar major depression, adult-onset hearing loss and alcohol use disorders) and delay of the age of death. Some causes of the burden of disease in the Region are expected to increase, however, such as HIV (mainly in low- and middle-income countries), unipolar depressive disorders, Alzheimer and other types of dementia and hearing loss with adult onset.

Challenges for the future

Although health has improved in the European Region in the past two decades, the agenda on the burden of disease is still unfinished. As data have shown consistently, inequality in health between countries is substantial and often present within countries. Some of this inequality has been linked to gender, socioeconomic factors, lifestyles and access to health care *(6)*. The low- and middle-income countries in the Region account for more than 65% of the burden of disease. Eight of the ten most frequent health conditions, causing nearly 40% of DALYs lost, tend to be avoidable and associated with three major risk factors: smoking, alcohol abuse and transport. The population-attributable fractions of these modifiable factors vary globally for males and females between 19% and 5% for smoking and 5.6% and 0.6% for alcohol abuse *(30)*, respectively. The overall fraction for transport is 2.8%, but no data are available by sex *(31,32)*. Positive dietary factors, including adequate micronutrient content, and physical activity may also play an important role *(22,30,33)*. In addition, the attributable fractions vary by type of disease and age. For example, for lung cancer and cardiovascular diseases among people aged 30–69 years, smoking contributes to almost 80% and 40% among men and 24% and 6% among women, respectively. Controlling these factors could reduce the burden of disease by a substantial fraction. When smoking rates decline, as in Poland, life expectancy at birth increases *(34)*. Again, health systems have to evolve to respond to different requirements.

Some CIS countries with high frequencies of these risk factors do not provide information to allow further analysis and thus may not recognize problems. For alcohol abuse, studies in CIS countries have shown that policies to limit access and reduce intake had important effects but were not sustained everywhere, and the mortality from cardiovascular diseases and injuries and violence therefore returned to a high level, in contrast with the EU12 countries *(16,35)*. Similarly, Estonia, Latvia and Lithuania, which experienced a burden of disease similar to that of the CIS countries, have been able to achieve higher and healthier life expectancy at birth than their CIS counterparts. This suggests that known public health policies and interventions can be effective but require stronger political will and concerted action in all sectors of society, with health considered in all policies, to realize them. The Tallinn Charter: Health Systems for Health and Wealth *(36,37)* provides a framework for public health action with proven health programmes and interventions; additional attention to country agendas and investment is required to achieve the Charter's goals.

Factors influencing health

This section integrates the main social, economic and environmental determinants of health and the key behavioural risk factors that influence health outcomes and distribution. Countries vary considerably in the distribution and severity of disease and thus in the total burden. For example, the health effects of the environment remain a common and growing concern – especially in relation to access to safe drinking-water and sanitation, air pollution, occupational safety and injuries – but the burden of disease due to known environmental factors varies up to fourfold between countries.

Such individual-level determinants of health as tobacco, alcohol, poor diet and insufficient physical activity, along with the growing levels of obesity in the Region, continue to exact a considerable toll. Insufficient attention or attempts at action do not usually cause lack of progress, but the interrelationships of lifestyles and behaviour have common root causes: the socioeconomic determinants of health. People with less education, lower occupational status or lower income tend to die earlier and to spend more years in ill health, with a higher prevalence of most types of health problems *(38)*. This arises in part from the conditions in which people are born, grow, live, work and age, and their exposure to a wide range of unfavourable material, psychosocial, environmental and behavioural risk factors. Indeed, relative deprivation and social inequality erode the emotional, spiritual and intellectual resources essential to well-being, with mental disorders continuing to rise, so that health-damaging behaviour may sometimes become a mechanism for coping with multiple problems *(39)*.

There are no easy answers. Daily living conditions need to be improved and the inequitable distribution of power, money and resources needs to be tackled *(6)*; social inequality and inequality in health run as threads through the next three sections. Addressing them requires a whole-of-government approach – not just the health sector – in collaboration with civil society, local communities, business, global forums and international agencies. Although evidence on individual interventions and potential policy options is plentiful, questions remain about the longer-term effectiveness of tackling such factors in isolation. Addressing such risk factors across the range of domains implicated – the environment, food safety, individual behavioural choices and the wider social determinants of health – clearly requires an integrated response. The requisite intersectoral action thus depends on a strong stewardship role for health ministries, to enable them to make the case for joint action with and beyond the health system.

Environment and health

More than 1.7 million annual deaths (18% of all deaths) are attributable to environmental factors in the European Region. The environment accounts for an estimated one third of the total burden of disease for children and adolescents aged 0–19. Well-designed environmental health interventions could reduce total mortality in the Region by almost 20% *(40)*.

The burden of disease due to known environmental factors is unevenly distributed between countries, varying up to fourfold across the Region (Table 2.15). This is due to multiple factors, including differences in exposure to a combination of risk factors such as unsafe drinking-

Table 2.15. Estimated deaths and DALYs lost due to environmental factors, WHO European Region, 2002

Subregion and country	DALYs		Estimated deaths	
	Per capita (thousands)	%	Number	%
Eur-A				
Andorra	17.6	14	91	23
Austria	16.3	14	11 424	15
Belgium	18.7	14	17 032	16
Croatia	23.0	14	8 374	17
Cyprus	17.5	13	1 363	26
Czech Republic	21.4	15	17 606	16
Denmark	19.1	14	9 235	16
Finland	19.1	15	8 167	17
France	17.2	14	80 107	15
Germany	17.1	14	132 169	16
Greece	20.0	16	19 966	19
Iceland	13.7	14	317	17
Ireland	17.8	14	5 286	18
Israel	14.1	13	5 594	15
Italy	16.0	14	90 809	16
Luxembourg	18.0	15	574	16
Malta	15.6	14	490	16
Monaco	15.5	14	42	8
Netherlands	15.8	14	21 830	15
Norway	16.1	14	7 502	17
Portugal	19.7	14	15 445	14
San Marino	16.3	15	44	24
Slovenia	19.8	14	2 926	16
Spain	17.3	14	58 495	16
Sweden	15.1	14	14 468	15
Switzerland	14.6	13	9 543	15
United Kingdom	18.1	14	101 335	17
Eur-B				
Albania	29.9	19	4 425	27
Armenia	26.3	16	4 712	18
Azerbaijan	35.7	19	12 927	28
Bosnia and Herzegovina	25.6	16	6 172	20
Bulgaria	28.6	16	18 469	16
Georgia	27.1	16	10 874	28
Kyrgyzstan	46.2	21	9 706	28
Poland	25.2	17	66 113	18
Romania	30.8	17	46 928	17
Serbia and Montenegro	26.8	15	21 023	19
Slovakia	25.1	16	9 315	18
Tajikistan	47.5	21	12 021	45
The former Yugoslav Republic of Macedonia	23.7	15	3 137	17
Turkey	30.4	19	86 712	20
Turkmenistan	48.5	22	9 108	31
Uzbekistan	30.1	18	33 479	24
Eur-C				
Belarus	43.4	20	29 712	20
Estonia	38.7	20	3 732	20
Hungary	28.0	16	21 740	16
Kazakhstan	49.3	20	39 274	26
Latvia	38.3	18	6 492	20
Lithuania	33.7	19	8 332	20
Republic of Moldova	34.5	17	8 952	21
Russian Federation	53.7	20	493 116	21
Ukraine	43.2	19	155 230	21

Source: Preventable environmental impact on mortality and morbidity in countries of the WHO European Region (2007) (41).

water, poor sanitation and hygiene and air pollution. In turn, countries' capacity and political determination to adopt effective interventions and legislation strongly influences this exposure. (This section introduces the country groups Eur-A, -B and -C.[3])

Known risk factors

Much of the burden attributable to the environment is due to established risk factors whose relationships to health are now well understood and for which reliable evidence is available on the effectiveness of the policies and interventions used in response. Important ones for countries in the European Region include (Table 2.16): access to safe water and improved sanitation, exposure to air pollution, exposure to persistent organic pollutants, mercury and pesticides, occupational risks and injuries.

Access to safe water and improved sanitation

Lack of access to safe drinking-water is still a leading cause of death among children aged 0–14 years in the Region. About 13 000 annual deaths (5.3% of the total mortality among children: 0.2% in Eur-A, 7.5% in Eur-B and 2.4% in Eur-C) are attributable to diarrhoeal disease related to exposure to unsafe drinking-water *(43)*. About 13 million people in Eur-B and 9 million in Eur-C do not have access to improved sources of water; 18 million in Eur-B and 32 million in Eur-C lack access to improved sanitation. Rural populations tend to have poorer access to safe drinking-water supply: 66% in Eur-B and 56% in Eur-C (Fig. 2.14) *(44)*. The slow progress in achieving universal access to safe drinking-water and improved sanitation, especially in rural areas in the eastern part of the Region, jeopardizes the achievement in the Region of MDG 7 (ensuring environmental sustainability) and the fulfilment of a basic human right. Action is needed to ensure safe drinking-water from source to tap, to improve the management of water demand and to take full advantage of supportive policy instruments, such as the WHO/United Nations Economic Commission for Europe (UNECE) Protocol on Water and Health to the 1992 Convention on the Protection and Use of Transboundary Watercourses and International Lakes *(45)*.

Exposure to air pollution

Outdoor and indoor air pollution is an important determinant of health, increasing mortality from cardiovascular and respiratory diseases and reducing life expectancy by about 8.6 months in EU countries. It reduces life expectancy by more than 13 months in the most polluted countries. In the past two decades, significant progress has been achieved in reducing the emissions of some air pollutants, such as sulfur, nitrogen oxides and lead. This is mostly due to improvements to industrial and energy production processes and increased energy efficiency and fuel quality. Nevertheless, nearly 90% of residents of urban areas are still exposed to air pollution concentrations exceeding WHO guideline levels *(46)*. The average exposure by country varies by a factor of three in the Region. On average, the concentrations of the main air pollutants (particulate matter, ozone and nitrogen dioxide) and related risks to health did not change or increased slightly from 2000 to 2006.

---

[3] Eur-A: 27 countries with very low child and adult mortality: Andorra, Austria, Belgium, Croatia, Cyprus, the Czech Republic, Denmark, Finland, France, Germany, Greece, Iceland, Ireland, Israel, Italy, Luxembourg, Malta, Monaco, the Netherlands, Norway, Portugal, San Marino, Slovenia, Spain, Sweden, Switzerland and the United Kingdom.
Eur-B: 17 countries with low child and adult mortality: Albania, Armenia, Azerbaijan, Bosnia and Herzegovina, Bulgaria, Georgia, Kyrgyzstan, Montenegro, Poland, Romania, Serbia, Slovakia, Tajikistan, the former Yugoslav Republic of Macedonia, Turkey, Turkmenistan and Uzbekistan.
Eur-C: 9 countries with low child but high adult mortality: Belarus, Estonia, Hungary, Kazakhstan, Latvia, Lithuania, Republic of Moldova, the Russian Federation and Ukraine.

Table 2.16. Deaths and DALYs lost attributable to environmental risk factors, WHO European Region, 2002

Country	Population (thousands)	Water, sanitation and hygiene				Indoor air pollution			Outdoor air pollution			
		Population (%) with:		Diarrhoea		Population using solid fuel (%)	Deaths per year	DALYs per 1000 population per year	Annual PM$_{10}$ (µg/m^3)[a]	Urban population (%)[b]	Deaths per year	DALYs per 1000 population per year
		improved water	improved sanitation	Deaths per year	DALYs per 1000 population per year							
Eur-A												
Andorra	69	100	100	–[d]	0.2	< 5	–	–	41	39	–	0.8
Austria	8 111	100	100	–	0.1	< 5	–	–	32	37	1 100	0.7
Belgium	10 296	100	100	–	0.2	< 5	–	–	41	34	2 000	1.0
Croatia	4 439	100	100	–	0.2	12	–	–	35	32	900	1.3
Cyprus	796	100	100	–	0.5	< 5	–	–	60	48	300	1.6
Czech Republic	10 246	100	98	–	0.1	< 5	–	–	42	24	1 700	1.0
Denmark	5 351	100	100	–	0.2	< 5	–	–	24	38	600	0.6
Finland	5 197	100	100	–	0.2	< 5	–	–	16	42	200	0.2
France	59 850	100	NA	–	NA[e]	< 5	–	–	25	42	4 800	0.4
Germany	82 414	100	100	–	0.1	< 5	–	–	29	32	10 400	0.6
Greece	10 970	NA	NA	–	NA	< 5	–	–	34	46	2 800	1.3
Iceland	287	100	100	–	0.2	< 5	–	–	21	59	< 100	0.4
Ireland	3 911	NA	NA	–	NA	< 5	–	–	15	32	< 100	0.1
Israel	6 304	100	NA	NA	NA	< 5	–	–	53	80	1 500	1.2
Italy	57 482	NA	NA	–	NA	< 5	–	–	37	27	8 400	0.7
Luxembourg	447	100	100	–	0.2	< 5	–	–	17	19	–	0.1
Malta	393	100	NA	–	NA	< 5	–	–	NA	NA	–	–
Monaco	34	100	100	–	0.2	< 5	–	–	NA	NA	–	–
Netherlands	16 067	100	100	–	0.2	< 5	–	–	38	52	3 600	1.2
Norway	4 514	100	100	–	0.2	< 5	–	–	22	33	400	0.3
Portugal	10 049	NA	NA	–	NA	< 5	–	–	27	56	1 900	1.0
San Marino	27	NA	NA	–	NA	< 5	–	–	19	NA	–	–
Slovenia	1 986	NA	NA	–	NA	8	–	–	44	21	300	0.7
Spain	40 977	100	100	–	0.2	< 5	–	–	30	42	5 800	0.7
Sweden	8 867	100	100	–	0.1	< 5	–	–	19	30	500	0.2
Switzerland	7 171	100	100	–	0.1	< 5	–	–	27	42	800	0.5
United Kingdom	59 068	100	NA	–	NA	< 5	–	–	26	53	12 400	1.0
Eur-B												
Albania	3 141	96	91	300	0.3	50	< 100	0.5	58	9	200	0.4
Armenia	3 072	92	83	< 100	1	26	100	0.8	84	54	1 600	4.0
Azerbaijan	8 297	77	54	800	3.9	49	1 800	7.2	64	23	1 400	1.4
Bosnia and Herzegovina	4 126	97	95	–	0.3	50	< 100	0.1	22	37	300	0.5
Bulgaria	7 965	99	99	–	0.2	17	< 100	0.1	59	37	3 400	3.0
Georgia	5 177	82	94	–	0.3	43	100	0.6	46	40	2 200	3.0
Kyrgyzstan	5 067	77	59	600	5	76	1 600	7.5	36	16	400	0.6
Poland	38 622	NA	NA	–	NA	< 5	–	–	40	32	6 000	1.1
Romania	22 387	57	NA	NA	NA	23	300	0.2	76	33	9 400	3.0
Serbia and Montenegro	15 035	93	87	–	0.6	NA	–	–	17	20	100	0.1
Slovakia	5 398	100	99	–	0.2	< 5	–	–	31	17	400	0.4
Tajikistan	6 195	59	51	1 800	10	75	1 600	7.9	57	11	500	0.6
The former Yugoslav Republic of Macedonia	2 046	NA	NA	NA	NA	30	–	0.1	29	29	200	0.7
Turkey	70 318	96	88	6 000	3	11	2 500	0.9	56	61	18 800	2.0
Turkmenistan	4 794	72	62	1 000	7	< 5	–	0.1	73	18	700	1.4
Uzbekistan	25 705	82	67	500	1	72	5 300	6.1	81	21	4 300	1.3
Eur-C												
Belarus	9 940	100	84	–	0.3	19	200	0.2	9	49	–	–
Estonia	1 338	100	97	–	0.2	16	–	–	19	37	100	0.5
Hungary	9 923	99	95	–	0.2	< 5	–	–	34	32	1 900	1.3
Kazakhstan	15 469	86	72	300	1	< 5	< 100	0.1	25	43	2 300	1.2
Latvia	2 329	99	78	–	0.3	10	–	–	17	42	< 100	0.2
Lithuania	3 465	NA	NA	–	NA	< 5	–	–	29	42	700	1.1
Republic of Moldova	4 270	92	68	100	0.4	63	200	0.7	41	27	900	1.5
Russian Federation	144 082	97	87	700	0.3	9	400	0.0	25	48	37 200	1.9
Ukraine	48 902	96	96	< 100	0.3	6	200	0.1	29	42	15 200	2.0

[a] Urban population weighted average for particulate matter less than 10 microns in diameter (PM$_{10}$) (estimate or monitored when available).
[b] Percentage living in cities with populations > 100 000 or national capitals.
[c] In this case, years of life lost to premature mortality.
[d] Zero of estimation or method not sensitive enough.
[e] Not available.
Source: Deaths and DALYs attributable to three environmental risk factors [online database] (42).

Fig. 2.14. Percentage of the population with access to an improved water supply, urban and rural areas, WHO European Region, 2006

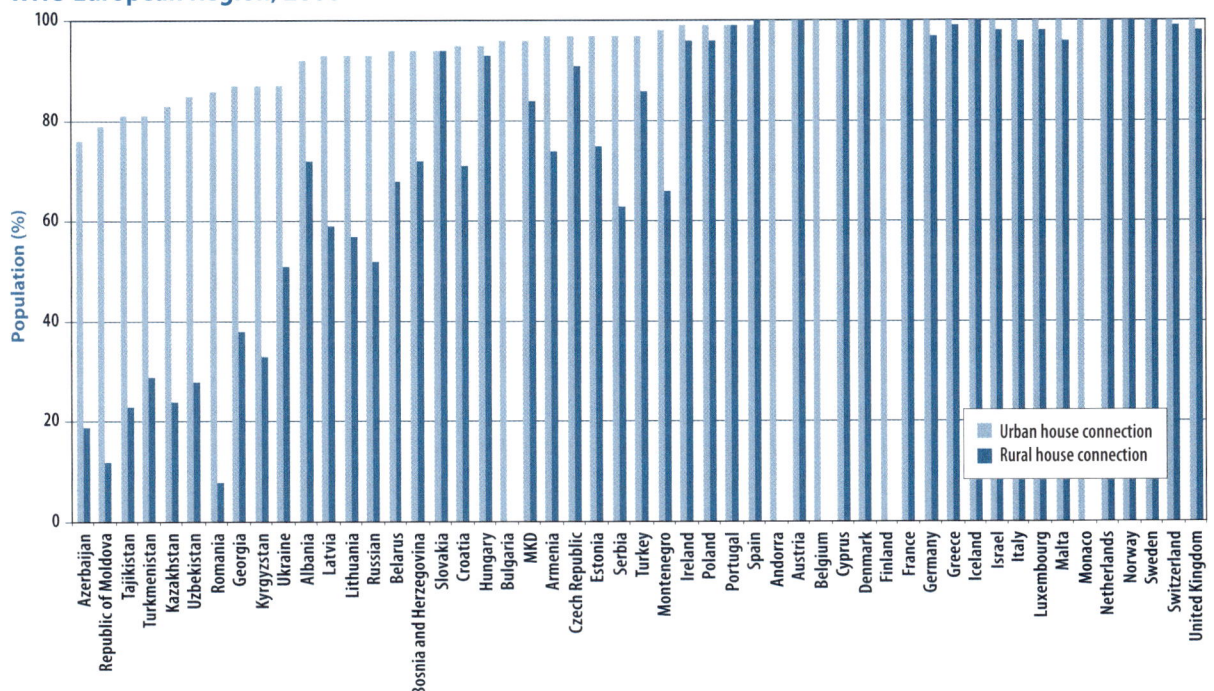

Note. MKD is the International Organization for Standardization (ISO) abbreviation for the former Yugoslav Republic of Macedonia.
Source: Joint Monitoring Programme for Water Supply and Sanitation (44).

Exposure to persistent organic pollutants, mercury and pesticides

The phasing out of lead in petrol, first in western Europe and later in central and eastern Europe, significantly reduced blood lead concentrations among children during the past two decades (47). Nevertheless, lead exposure is still considerably higher in the south-eastern part of the Region than the northern and western parts. As children have no known safe exposure level, the concentrations of lead in blood need to be further reduced. In many countries, the legislative basis of the air quality management system and air quality monitoring needs to be updated to better reflect the WHO air quality guidelines (46). Moreover, clearer guidance on indoor air quality is required. The WHO Regional Office for Europe is developing guidelines on indoor air quality.

A few countries have provided data on persistent organic pollutants in human milk. These data indicate that population exposure to certain persistent organic pollutants, such as dioxin, has declined in the past decade, although countries differ (48). New compounds have emerged: polybrominated and polyfluorinated compounds. Mercury and its compounds are highly toxic to humans, ecosystems and wildlife. Even relatively low doses can have serious neurotoxic effects on adults and children. In some countries in the Region, consuming contaminated fish or large amounts of uncontaminated fish results in hazardous intake of methylmercury. As this counteracts the otherwise beneficial health effect of fish consumption, reducing the concentration of mercury in fish should be a high priority. Reducing emissions to the atmosphere and avoiding soil contamination are means of achieving this aim.

Although most countries in the Region regulate pesticides, they can harm health and the environment, and careless use and overuse can exacerbate the effects. The use of obsolete pesticides remains a problem in some of the countries in central and eastern Europe and the Caucasus. Some countries are addressing this problem, but others need to strengthen action.

Occupational risks

Hazardous exposure at the workplace is among the 10 most important risk factors affecting the burden of disease in Europe. Each year about 300 000 people die from occupational diseases and 27 000 from occupational injuries in the Region. Occupational diseases and injuries result in a loss of about 4% of GDP. The incidence and mortality rates vary significantly between countries, largely owing to differences in the reporting systems. Nevertheless, the absence of a clear overall decline in work-related injuries indicates that progress is not adequate. Action is needed to fully implement World Health Assembly resolution WHA60.26 *(49)*, which highlights opportunities for combining health protection from occupational hazards with health promotion interventions at the workplace.

Injuries

Unsafe environmental conditions play a major role in determining injuries. For example, an estimated 25% of road traffic injuries in western Europe is attributable to environmental conditions, such as road infrastructure and the availability of pavements and facilities for cyclists and pedestrians *(50)*. Injuries represent the third leading cause of death in the Region, with almost 800 000 lives lost annually; 66% of these deaths are preventable *(51)*, and the costs are an estimated 2% of GDP. The political and economic transition in the Region has resulted in increased inequality in injuries. Differentials between countries are high and increasing (Fig. 2.15).

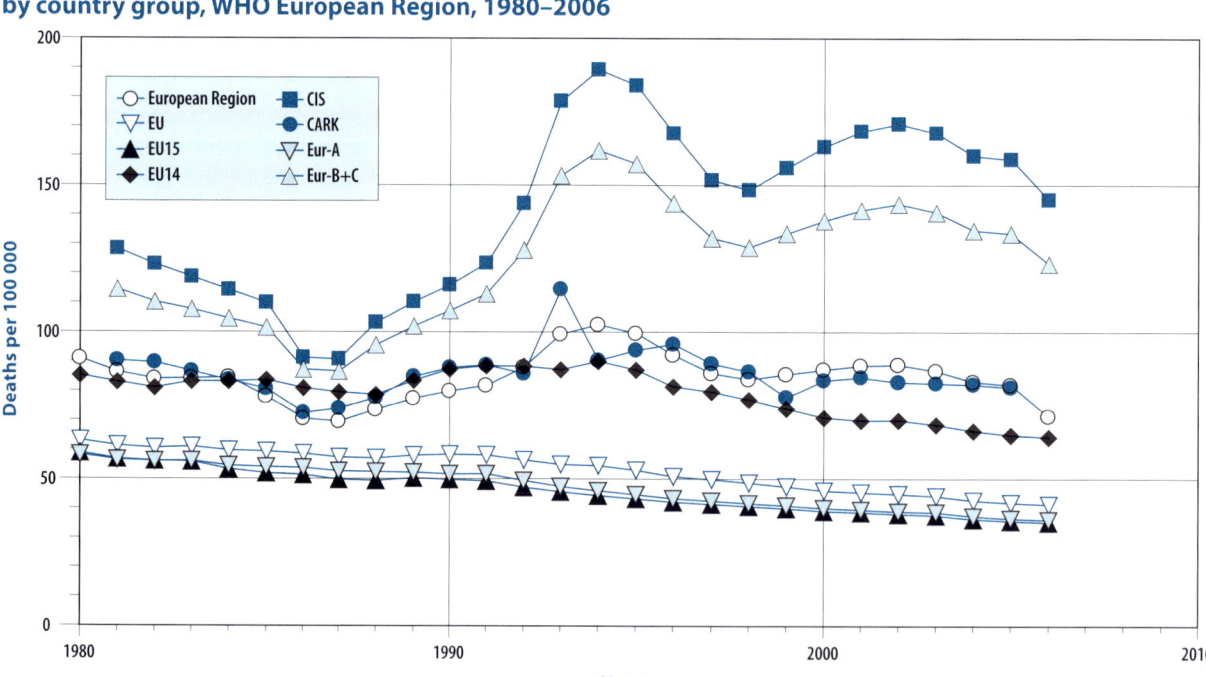

Fig. 2.15. External causes of death (injury and poisoning): SDRs per 100 000 population by country group, WHO European Region, 1980–2006

Source: European Health for All database *(4)*.

The ratios of mortality rates vary between low- and middle-income countries and high-income countries in the Region by individual injury cause, ranging from 16.9 for poisoning to 1.3 for falls. Within countries, the rates for road traffic deaths are 3.5 times higher among children of lower social class than those of higher social class; for poisoning, this ratio is 18. Through resolution EUR/RC55/R9, the WHO Regional Committee for Europe advocates reducing violence and unintentional injury by promoting an evidence-based and multisectoral public health approach *(52)*.

Emerging concerns

In recent years, several other risk factors have emerged that are less well known but cause concern because of their likely impact, upward trends, uncertainty surrounding the extent and severity of their effects, or potential for long-term health effects. These include: climate change, waste-related exposure, foodborne disease and energy insecurity.

There is now strong consensus that the climate is changing. If current trends continue, rising temperature and sea levels and more frequent extreme weather events could increase mortality and morbidity and worsen the determinants of health. Potential health threats include shortages of food and water, loss of shelter and livelihoods, outbreaks of vector-borne disease and increasing inequality within and between countries *(53)*. Some of these effects have already increased in Europe; for example, the 2003 heat-waves caused more than 70 000 excess deaths *(54)*. Heat-related mortality is estimated to increase by 1–4% for each 1 °C rise in temperature, meaning that it could rise by 30 000 annual deaths by the 2030s and 50 000–110 000 annual deaths by the 2080s *(55)*.

Climate change will be a main challenge for environmental health in the foreseeable future *(56)* and is a WHO priority *(57)*. Issues include:

- temperature-sensitive infectious disease, such as foodborne infections, which could lead to an extra 20 000 annual cases by the 2030s and 25 000–40 000 annual cases by the 2080s *(58)*;
- changes in infectious disease transmission by vectors such as mosquitoes and ticks, as a result of changes in their geographical ranges, seasons of activity and population sizes *(53)*;
- heavy precipitation, linked to some outbreaks of waterborne diseases, from mobilizing pathogens or extensive water contamination from overflowing sewage pipes; and
- important effects on the concentrations and dispersion of air pollutants: for example, the United Kingdom could have about 800 additional annual ozone-related deaths by 2020 *(59)*.

Despite the lack of unequivocal evidence on the health implications of current practices for waste management, there are concerns about the health effects of several options, including landfilling, incineration and disposal of health care and other hazardous waste. Given the growing generation of waste, policy-makers must increasingly choose the most appropriate policies for safely disposing of it. A review of European case studies on the health effects of landfills and incinerators reaffirmed the importance of the EU's waste management hierarchy, favouring the minimization of waste generation, followed by the reuse of goods, value recovery through recycling and composting and, finally, incineration and landfilling, preferably with energy recovery *(60)*. Further developing and applying economic assessment of waste management options and of participatory approaches for identifying health-friendly policy responses is a priority. Special attention should be paid to the illegal practices and toxic waste dumping documented in the eastern part of the Region, which can have potentially serious health implications, and as already seen in the Campania region in Italy *(61)*.

Foodborne disease constitutes a considerable public health burden and challenge throughout the Region. Due to insufficient reporting systems, the available data are not systematic and do not allow reliable comparisons. The incidence of foodborne diseases, however, is estimated to be many times higher in the eastern than in the western part of the Region *(62)*.

Diseases of zoonotic origin are of particular concern. These include commonly reported diseases such as salmonellosis, campylobacteriosis and brucellosis. Botulism and zoonotic parasitic diseases (such as trichinellosis and echinococcosis) are reported in some parts of the Region. The food chain can be contaminated by various chemical hazards, such as dioxins, persistent organic pollutants and heavy metals. Although many of the traditional hazards remain, problems are also emerging as a result of changing risk factors, including:

- the centralization, industrialization and globalization of the food chain;
- changing consumer behaviour such as eating more outside the home and eating more raw food;
- changes in pathogens; and
- antimicrobial resistance, an increasing public health problem that is partly related to the use of antimicrobial agents in animals.

The second WHO European Action Plan for Food and Nutrition Policy *(62)*, developed to support countries in implementing national plans, addresses the main public health challenges in nutrition and food safety and security.

Securing access to safe, clean, reliable and affordable sources of energy for households for heating and cooking is an important new concern. This has been prompted by a combination of increasing evidence of the health effects of indoor air pollution caused by solid fuel, several cold spells that were particularly dramatic in the CARK and crises in the international trade of natural gas. These highlight the need to protect the most vulnerable segments of society and to ensure a continuous supply of energy to the health care infrastructure, including during extreme weather events.

Evolving response to old and new challenges

Environmental health risks are increasingly complex and multifactorial. The traditional approach, based on risk assessment, has important limitations. As underlined by recent international discussion, much work is still required to close the gap between science and policy, to ensure that the achievements of research inform policy-making, even under conditions of high uncertainty *(63)*. Many tools and institutional structures are needed, including adopting precautionary approaches. The WHO Regional Office for Europe has long promoted the precautionary principle as a tool for protecting health, the environment and the welfare of future generations.

In addition, WHO and other health agencies have expanded the scope of their work in environment and health and broadened the subject to include upstream determinants of health, such as development plans and policies. As part of their stewardship role in the health system, European governments – especially health ministries – are increasingly taking the health-in-all-policies approach, which considers the health implications of policies and decisions of various sectors such as transport, energy, industry, housing and tourism *(64)* (see the section on stewardship for healthy public policies in Part 3). Member States recognize the importance of addressing environmental health risks at the national level through multisectoral policy action, using consultative processes such as environmental health performance reviews and capacity-building activities.

The environment and health process in the European Region, with its series of ministerial conferences on environment and health, the WHO/UNECE Protocol on Water and Health *(45)* and the Transport, Health and Environment Pan-European Programme (Box 2.1) are examples of processes that facilitate the direct engagement of sectors to better protect health.

Box 2.1. Working with other sectors: the Transport, Health and Environment Pan-European Programme (THE PEP)

THE PEP was set up in 2002 as a joint policy platform of the WHO Regional Office for Europe and UNECE to achieve more sustainable transport patterns and more closely integrate environmental and health concerns in transport policies.

In January 2009, at the Third High-level Meeting on Transport, Health and Environment, representatives of all three sectors adopted the Amsterdam Declaration – Making THE Link: Transport choices for our health, environment and prosperity *(65)*. It recognized the opportunity provided by the current economic downturn to rethink investments in transport policies and to leverage opportunities for economic growth provided by investment in sustainable transport policies. In particular, the Amsterdam Declaration set four priority goals:

- contributing to sustainable economic development and stimulating job creation by investing in environment- and health-friendly transport;
- managing sustainable mobility and promoting a more efficient transport system;
- reducing emissions of transport-related greenhouse gases, air pollutants and noise; and
- promoting policies and actions conducive to healthy and safe modes of transport.

The adoption of the Tallinn Charter *(36)* and the preparation of the Fifth Ministerial Conference on Environment and Health, to be held in Parma, Italy in 2010 *(66)* represent important milestones in achieving strong political consensus on and support for enhancing the stewardship role of health systems in addressing the environmental effects on health in the Region.

Lifestyle and behaviour

Seven lifestyle and behavioural risk factors are responsible for about 60% of the burden of disease in the WHO European Region: high blood pressure, tobacco use, harmful use of alcohol, high serum cholesterol, overweight, unhealthy diet and insufficient physical activity *(13)*. These are the same leading risk factors in all subregions of the Region (Eur-A, -B and -C) and in most countries, although the rank order may differ. In most countries in the Region, the leading risk factor for deaths is high blood pressure, while tobacco is the leading risk factor for burden of disease *(13,67)*. Alcohol is the leading risk factor for both disability and death among young people in Europe *(68)*. This section focuses on four main lifestyle-associated risk factors: tobacco use, the harmful use of alcohol, unhealthy diets and insufficient physical activity, with obesity as a thread common to the last two.

Situation assessment

Tobacco use
In 2005, the prevalence of tobacco use among people aged 15 years and more in the European Region was 34.1%, and almost twice as high among men (44.4%) as women (23.2%) *(12)*. The prevalence of smoking among men and women has stabilized or is decreasing in most

countries in the western part of the Region *(69)*. It has started to decrease in some countries in the eastern part of the Region, although in general it is only stabilizing among men, with no clear trends overall, and has risen slightly in some cases among women *(69)*.

Almost one fifth of adolescents (19.9%) aged 13–15 years use tobacco: slightly more boys (22.7%) than girls (16.8%) *(12)*. In the eastern part of the Region, smoking among 15-year-olds tends to be higher among boys than girls; the opposite is true in many western European countries *(69)*.

Tobacco use is the single most preventable cause of death: a tobacco-related disease will kill half of all users, and lung cancer mortality reflects smoking prevalence *(70)*. Across the Region, the standardized death rates for lung cancer among men have declined, while lung cancer is steadily increasing among women in Eur-A countries *(20)*.

Tobacco is the leading contributor to the burden of disease in more than half the countries in the Region and one of the three leading contributors in the vast majority of countries *(70)*. A particular concern is the growing concentration of smoking in groups with lower socioeconomic status throughout the Region, widening the gap in current and future health outcomes *(70)*.

Harmful use of alcohol
In 2003, alcohol consumption among people aged 15 years and more in the WHO European Region was 8.84 litres per person: the highest of any WHO region *(12)*. Trends for alcohol consumption differ across Europe *(68,71)*. In northern Europe, it is high and continues to rise. In south-western Europe, the decline of past decades seems to be ending. In the eastern part of the Region, consumption in general remains at the very high level reached in the mid-1990s, although religious belief leads to very low levels in some areas *(68)*.

Women account for 20–35% of overall consumption in the European Region: the highest proportion of any WHO region. Youth intoxication continues at a very high level in the western part of the Region, has increased to a similar level in the eastern part of the Region and has become a concern in the southern part of the Region *(68)*.

Alcohol-related deaths and diseases in a society rise and fall in accordance with overall consumption. Overall, alcohol-related deaths increased by about 15% between 2000 and 2002, representing 6% of all deaths and 11% of the burden of disease in the Region. Alcohol also contributes significantly to social problems, including crime and problems in the family and at work *(68)*.

Men have considerably higher alcohol-related mortality and burden of disease than women. Alcohol is the most important risk factor for mortality and morbidity among young people. Among those aged 15–30 years, more than one third of the burden of disease among men and about 14% of that among women is attributable to alcohol *(68)*.

Drinking patterns are important determinants of public health. The extent to which the predominant drinking patterns are detrimental increases in general towards the north and towards the east of the Region. The northern part of the Region has a greater proportion of binge drinking; any given increase in alcohol consumption in this part is associated with more homicide, suicide and unintentional injury than in the southern part of the Region. The gradient is similar for some chronic diseases, such as cirrhosis of the liver *(68)*.

Unhealthy diets, insufficient physical activity and obesity
Poor nutrition accounts for 5% of the total burden of disease in the European Region. Undernutrition may be acute in areas facing food insecurity and more chronic among people living in poverty or among vulnerable population groups such as older people or those with chronic illness or disabilities. Micronutrient deficiencies are also a concern for the Region, and the rate of exclusive breastfeeding at 6 months of age is low everywhere (ranging from 1% to 46%), even in countries with high initiation rates *(62)*.

The proportion of total fat in adult diets in countries in the Region ranges from about 30% to more than 40% of energy intake: the recommended level is 15–30%. It is high in all countries in the Region, especially Belgium and Greece (adults) and France and Spain (children). In addition, the intake of sugar is also greater than the recommended 10% of total energy in most countries *(72)*. The availability of sugar-sweetened beverages (such as soft drinks) has increased in the past decade in almost all countries in the Region, with consumption higher in the northern than in the southern part and among men more than women *(72)*.

In many countries, mean individual fruit and vegetable consumption is substantially below the recommended minimum of 400 g per day. Intake of dietary fibre is uniformly low in countries in the Region (1.8–2.4 g/MJ for men and 2.0–2.8 g/MJ for women), related to low fruit and vegetable intake and inadequate levels of whole-grain cereals. The recommended intake is 2.5–3.1 g/MJ. The traditional (and advantageous) Mediterranean diet, with higher consumption of plant food, vegetable oil and fish, is gradually disappearing, especially among young people *(72)*.

Insufficient physical activity is a key risk factor for a wide range of noncommunicable diseases and for poor well-being and quality of life. One in five people in the Region takes little or no physical activity (less than the recommended minimum), and southern and eastern countries in the Region seem more strongly affected. There are no comparable data for the Region to assess trends but, based on national data, trends are worsening, with a few exceptions. Physical activity seems to be disappearing from daily life as Europe becomes more urbanized, people drive more, jobs become more sedentary, tasks become more mechanized and leisure time is increasingly spent on sedentary activities *(73)*.

There is substantial inequality both within and across countries. Access to leisure and exercise opportunities tends to be unequal across the social spectrum: poorer people are more likely to live in environments that do not support physical activity and are less likely to have access to transport to reach some facilities *(74)*. Nevertheless, the situation is complex, as people with lower socioeconomic status tend to have more active jobs and to commute more actively, as they own fewer cars. Certain population groups are especially vulnerable to physical inactivity: people who are very young, very old or disabled; families in precarious circumstances; migrants; members of ethnic minorities; and women *(75)*. Given the ageing of many populations in the Region, the lack of physical activity among older people is a particular concern, as it will have major effects in loss of independence and related costs for health care systems and reduction of years of healthy life.

Physical inactivity causes an estimated 600 000 annual deaths in the Region (5–10% of total mortality depending on the country) and the annual loss of 5.3 million years of healthy life due to premature mortality and disability. Based on two studies, in Switzerland and the United Kingdom, insufficient physical activity is estimated to cost each of the Region's countries about US$ 150–300 per person per year *(73)*.

Diets in the Region are increasingly characterized by high energy intake and low satiety, and consumption of sugar-rich and alcoholic beverages is increasing. Along with low levels of physical activity, these factors are leading to rising obesity (a body mass index (BMI) ≥ 30 kg/m^2) in virtually all parts of the Region *(72)*; 30–80% of adults in the Region and up to one third of children are overweight (BMI ≥ 25 kg/m^2) (Fig. 2.16). More than 60% of children who are overweight before puberty will be overweight in adulthood, reducing the age at which some noncommunicable diseases, such as diabetes mellitus, become apparent *(72)*.

Fig. 2.16. Overweight among school-aged children based on surveys in selected countries, WHO European Region, 1958–2003

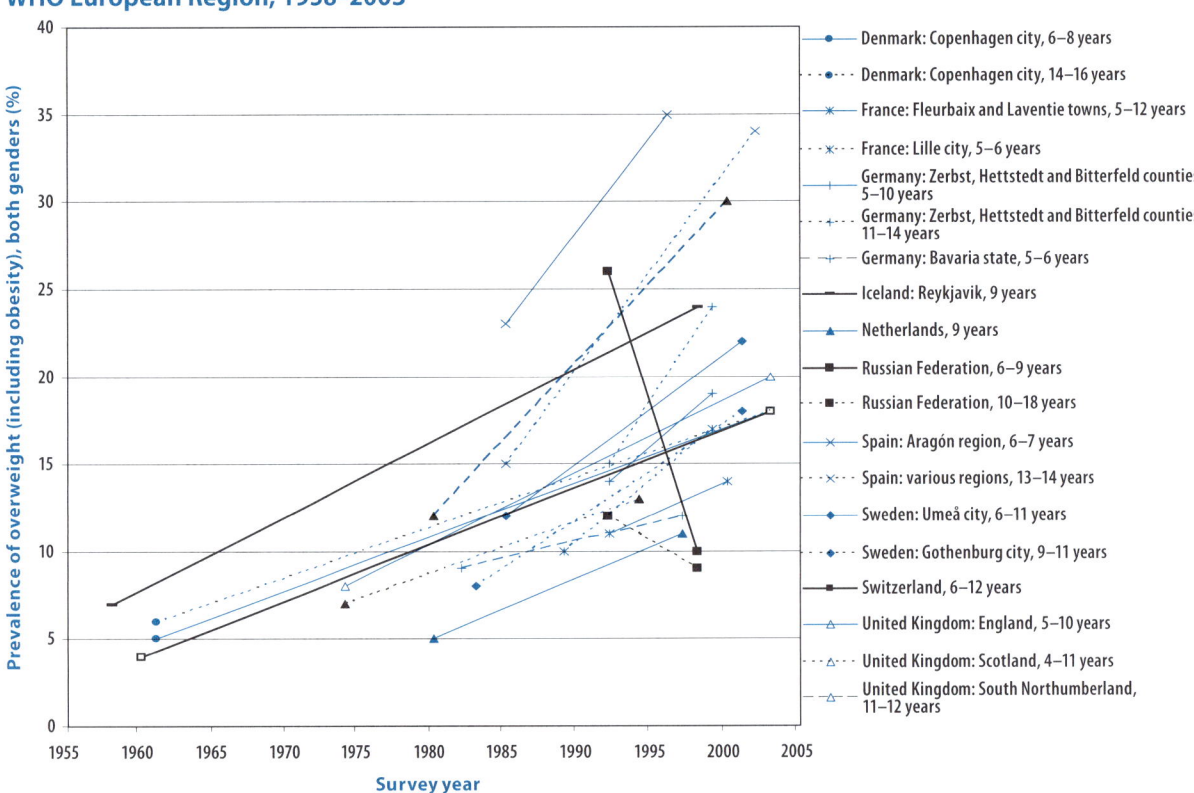

Source: The challenge of obesity in the WHO European Region and the strategies for response. Summary (72).

The combination of poor diet, insufficient physical activity and the resulting obesity and its associated illnesses is responsible for as much ill health and premature death as tobacco smoking. The costs of treating the resulting ill health are estimated to account for up to 6% of total health care expenditure *(72)*. In response to the emerging challenge of the obesity epidemic, the Regional Office organized the WHO European Ministerial Conference on Counteracting Obesity in 2006, which adopted the European Charter on Counteracting Obesity *(76)*.

Issues, challenges and responses

Role of government, regulatory and fiscal measures

The term "lifestyles" in relation to these risk factors can sometimes be misleading, implying that change is entirely the responsibility of individuals. Government and society have important roles. Some of the most effective policy measures to tackle risk factors are fiscal, regulatory or legislative, to be implemented and enforced by government. For alcohol, as emphasized by the *Framework for alcohol policy in the WHO European Region (77)*, effective policy and legislative interventions would include: taxing alcohol sales, imposing laws on drink–driving with enforcement measures (such as random breath testing of drivers), restricting retail outlets and controlling advertising.

Similarly, cost-effective measures for tobacco control would be: taxing tobacco products, thereby increasing consumers' costs by at least 33%, to curb smoking; restricting smoking in public places and workplaces; and banning tobacco advertising *(78)*. From 2001 to 2005, the price of tobacco products rose by an annual rate of 6.8% above inflation in the EU countries, showing good progress compared with the 2.7% annual rate of increase during 1997–2001 *(69)*. In 2006, excise tax was reported as comprising more than half the price of tobacco products in 28 countries in the Region, although ranging from 8% (the Republic of Moldova) to 69% (Israel) *(70)*. The WHO Framework Convention on Tobacco Control *(79)*, which entered into force in 2005, was the first international treaty negotiated under the auspices of WHO and represented a paradigm shift in addressing a major public health challenge through an international regulatory strategy (see also the section below on improving health outcomes).

Although regulatory measures can be among the most effective tools available to public health, caution needs to be exercised to ensure that they are not undermined. Within the EU, very large traveller's allowances for alcohol for personal use have restricted several national governments' ability to control sales to residents, and have forced some governments to lower alcohol tax rates. Further, the price differential between duty-paid and duty-free tobacco products has contributed to an increase in smuggling since the early 1990s. International cooperation, for example on cross-border and illicit trade, and strengthening and enforcing legislation have met with some success *(69)*.

Urban environment and other settings
A complex set of factors affects diet and lifestyle behaviour in modern society. Many are outside the direct control of the health sector and require action in conjunction with transport, environment, urban planning, agriculture and other sectors to create health-supporting environments and health-promoting opportunities.

Urban design often discourages safe, active transport: countries with urban environments less supportive of cycling and walking report lower levels of physical activity. Safe environments for cycling and walking can provide opportunities for exercise at reasonable cost and as part of people's daily transport routine. The health sector can work with:

- urban planners to ensure that services and jobs are located within distances that can be covered on foot or by bicycle;
- employers to facilitate regular physical activity within the workplace; and
- local governments and leisure services to improve access to recreation facilities for low-income neighbourhoods and to provide an example by promoting active transport for their employees.

Growing evidence and examples from intersectoral initiatives are available through the work of the Transport, Health and Environment Pan-European Programme (THE PEP) *(80)*, the WHO European Healthy Cities Network *(81)* and the European network for the promotion of health-enhancing physical activity *(82)*.

Schools provide a good setting for health-promoting opportunities. Strong evidence indicates that school-based physical education increases levels of physical activity and fitness, but the amount of physical education provided and its organization vary between countries. Providing safe routes to school can develop active commuting by such means as "walking school buses" *(75)*, instead of using cars. Removing vending machines selling confectionery and sugary drinks from schools and ensuring the provision of safe drinking-water can promote water over soft drinks. Further, planning and subsidizing healthy menus can be used to influence food-related behaviour and the choices made in school canteens *(62)*.

Surveillance

Surveillance systems for risk factors have shortcomings. Standardized instruments have not been commonly used across the Region, which makes monitoring within-country trends and patterns and making cross-country comparisons more difficult. Internationally comparable data on levels of physical activity across the Region, for example, have only begun to be collected in recent years. Half of countries worldwide do not have minimal information about young people and tobacco use *(70)*. Alcohol consumption and dietary patterns are estimated from a range of sources.

Investment in risk surveillance systems is needed so that they can collect reliable national data on risk factors and enable trends to be monitored, interventions evaluated, evidence for policy development compiled and international comparisons made. Initiatives such as the new European Information System on Alcohol and Health, which form part of and use the same indicators as the new Global Information System on Alcohol and Health, are therefore welcome. The System will be made public from late 2009 and include data on consumption, harm and policies.

Social determinants of health

The social determinants of health are the social conditions in which people are born, grow, live, work and age *(83)* that shape their health and disease exposure, vulnerability and outcomes. These social factors may include employment and working conditions, living environments, the availability of and access to health and social protection services, education and social cohesion or connectedness. They include how social class, gender, age and ethnicity norms, values and discrimination relate to other determinants of health to increase the vulnerabilities and risks that lead to inequity in health *(84)*.

Pandemic (H1N1) 2009 influenza, the severe economic downturn, acute effects of climate change and the 2008–2009 food crisis have strongly highlighted the need to address socially determined inequity in health. Socially disadvantaged people are at higher risk for pandemic illnesses. More people have been thrown into poverty, food insecurity and unemployment; the International Labour Organization estimated that unemployment would increase in Europe and central Asia by 8 million people in 2009 *(85)*. The unemployment rate in the EU rose from 6.8% in April 2008 to 8.9% in May 2009 *(86)*.

The long-standing interest in and commitment to acting on the social determinants of health arose because of their influence on health and, in particular, people's opportunities to lead healthy and longer lives *(87)*. The principles and functions of the WHO Constitution *(88)* reflect this. WHO's work with other specialized United Nations agencies, when necessary, to improve nutrition, housing, sanitation, recreation and/or economic or working conditions is critical to achieving its objective of all people attaining the highest level of health. WHO's work to strengthen primary health care, its Health for All strategy and health promotion and many other programmes draw on this mandate.

While overall health status in the Region has improved *(39)* (see the section above on key health status indicators), this improvement is not shared equally across the population. Socially determined gaps exist both between and within countries. Within countries, rural and remote population groups have higher mortality than their urban counterparts, and rates vary by ethnicity and socioeconomic status *(85)*. Inequality resulting from the social determinants of health includes not only decreased life expectancy and higher mortality rates but also morbidity as measured by self-rated health status, number of years lived in good health, prevalence of noncommunicable diseases, health behaviour and access to health care *(89,90)*. Unfortunately, inequity in health has increased both overall and between population groups in the same countries *(38,91)* (Fig. 2.17).

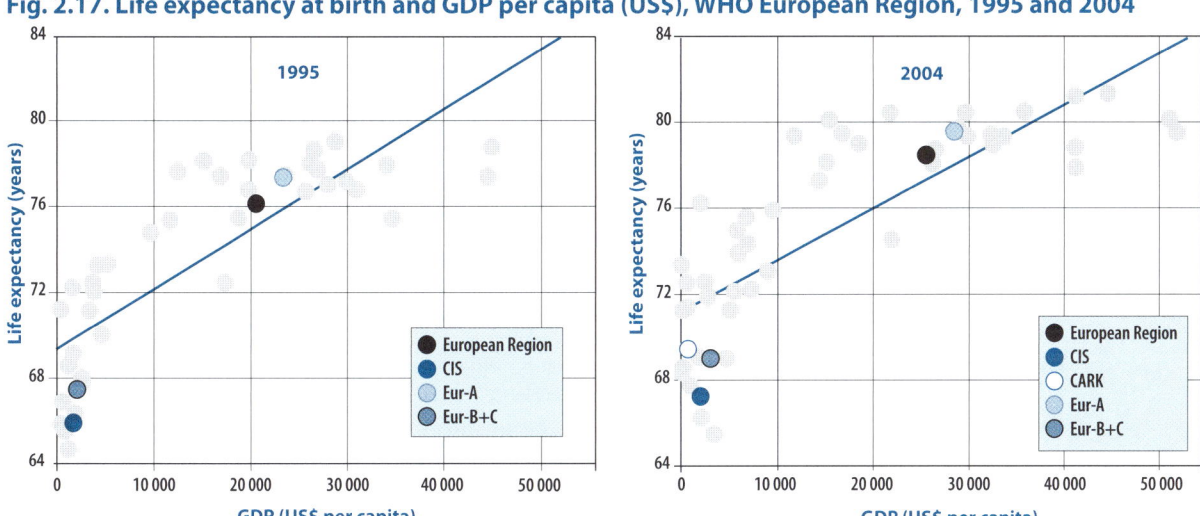

Fig. 2.17. Life expectancy at birth and GDP per capita (US$), WHO European Region, 1995 and 2004

Source: European Health for All database *(4)*.

Social and life-stage conditions affecting health

Poverty is a key social determinant and explains inequality in health between the most and least affluent countries and population groups. Differences in health also follow a strong social gradient, which reflects the position of an individual or population group in society and subsequent differences in health outcomes. These differences are associated with lower educational and employment status, poorer housing and reduced participation in civic society and sense of control over life *(6)*. These patterns of differences in health opportunity affect countries with both higher and lower incomes *(92)*.

For countries in the eastern part of the Region, available data on the health-related MDGs *(16)* and the burden of noncommunicable diseases show differences by socioeconomic level, sex and geographical location *(93,94)* (Fig. 2.18).

These data suggest that people living in poverty, migrants, internally displaced people and members of ethnic minorities are systematically disadvantaged *(94,95)*. Limited access to

Fig. 2.18. Ischaemic heart disease among people aged 0–64 years: SDRs per 100 000 population and GDP per capita (international dollars), WHO European Region, 1995 and 2005

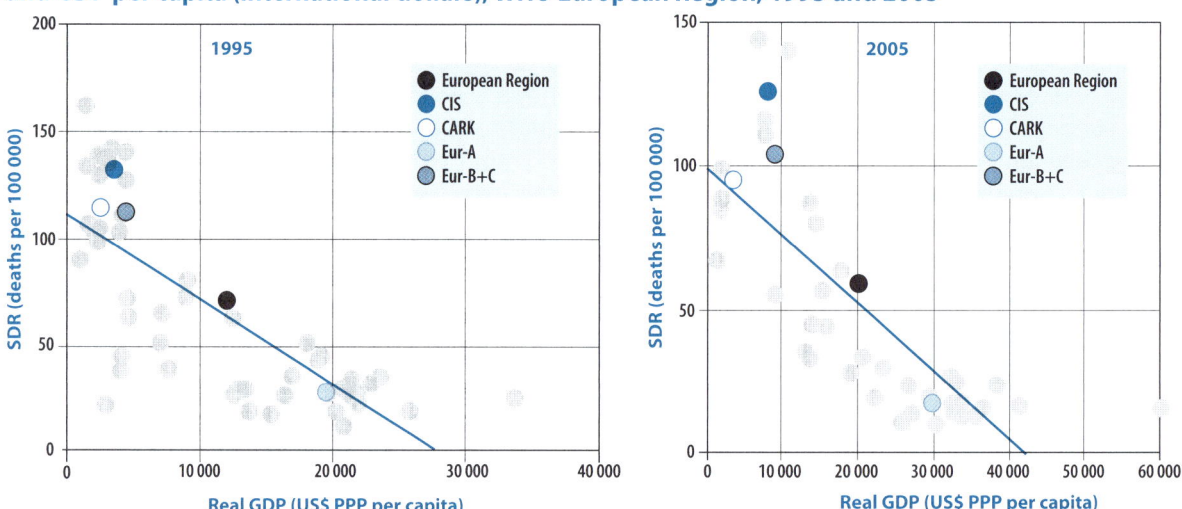

Source: European Health for All database (4).

health services and weak social health protection contribute to this inequity in health. Where social health protection is weak and health systems rely heavily on out-of-pocket payments, catastrophic health expenditure has been shown to increase the fraction of the poor population by 3–9 percentage points (96).

Unemployment, unsafe working conditions and precarious work – including informal, temporary and contract work, child labour and slavery or bonded labour – are associated with poorer health status. Workers in occupations with lower status are more exposed to a cluster of work-related health hazards, affecting physical and mental health. Stress at work is associated with a 50% excess risk of coronary heart disease, and consistent evidence indicates that high job demand, low control and imbalance between effort and reward are risk factors for mental and physical health problems (7). Such findings have been consistently reported across the Region. For example, data in Sweden indicate that mortality and ill health are much greater among blue-collar workers than white-collar workers in managerial positions (97). In Hungary, variation in cardiovascular mortality rates for people aged 45–64 was largely attributable to unfavourable working and other psychosocial stress conditions (98).

Increasing globalization has increased the use of flexible employment options. This is usually reflected in less secure employment conditions, including fixed-term and temporary contracts and people working without contracts. Such conditions are associated with negative mental health effects and more frequent among women and manual male workers (99).

Changes in employment structure differentially affect women and men depending on the gender-related job segregation in a country. Men are usually more severely affected in economies dominated by construction and durable goods manufacturing, whereas public-sector cutbacks can be expected to raise women's joblessness disproportionately (100). Improving occupational health and using the workplace to promote health and education can reduce the amount of sick leave taken, improve health outcomes for all socioeconomic groups and help to reduce inequity in health (97).

An estimated 72 million international migrants live in the European Region *(101)*; the global total is estimated to be 210 million *(102)*. Migrants experiencing socioeconomic disadvantage and other adverse conditions can face numerous factors that harm health. Migrants can be especially vulnerable to health problems, including occupational health issues, respiratory diseases, communicable diseases (such as TB or hepatitis), poor nutrition, poor reproductive and sexual health and mental disorders. All of these are made worse by limited access to the health system and other social services *(103)*.

Although the European Region has the highest score on the Gender-related Development Index *(104)* of any WHO region, gender inequity is deep, as reflected by women's disadvantaged position in decision-making bodies. For example, men occupy 76% of national parliament seats and 85% of membership of high-level decision-making bodies in employer and trade union organizations taking part in discussions, negotiations and joint action with each other and with EU institutions *(105)*. As mentioned, inequity in health may disadvantage men for mortality from all causes, cancer and external causes, and women for mortality from cardiovascular diseases *(106)*. Differences between men and women in access to health care and treatment are also widespread. In Sweden, the top-ranking country on the Gender-related Development Index, women have less access to: dialysis and kidney transplantation, referrals for bronchoscopy, operations for knee and hip arthritis, cataract operations, certain areas of cardiovascular care, light therapy related to psoriasis and eczema, special stroke units and new and more expensive medication. Further, women have longer waiting times for an appointment with a general practitioner (GP) for both acute and non-acute health conditions *(107)*. In addition, there may be considerable gender differences in individual illness groups across the range of specific conditions. Fig. 2.19 shows differences in hospital admission rates between women and men for mental health conditions in Spain *(108)*.

Fig. 2.19. Percentage distribution of hospital admissions by diagnosis and sex for mental health conditions in Spain

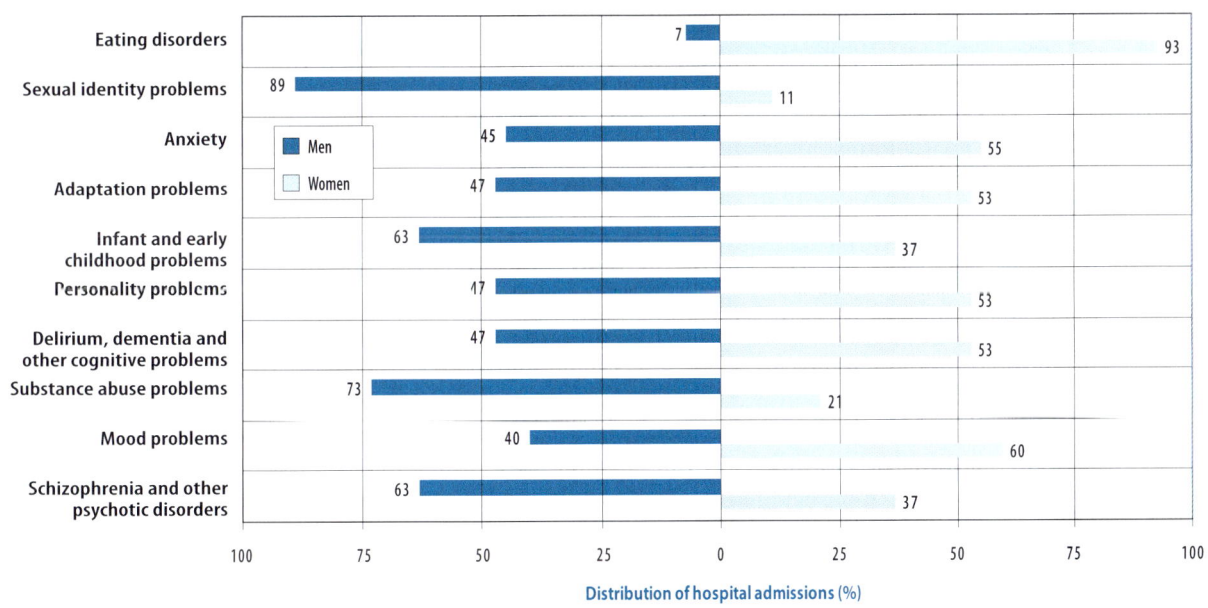

Source: National Health Survey 2006 [web site] *(108)*.

A study of 22 countries in the Region found that mortality is higher among people with less education, although this inequality varies greatly between countries. For example, the relative index of inequality among men in EU15 countries is 2 between the men with the least and the most education. For three EU12 countries, the relative index of inequality for men is 4 or higher *(109)*.

Inequality in health persists throughout life *(110)*. A life-course approach is relevant for measuring the social determinants of health. Do they have greater effects during certain stages of life? Further, interventions to address the social determinants of inequality in health need to be selected to determine the best time to intervene *(111,112)*.

A 1958 British cohort study examined the relationships between adult health and socioeconomic status as measured by occupational class at birth at four life stages (birth, 16, 23 and 33 years of age) and using self-rated health as an outcome. Although a change in adult socioeconomic status, such as higher level of education, has some effect, improved socioeconomic status in adulthood does not fully compensate for disadvantaged beginnings *(113)*. The study found that no particular life stage dominates but that the cumulative effect or duration of exposure strongly predicts health status in early adulthood. More recent evidence, however, indicates that, although the duration of exposure matters, the social determinants of health (including gender) exert a particularly powerful effect in early childhood *(112)*.

Early childhood is considered the most important stage of development. Healthy early child development includes the physical, social (emotional and language) and cognitive domains, each of which is equally important. Early child development strongly influences well-being, obesity or stunting, mental health, heart disease, literacy and numeracy, criminality and economic participation throughout life. What happens to children in their early years is critical for their developmental trajectory and life-course *(114)*. External influences such as poverty affect cognitive, social and emotional development with lifelong effects. This process starts in the womb: social determinants such as maternal level of education, household income and poverty affect early child survival and development *(115)*.

Despite overall improvements in child mortality, early child mortality and health differ significantly between and within countries in the European Region. For example, despite the known data limitations *(91)*, the mortality rate for children younger than 5 years differs 40 times between countries. A child born in a CIS country is three times as likely to die before the age of 5 as a child born in an EU country. Within countries, rural and remote populations have higher mortality than their urban counterparts, and rates vary by ethnicity and socioeconomic status *(95)*, including poverty.

A child's ability to participate in and benefit from education can have lifelong effects on cognitive, emotional and social development and capacity. Factors determining this include early undernutrition, iron deficiency, environmental toxins (such as fuel used for cooking that affects indoor air quality), stress and poor stimulation and social interaction *(116)*. These biological and psychosocial risk factors are not only hazards that can compromise development but are also often determined by social factors such as gender inequity, low maternal education, reduced access to services and poverty *(117)*. Although exposure to all these risk factors has significant effects, early interventions can make a difference – both by tackling risk factors such as malnutrition and iodine deficiency directly and by addressing the social determinants of risk factors, especially poverty and gender inequity. In general, the earlier the action or intervention, the greater the benefit *(116)*.

Tackling child poverty and stopping the transmission of poverty and exclusion from one generation to the next *(118)* are important because a 20% deficit in adult income will influence national development *(116)*. Investment in early child development can help enable more children to grow into healthy adults who can contribute positively to society. Societies that invest in children and families in the early years have better health status and less inequity in health *(6,114,115,119,120)*.

Nevertheless, children continue to be disproportionately exposed to poverty throughout the Region. For instance, in the EU, 19% of children are at risk of poverty, defined as living in a household with equivalized income below 60% of the national equivalized median income *(118)*. In addition, malnutrition and micronutrient deficiencies among children in some countries in the Region remain high and an immediate public health concern, given their links to poor health and development outcomes and the long-term loss of development potential *(95)*.

Social exclusion has been identified as an important social determinant of health in the European Region based on its effects on health, well-being and life opportunities. Wilkinson & Marmot *(121)* concur with the conclusion that, "By causing hardship and resentment, poverty, social exclusion and discrimination cost lives" *(122)*. Social exclusion is strongly related to, but more than, low income, poverty or financial barriers to accessing services. It is also determined by factors such as sense of control (Fig. 2.20) *(123)*. Farrell et al. *(124)* say that: "It is about isolation from participation in social life, and from power and decision-making. It is harmful to the individuals and communities affected; it is harmful to society as a whole and it is linked to poorer health outcomes.". For example, homeless people may defer seeking health care services for essentially preventable conditions not because of financial barriers to access but because they experience the system and providers as discriminatory and excluding or are concerned about this *(125)*.

Fig. 2.20. Distribution of social capital as measured by perceived control over life by asset quintiles in eight CIS countries

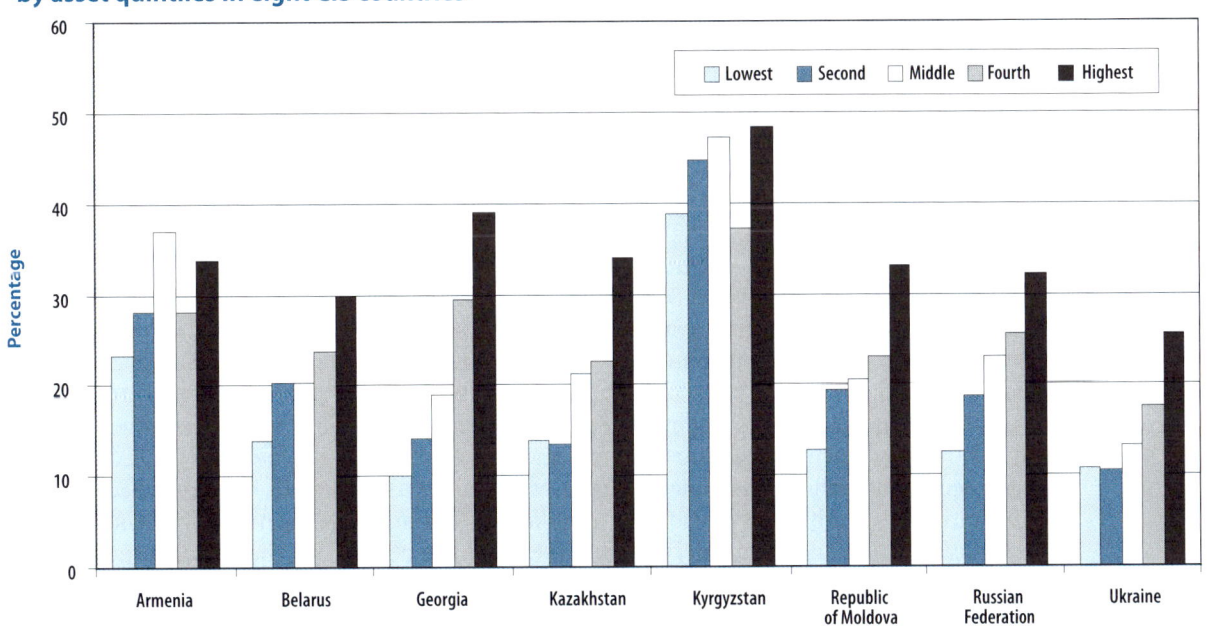

Source: data from Suhrcke et al. *(123)*.

According to research commissioned by the European Commission for 2004 and based on the currently observed patterns of mortality by educational level, societal losses due to inequality in health are significant *(126)*. For example, 707 000 annual deaths were attributable to inequality in health in the current EU countries, except Bulgaria and Romania. About 11.4 million life-years were lost annually due to these deaths. Similarly, more than 33 million cases of ill health annually were attributable to inequality in health. It was estimated to reduce life expectancy at birth in the current EU countries (except Bulgaria and Romania) for adults by 1.84 years and life expectancy in good health by 5.14 years. In addition, socioeconomic inequality in health is likely to have substantial economic effects. The estimates of inequality-related losses to health as a capital good (leading to lower labour productivity) seem modest in relative terms (1.4% of GDP) but are large in absolute terms (€141 billion annually) *(126)*.

The capacity to act on the social determinants of health is increasing. Challenges and gaps in the evidence remain, especially in measuring inequality in health across the life-course and obtaining better data on gender and ethnicity *(6,91,92)*. Nevertheless, approaches to measurement and evidence in this field have improved significantly in recent years, and evidence is increasing not only on the need to act but also on what can be done *(6,125)*, as shown by the final report and work of the Commission on Social Determinants of Health *(6)*.

WHO Executive Board resolution EB124.R6 on reducing health inequities through action on the social determinants of health *(127)* draws on the Commission's final report and is rooted in WHO's longstanding commitment to equity and action on the determinants of health. It synergizes with the Tallinn Charter *(36)*, which embodies European Member States' commitment to strengthening health systems that address socially determined inequity in health through measures based on the shared values of solidarity, equity and participation: fostering investment across sectors that influence health, using primary health care as a platform for intersectoral and interprofessional cooperation, paying due attention to the needs of the poor and preventing impoverishment as a consequence of ill health.

The need to address the social determinants of health and inequity in health is high on the agenda for both WHO and European countries. This is particularly important in the current economic environment, in which decision-makers want to determine how to invest to best address the key social determinants and to prevent inequity from increasing *(128)*.

Current and future challenges

Although the overall health situation in the European Region has continued to improve in the past decades, countries are experiencing significant demographic, epidemiological and health care changes that will shape forthcoming health conditions and challenge the future of health systems in the Region.

Controlling communicable diseases, delaying the emergence of chronic noncommunicable conditions and reducing premature mortality from both have had positive health effects and increased longevity. Nevertheless, despite newer and more effective medical technology and treatment that limit acute effects and mortality, the incidence and prevalence of noncommunicable diseases have decreased for some conditions but not overall, leading to increased disability. Combined with the need for longer-term care and rising health care costs, these aspects can create additional demands on the health system and a need to adjust it. If the trends continue or deteriorate, the stress on the health systems will generate a complex situation difficult to overcome. In contrast, alternative, more encouraging scenarios – resulting from improved long-term care and changes towards healthier lifestyles and behaviour starting early in life – may actually reduce the demands on the health system.

This section highlights some of these challenging features and suggests their interrelationships. Such knowledge and evidence are necessary for making decisions on the health system interventions needed to continue improving the health of the Region's population.

Changing demographics in the European Region

The countries in the Region are undergoing an important demographic transition characterized by slower growth and increasing life expectancy of their populations. Compared with other WHO regions, Europe is considered to be at a stage of relative stability, in which fertility and mortality balance natural population growth. Nevertheless, certain conditions – including very low fertility levels, increasing ageing and immigration – are creating additional demographic pressure that requires attention and policies for managing the potential effects on health and welfare systems.

Population change and distribution

In 2007, the population of the 53 countries in the WHO European Region was 883.5 million, an increase of nearly 9 million (1%) since 2003 *(4)*. Fertility continued to decline, with an average of 1.6 children per woman of childbearing age in 2007. Fertility varied among country groups, however, from 1.3 in EU12 countries to 2.4 in the CARK. Overall population growth in the Region is therefore slowing to an annual average of 0.1%, with 17 countries, mostly in the eastern part, already having a natural decline of 0.1% or more (Fig. 2.21). If current growth trends continue, population size, according to the medium fertility variant *(129)*, is projected to increase slightly, peaking at 904.7 million by 2030 (an increase of 2%), and then to decline to 886.3 million by 2050.

In 2005, 70% of the population of the European Region lived in urban areas *(130)*. This proportion is larger in the EU15 countries (76%) than in the CIS countries (64%) and CARK (41%). Urbanization is projected to continue at an annual rate of 0.2 percentage points until 2030, which will result in 80% of the population living in urban areas. In general, urban and rural areas differ according to population structure, educational levels, lifestyles, occupational backgrounds and exposure to environmental factors, all of which may affect populations' health status and access to health care *(131)*.

In the past two decades, the Region has undergone additional important changes in population due to migration, a trend that is expected to continue. Although precise information on migration flows is difficult to obtain because migration is sometimes illegal, nearly 1 million immigrants are estimated to reach the EU every year from neighbouring areas, especially higher-income countries *(102,132)*. This population inflow has sustained nearly 70% of population growth and, to a lesser extent, employment levels. Although the long-term effects of immigration on population growth and structure are still uncertain, the health system and other social sectors will have to focus additional attention on the current and future needs of this population, which is usually characterized as younger, less affluent and having more illnesses and limited access to health care *(131)*.

Fig. 2.21. Population growth, WHO European Region, 2006 or latest available year and projection for 2050

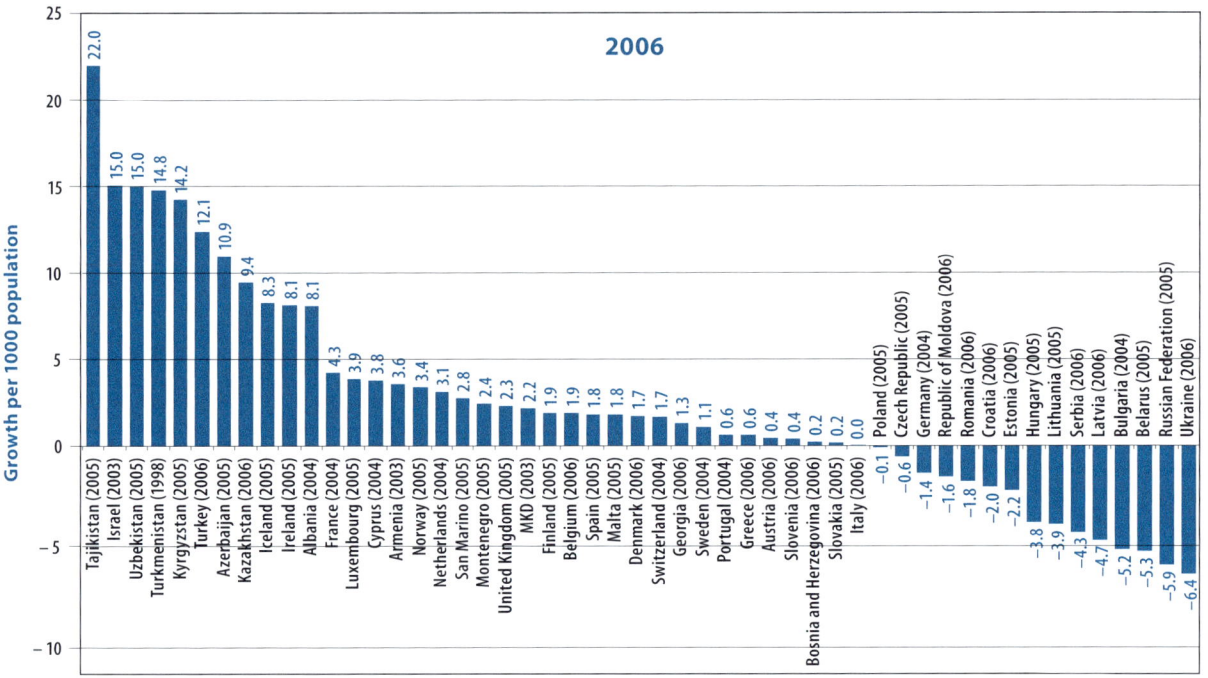

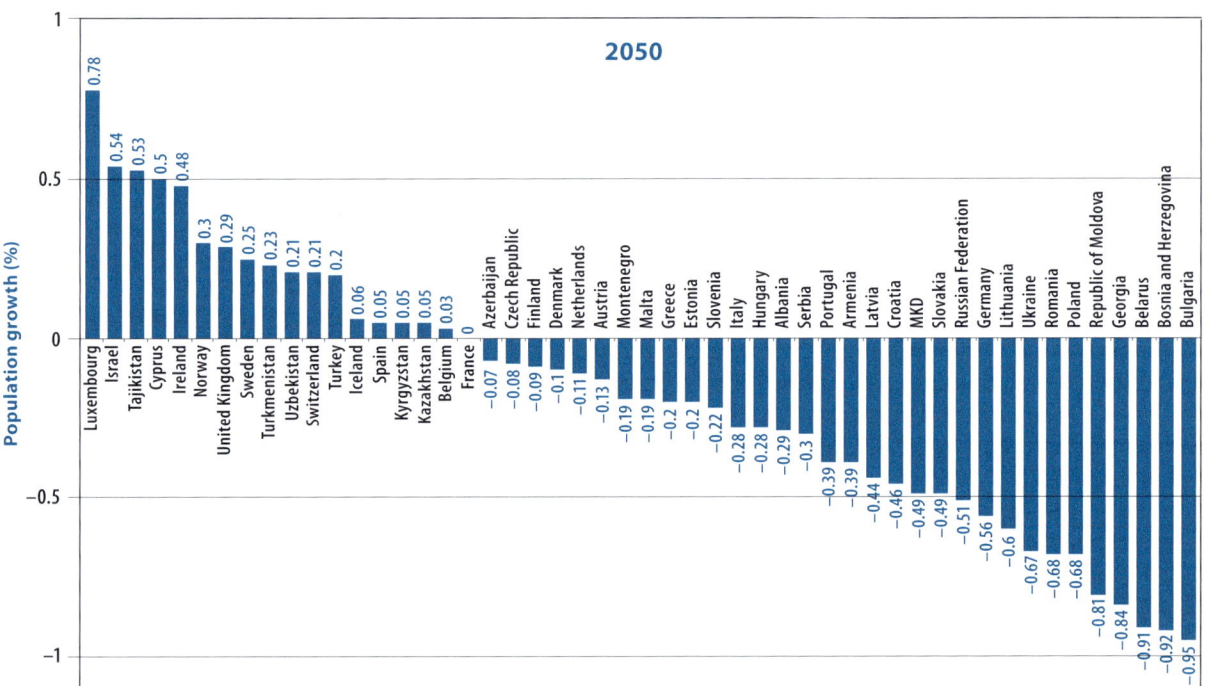

Note. MKD is the International Organization for Standardization (ISO) abbreviation for the former Yugoslav Republic of Macedonia.
Source: European Health for All database *(4)* and United Nations Population Division *(129)*.

The increased longevity in the Region has been associated with reduced incidence of some chronic noncommunicable diseases, improved health care and rapidly declining fertility (as mentioned above, except in some countries) *(133)*. Overall, the fertility rate is now well below the replacement level of 2.1 children per woman of childbearing age. Together, these factors have led to decreased growth and increased ageing. Today, less than 17% of the population of the Region is younger than 15 years and nearly 16% (about 138 million people) is older than 65 years (Fig. 2.22). The number of people older than 65, however, is growing more rapidly than the rest of the population. By 2050, more than 27% of the population (nearly 240 million people) is expected to be 65 years and older. Derived from the above figures, the total dependency ratio[4] in the Region is expected to increase from 47% in 2007 to 74% in 2050 *(128)*.

Fig. 2.22. Percentage of the population aged 65 years and older by country group, WHO European Region, 1970–2005

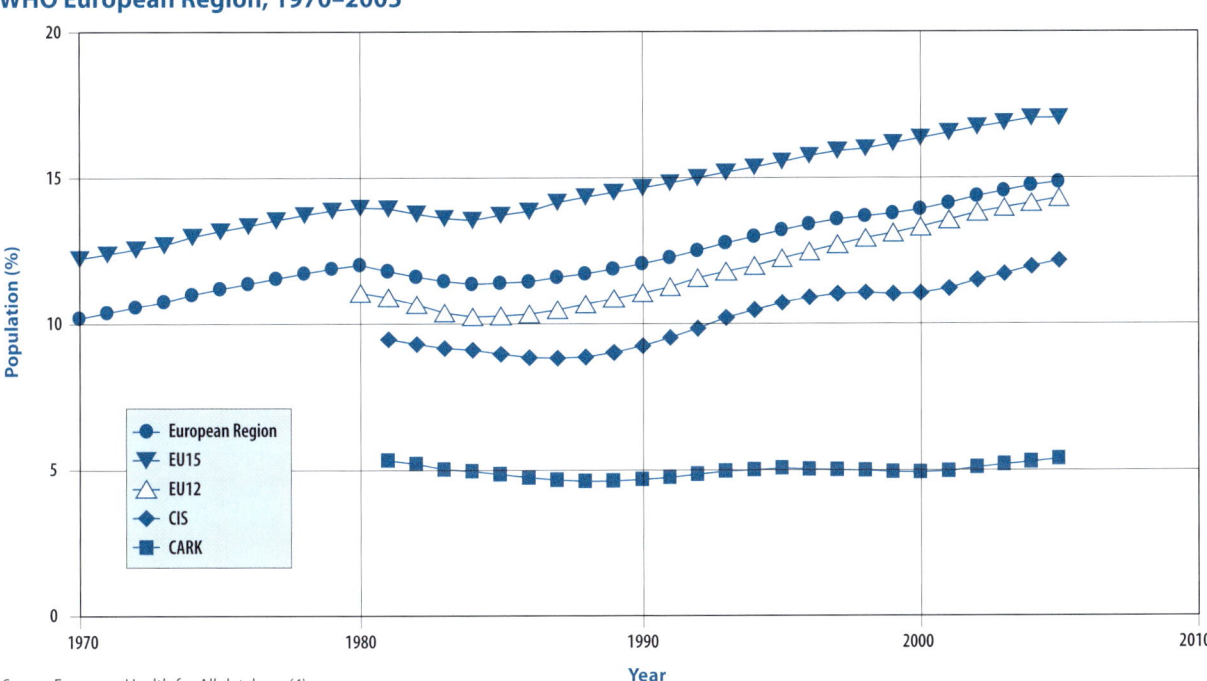

Source: European Health for All database *(4)*.

The ratio of males to females in the Region was close to 1.0 in 2006, but varies with age: from 1.1 for those under 15 years to 0.7 at 65 years and above and 0.4 at 85 years and above (or 2.5 women for each man). The ratios for the groups aged 0–14 and 65 years and more are projected to remain similar by 2050, but that for those aged 85 years and more is projected to increase to 0.5 *(129)*.

The current situation and projected growth and ageing trends of the population often vary markedly across countries. For example, the population age structure in the CIS countries in 2005 shows a narrow base under the age of 10 years, followed by a sharp increase at age 15 and fluctuations among the working-age groups; the proportions of older age groups decrease rapidly at 70 years (Fig. 2.23). EU15 countries have a smoother transition. When the

---

[4] The dependency ratio is the ratio of the total population aged 0–14 years and 65 years and more to the population aged 15–64 years – supposedly the economically active group. It is presented as the number of dependants per 100 people 15–64 years old.

Fig. 2.23. Population age structure, CIS and EU15 countries, 2005 and 2050 (projected)

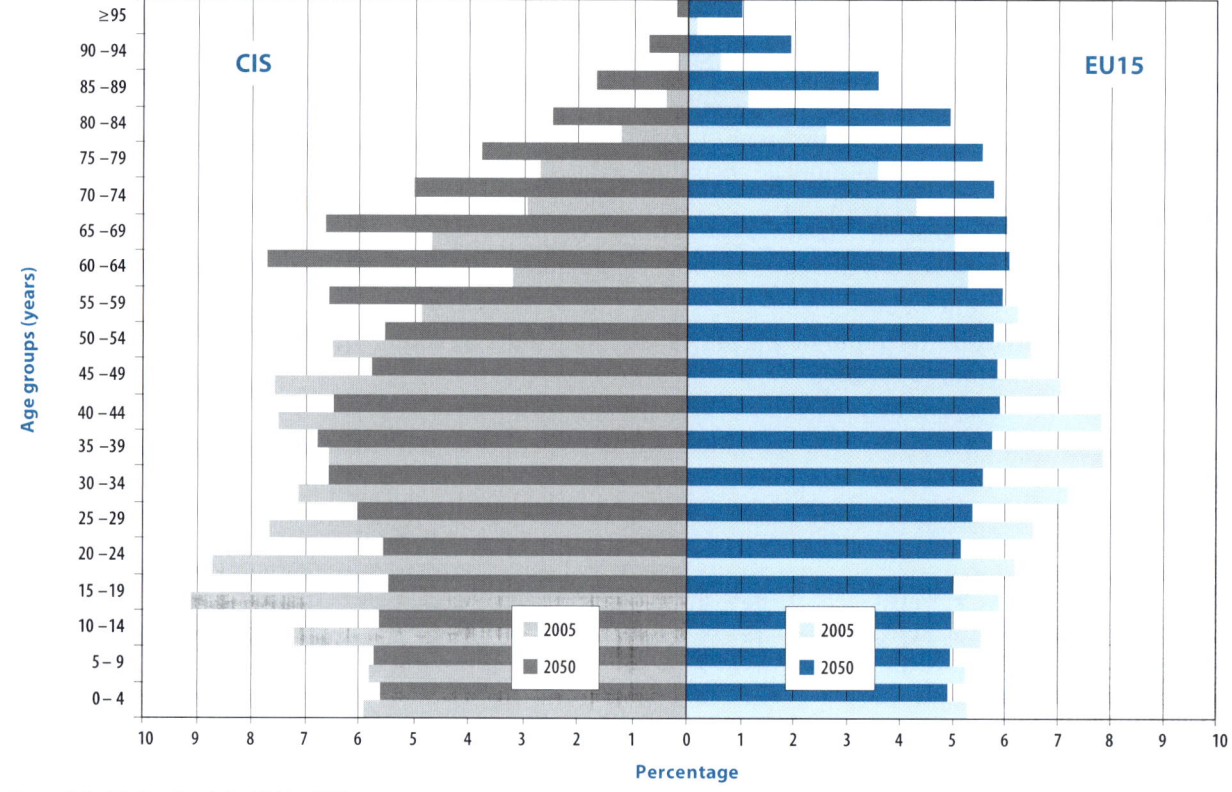

Source: United Nations Population Division (128).

projections to 2050 are considered, the CIS countries have fewer older people: 20% aged 65 years and older, in marked contrast with the EU15 figure of nearly 30%. The male-to-female ratio in the EU15 countries in 2006 was an estimated 1.1 for people under 15 years and 0.8 for those aged 65 and older. In the CIS countries, these figures were 1.2 and 0.8, respectively.

Challenges and implications for the future

The ageing of the population of the Region during the past decade (with an increase of 13% in the number of people 65 years and older) reflects longer life expectancy at birth of 2.5 years since 1990 (3% increase) and improved overall living and health conditions. Nevertheless, the increase in the older population may have negative effects. During the coming years, population ageing, low fertility and delays in the onset of chronic noncommunicable diseases will change or increase the demands on countries' health systems. Since the health trends among older people are complex, how ageing will affect health systems and population health in general is still very uncertain (134). For example, an estimated 20% of the population in the EU reported a long-term illness or disability, but the highest and the lowest country proportions differed threefold (135). Evidence indicates that the proportion of older people with a disability in the EU is decreasing, but the absolute numbers will increase since the older population will grow. Meanwhile, the prevalence of most chronic conditions continues to rise with age, and nearly 75% of people 65 years and older will die from cardiovascular diseases or cancer in most countries in the Region.

These trends at the country level also apply within countries, thus compounding the interpretations and predictions. Possible scenarios have been outlined considering broad changes in illness, disability and vulnerability that determine the quality of life. A first scenario comprises people living longer but with chronic diseases or their consequences, thus accumulating poor health, which in turn increases the demand for health services. A second scenario, generally accepted to be more likely, envisions a decline in the severity of disabling conditions during working age accompanied by an increase in mild disability. Since morbidity may be compressed – squeezing the burden of disease and disability into the final few years of life by delaying the onset of disease – this may not affect the overall demand for health services. A final and more optimistic alternative is that improved population lifestyles and delayed illness and disability would create conditions for reducing the demand for health services: validating the hypothesis of compressed morbidity, which would save costs for the health system.

Despite the decrease in chronic diseases, the economic burden of increased ageing on health systems may result in some countries doubling their current expenditure because of increasing health care costs *(133,136,137)*. Nevertheless, although aggregate costs for the older population may be higher, this is not true for the individual; for the same condition, older people incur lower health care costs than younger ones, partly because they receive less intensive treatment *(138)*. In addition, the imminence of death, not necessarily ageing, has been suggested to drive health expenditure. Again, the available evidence (or its measurement) is still too contradictory to allow any accurate predictions.

A decline in the economically active population, with total dependency ratios projected to increase to nearly three quarters of the population by 2050, may affect the funding and sustainability of the health and welfare systems in many countries. According to the European Commission, ageing will reduce the economically active population, thus causing the annual GDP growth rate in EU countries to decline from 2.4% in 2004–2010 to 1.2% in 2030–2050. In addition, public spending related to pensions and services for the older population is expected to increase by 3–4 percentage points of GDP between 2004 and 2050 *(134)*.

Several policy approaches have been proposed to reduce the impact of ageing on the health system, from health-system-specific interventions to wider social and economic policies. The former include:

- emphasizing the prevention of the most important chronic diseases and risk factors by following healthy lifestyles, at least from early mid-life, if not over the whole life-course;
- targeting health care interventions to postpone the onset of cardiovascular diseases, obesity, hypertension and dementia;
- promoting self-care and improving long-term care with more efficient use of resources, including formal and informal care; and
- involving older people directly in more decisions and activities (including economic choices) that affect their care *(132,134,139)*.

In addition, special attention should be paid to gender and to lower-income groups. Currently, nearly 40% more women than men live to be 65 years or older and three times as many, 85 years and older. Further, poor and older people have a 30–65% higher risk of almost all chronic diseases than affluent and younger people *(135)*. As noted above, women also experience longer life with poorer health than men, especially because of multiple conditions, thus requiring more integrated care approaches. In addition, as women tend to have poorer access to health services than men, greater access needs to be facilitated.

Social and economic policies suggested to limit the impact of ageing on society include: increasing overall employment, deferring the age of mandatory retirement and improving older people's participation in the workforce, increasing tax receipts by increasing economic growth and reducing public-sector expenditure now to cover increases in future expenditure *(140)*. Facilitating older people's participation in employment will require upgrading skills and retraining *(141)*. No single policy or set of policies will suffice for the whole European Region, and decisions will have to be adjusted to respond to different circumstances.

Mitigating the burden of communicable diseases

Communicable diseases significantly threaten human health and international security. Vaccine-preventable, foodborne, zoonotic, health-care-related and chronic communicable diseases contribute considerably to health care costs *(142)*. Although communicable diseases are not among the leading causes of death and illness in the European Region, substantial and sustainable resources are needed to maintain preparedness and to enable countries to respond to and control outbreaks.

Emerging and re-emerging epidemic-prone infections are of great public concern to countries and the Region as a whole. Preventing and controlling them remain the fundamental public health functions of national health systems. The WHO Regional Office for Europe develops norms and standards, guidance and other tools to help countries implement effective disease control programmes. Further, the Regional Office supports countries in designing and implementing evidence-based interventions, assessing the burden of disease and risk factors and monitoring progress towards reducing death and disability. It does this by integrating these activities with managing and disseminating technical knowledge to strengthen communicable disease surveillance and response systems and public health programmes and services.

Communicable disease trends in the European Region

TB

The European Region had 431 518 new cases and 63 765 deaths from TB in 2007: 49 new cases and 7 deaths every hour. Countries reported 350 529 new and relapse cases, representing a notification rate of 39 per 100 000 population, with a slight decrease from 43 per 100 000 population in 2002 to 39 per 100 000 population in 2007. TB prevalence declined from 54 per 100 000 population in 2006 to 51 per 100 000 in 2007; the target is 27 per 100 000 population by 2015. TB mortality was stable: 7.0 per 100 000 population in 2006 and 2007 versus a target of 3 per 100 000 by 2015. Coverage with the WHO-recommended DOTS TB control strategy was reported to be 75% in 2007, with 39 countries reporting 100% coverage, including all 18 high-priority countries in the European Region: Armenia, Azerbaijan, Belarus, Bulgaria, Estonia, Georgia, Kazakhstan, Kyrgyzstan, Latvia, Lithuania, the Republic of Moldova, Romania, the Russian Federation, Tajikistan, Turkey, Turkmenistan, Uzbekistan and Ukraine *(143)*.

TB control in the Region is far from optimal, however. The overall case detection rate (all cases from all sources) was 75%, but the rate of new smear-positive cases is 55%, falling short of the global target of 70%. Nevertheless, the overall case detection rate shows that 75% of the people with TB in the Region are diagnosed, some by means other than smear microscopy, such as culture and X-ray.

The proportion of people with new smear-positive TB cases who started treatment in 2006 and were cured was 70% (the global target is 85%). Among the high-priority countries of the Region, the least treatment success was reported in the Russian Federation (58%), followed by Ukraine (59%) and Azerbaijan (60%). Turkey (91%), Kyrgyzstan (82%) and Uzbekistan (81%) have the most successful treatment programmes.

Worryingly, multidrug-resistant TB (MDR-TB) strains were considered to account for 43 600 (about 10%) of the new TB cases and 43% of re-treated cases, and an estimated 42 300 of the people with new TB cases were also living with HIV (see Box 2.2 for an example of WHO's response). A high rate of MDR-TB – the highest in the world – is the main challenge for TB control in the Region. Among the 27 high-priority countries collectively accounting for 85% of estimated MDR-TB cases globally, 15 (listed by the estimated total of cases) are in the European Region: the Russian Federation, Kazakhstan, Ukraine, Uzbekistan, Tajikistan, Azerbaijan, the Republic of Moldova, Kyrgyzstan, Belarus, Georgia, Armenia, Lithuania, Bulgaria, Latvia and Estonia *(144)*.

Box 2.2. Combating TB and HIV in Baltic countries

The numbers of people reported to have new HIV infections and MDR-TB in Estonia, Latvia and Lithuania are increasing. To address this problem, the Regional Office established a project to scale up treatment and care for HIV/AIDS and TB and accelerate prevention within the health system in these Baltic countries. Its goal is to reduce HIV and TB transmission and vulnerability from and impact of HIV and TB by strengthening national interventions, developing collaboration between national programmes and enabling the health systems to adapt to the challenges of controlling HIV in a sustainable manner. National working groups for TB, HIV and health system strengthening have recently been established, and the national HIV and TB policies were reviewed.

Further, action plans and policy documents for collaborative TB/HIV interventions were developed and work was done to improve TB/HIV surveillance systems. In each country, a detailed cost analysis and flow-of-funds assessment were made with the support of the Regional Office to highlight potential areas for and the economic implications of collaborative TB/HIV interventions. Regular workshops attended by the three national working groups and WHO experts were held to assess and discuss the progress, achievements and challenges of each country.

A ministerial meeting co-organized by WHO and focusing on countries with a high burden of MDR- and extensively drug-resistant TB was held in Beijing, China in April 2009. It aimed at building the commitment – through a call for action *(145)* – needed to dramatically expand action to address these problems. This includes better and more rapid diagnosis, stronger laboratory networks and proper first- and second-line drug management. The meeting built on the WHO European Ministerial Forum "All against Tuberculosis", held in October 2007 *(146)*. In the resulting Berlin Declaration on Tuberculosis *(146)*, the Member States committed themselves to adopting the Stop TB Strategy *(147)*, to try to secure sustainable financing for TB prevention and control and to assess progress in implementing the Declaration along with the Regional Office, the EU and other relevant institutions and organizations.

HIV

An estimated 2.4 million people in the European Region are living with HIV. Fig. 2.24 shows the annual number of newly reported cases in the Region and the disturbing trends in AIDS cases and AIDS-related mortality *(148)*. In signing the Dublin Declaration on Partnership to Fight HIV/AIDS in Europe and Central Asia in February 2004, the countries of the Region committed themselves to providing universal access to effective, affordable and equitable HIV prevention, treatment and care. In 2007 and 2008, the WHO Regional Office for Europe led a review of countries' implementation of the Declaration involving more than 100 experts from across the Region *(149)*.

Fig. 2.24. Annual number of newly reported HIV and AIDS cases, WHO European Region, 1985–2007

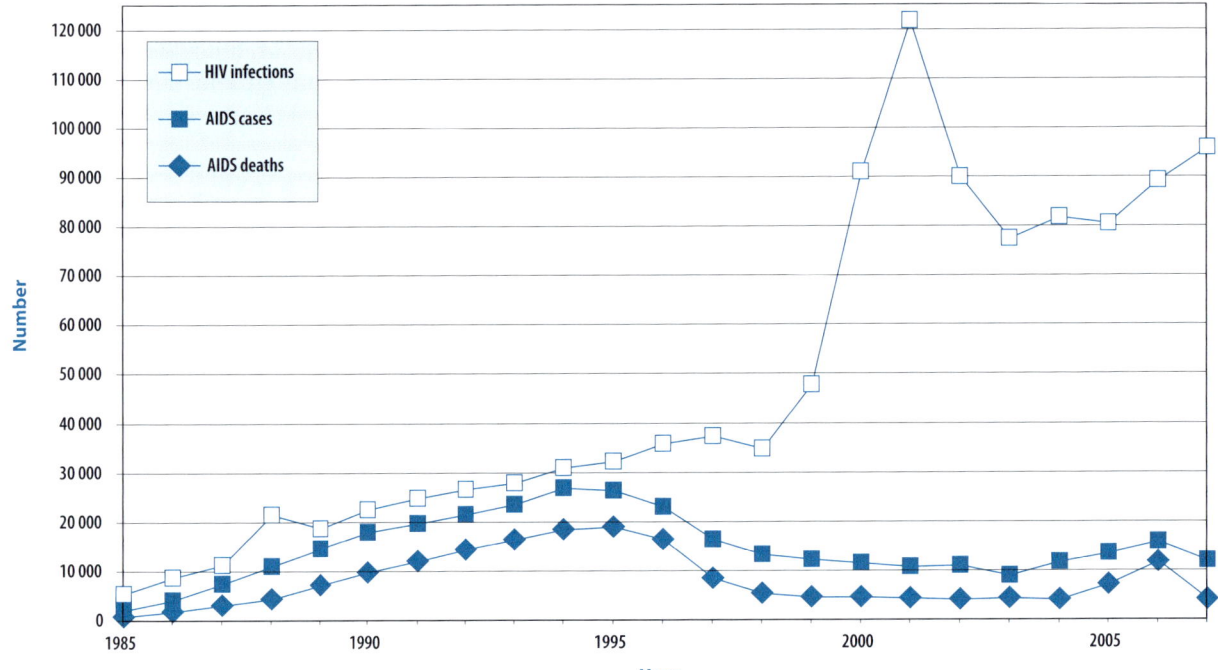

Source: European Centre for Disease Prevention and Control and WHO Regional Office for Europe (148).

The report showed substantial progress in treatment coverage (149). The number of people receiving antiretroviral therapy increased from 282 000 in 2004 to about 435 000 by the end of 2007. Treatment gaps in countries in the eastern part of the Region, however, are still significant and increasing. Further, injecting drug users, the most severely affected group in this part of the Region, face major challenges in access to prevention (especially needle and syringe exchange programmes, and opioid substitution therapy) and treatment services. WHO has developed new guidance to assist countries in addressing these issues in the context of reaching universal access to HIV prevention, treatment and care (150) and continues to work closely with national authorities to improve access and internationally to advocate for such prevention interventions.

Treatment access is also a problem in western Europe, where many migrants from countries with a high HIV prevalence do not receive the services they need. Further, with the recent increase in newly reported cases among men who have sex with men, the Regional Office held a consultation on the issue in Bled, Slovenia while Slovenia held the EU Presidency. Participants stressed the importance of targeted prevention, especially condom use (151), given that the epidemic has not yet spread to the general population. The targeting of HIV efforts still urgently needs to be scaled up and improved to reduce inequity and to promote greater harmonization of the highest standards of prevention and treatment programmes and policies. This requires strong European political leadership and accountability if the Dublin Declaration (149) and the MDGs (17) are to be achieved.

Hepatitis

Hepatitis B and C are the underlying cause of about 1.5 million annual deaths globally; 500 million people are currently infected with chronic hepatitis B or C. One in three people worldwide has been exposed to one or both viruses. These viruses affect millions in the European Region but are not yet universally recognized as a public health priority because:

- health care officials lack awareness;
- strong advocacy is lacking at the international and national levels;
- surveillance of chronic hepatitis B and C infection is inadequate throughout the Region; and
- hepatitis B vaccine and hepatitis treatment are unavailable or unaffordable.

These deficiencies have led to premature mortality and increased public health spending.

The Regional Office works to make hepatitis B immunization more accessible, especially to high-risk groups; internationally, it advocates addressing viral hepatitis B and C as one of the major public health challenges in the Region. Improving bloodborne hepatitis surveillance is a top priority of the Regional Office. This is crucial for obtaining reliable information on the prevalence of hepatitis infection and the burden of disease in the Region. Other key priorities are providing universal access to treatment for hepatitis B, hepatitis C and HIV while developing strategies to reduce the price of such treatment and improve hepatitis surveillance. Further, in recent years the Regional Office has worked closely with patient groups to raise awareness about hepatitis testing and treatment.

Vaccine-preventable infections and diseases

Vaccination is one of the most cost-effective health interventions, saving millions of people from illness, disability and death each year. For example, all 53 Member States were certified as polio free in June 2002. Effective and safe vaccines against more than 20 serious diseases are available, and many promising new vaccines are being developed. WHO is working to establish surveillance systems for collecting and using high-quality evidence-based data in order to introduce new vaccines.

Although today's vaccines are highly effective and safe, new challenges are emerging. As vaccine-preventable diseases still pose significant threats in the Region, strengthening immunization remains vital. The Regional Office's most public effort in this field is European Immunization Week, held every April (Box 2.3) *(152)*.

Box 2.3. Fourth European Immunization Week 2009: an online strategy

The main challenges faced by the European Region's immunization programmes are changing. National programmes still have problems delivering services to geographically and socially marginalized populations, and the effectiveness of vaccinations in reducing the incidence of once common diseases has led to broader public misapprehension. Complacency and scepticism have enabled the persistent propagation of misinformation. This has resulted in a stagnation or decrease in immunization coverage in many countries and contributed to recent outbreaks of disease that threaten the health of this and other WHO regions.

To counter this, the WHO Regional Office for Europe launched a Region-wide initiative, European Immunization Week. Its main goals are to raise public awareness, to highlight the benefits of immunization, to support national immunization systems and to provide a framework for mobilizing public and political support for efforts to protect the public through universal childhood immunization. On 22 April 2009, the fourth European Immunization Week went viral; an online campaign targeted millions of people in the European Region with information about vaccination in their countries and outbreaks in Europe, and a video about the potential perils to young children.

Major achievements have been made in reducing measles incidence across the Region and reaching the target of 95% coverage with the first dose of measles-containing vaccine (MCV1) (Fig. 2.25).

Fig. 2.25. Measles vaccine coverage and reported measles cases, WHO European Region, latest available year

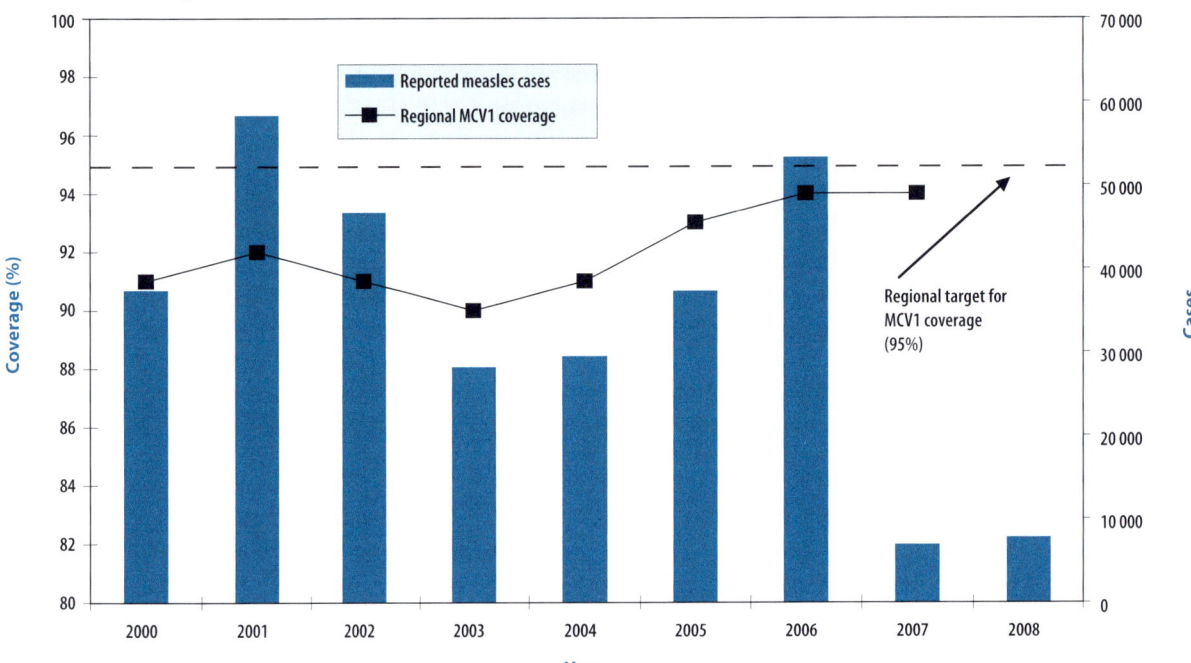

Sources: data from *WHO vaccine-preventable diseases: monitoring system – 2008 global summary (153)* and Centralized information system for infectious diseases (CISID) [online database] *(154)*.

During 2005–2008, nationwide supplementary immunization activities were implemented in eight countries in the eastern part of the European Region, reaching about 27 million people. Some countries with measles outbreaks promoted vaccination through enhanced health communication and accelerated routine immunization activities. Nevertheless, measles outbreaks occurred in the Region throughout 2008 and 2009, especially in the western part, threatening progress towards the 2010 regional goals for eliminating measles and rubella. At this critical juncture, re-emphasizing WHO Regional Committee for Europe resolution EUR/RC55/R7, urging Member States to give high priority to achieving these goals *(155)*, is important.

Since 2006, the Region has had no human cases of H5N1 avian influenza. Nevertheless, countries bordering the Region are experiencing cases, and case fatality remains high (62%). More and more countries in the Region have H5N1 avian influenza contingency plans, and some have conducted tabletop and field simulation exercises and trained relevant staff in outbreak detection and case management, with support from WHO.

Pandemic preparedness continues to be in focus in the Region, as some countries are not readily prepared. Since early 2008, the Regional Office has organized intercountry workshops to stress the persistent risk of pandemics and thus the necessity for preparedness. Its staff made assessment visits to eight countries in south-eastern Europe in 2008 to assess the current level of pandemic preparedness and raise awareness about the need for and scope of pandemic preparedness.

On 13 February 2009, the Regional Office joined the European Centre for Disease Prevention and Control (ECDC) in launching the first regional influenza bulletin, using the European Influenza Surveillance Scheme *(156)*. This marks a new phase in influenza surveillance in the Region, significantly increasing its geographical coverage and providing all European countries with a sophisticated and user-friendly platform.

The number of reported malaria cases has declined from 90 712 in 1995 to 593 in 2008 as a result of intensive antimalaria interventions *(157)*. Owing to local transmission, malaria is still reported in Azerbaijan, Georgia, Kyrgyzstan, the Russian Federation, Tajikistan, Turkey and Uzbekistan. The Regional Office works closely with these countries towards certifying them as malaria-free.

In 2005, all malaria-affected countries in the Region endorsed the Tashkent Declaration: "the Move from Malaria Control to Elimination" in the WHO European Region *(158)*. Although the ultimate goal is to interrupt malaria transmission by 2015 and eliminate the disease from the Region, successful malaria elimination will help strengthen national health systems through the integration of targeted disease-specific programmes into their existing structures and services.

In its efforts to eliminate malaria, WHO particularly emphasizes situations in which the disease might spread between neighbouring countries and regions. Countries in the European and the Eastern Mediterranean regions have similar epidemiological situations and problems with malaria. WHO therefore promotes closer cross-border cooperation by organizing border meetings, improving malaria notification in these areas, developing joint projects and international training courses and arranging visits from national malaria programme counterparts and WHO staff.

WHO is coordinating the global response to the influenza pandemic (H1N1) *(159)*. On 27 April 2009, the national focal points for the International Health Regulations informed the Regional Office about the detection of four laboratory-confirmed cases of pandemic (H1N1) 2009 virus infection: two each in Spain and the United Kingdom. Israel reported two additional confirmed cases the next day. By late November 2009, countries throughout the European Region reported high or very high intensity of influenza-like illnesses and/or acute respiratory infections and 17 countries had started vaccination campaigns. Reports of adverse events are fewer than for seasonal influenza vaccination, and most are mild. Eight countries in the Region are eligible to receive vaccine donated to WHO.

The WHO Director-General's determination that pandemic (H1N1) 2009 was a public health emergency of international concern under the current Regulations, on 25 April 2009, included advice that countries intensify surveillance for early case detection. National authorities took important steps to ensure an effective response. On 27 April 2009, the WHO Regional Director for Europe, Dr Marc Danzon, contacted the health ministers, chief medical officers and national focal points in the Region to describe the Regional Office's initial response. He emphasized that cooperation between WHO and national and international counterparts would be crucial in preparing for and responding to the potential spread of the virus in the Region.

Between 27 and 29 April, WHO raised the pandemic threat level from phase 3, through phase 4 to phase 5, reflecting sustained human-to-human transmission at the community level in at least two countries of one WHO region. On 11 June, WHO declared a pandemic (phase 6), reflecting the geographical spread and reach of the virus to more than one region of WHO, rather than its severity. This was a clear call for countries to reshape their pandemic response strategy, moving from containment to mitigation.

On 7 July, WHO announced the revision of reporting requirements to WHO for monitoring the pandemic. These included the discontinuation of reporting of confirmed cases and the introduction of qualitative indicators of influenza-related activity: geographical spread, trend, intensity and impact on the health care system. In the WHO European Region, countries share data and information with WHO through the Regional Office's influenza surveillance web site *(160)*. The information collected is the basis for a weekly European regional influenza bulletin published on the site in English and Russian.

The pandemic is characterized as of "moderate" severity, but it has spread internationally with unprecedented speed. Most cases are mild and have resolved without complications, but some groups appear to be at higher risk of severe disease and death. By 20 November 2009, 652 deaths had occurred in the European Region.

Where possible, countries should monitor the virological characteristics of the virus and where appropriate any unusual events, such as clusters of severe illness. In addition, WHO recommended three objectives that countries could adopt for their pandemic vaccination strategies:

- protecting the integrity of the health care system and the critical infrastructure of the country;
- reducing morbidity and mortality; and
- reducing transmission of the pandemic virus within communities.

For countries in the Region that are not eligible for donated vaccine, do not produce vaccine, or do not have an advance vaccine purchase agreement, WHO and the United Nations Children's Fund (UNICEF) are working to procure supplies of vaccine through UNICEF's supply division. Further, the WHO Regional Office for Europe organized a series of subregional workshops including: two on the deployment of pandemic influenza vaccine (August and October 2009), one on the public health response to the pandemic (August 2009) and three on hospital preparedness (September and October 2009).

The Regional Office works directly with its Member States, through the national focal points for the International Health Regulations and the network that contributes to the influenza surveillance web site, by providing supplies, training, tools, and technical assistance in preparedness plans. The Regional Office is working closely with the Directorate-General for Health and Consumers of the European Commission and ECDC. Similarly, WHO consults closely with United Nations agencies and other international organizations (including those involved in trade and travel) and manufacturers of vaccines, drugs, diagnostic equipment and personal protection equipment. The Regional Office web site offers updates and further information *(159)*.

The revised International Health Regulations, adopted in 2005, entered into force in June 2007. They constitute the global framework for epidemic alert and response at the international level and reflect the commitment of WHO and the 194 States Parties to establish core capacities for surveillance and response at the national and subnational levels and to detect, assess, notify, report, verify and respond to events of potential international public health concern. Similarly, each State Party is required to designate a functional national focal point and authorities responsible within its respective jurisdiction for implementing the Regulations. WHO's mandate includes seeking to verify unofficial reports of events with potential international implications.

From the time the Regulations entered into force in June 2007 until December 2008, the national focal points reported 46 of the 161 events of potential international public health concern assessed in the European Region. Nearly half the events assessed were initially identified as being potentially infectious in nature.

By 14 June 2009, each State Party was required to assess national structures and resources for their ability to meet the minimum core capacity requirements for surveillance and response and to develop a national action plan. The national action plan must be implemented to ensure that the core capacities are present and functioning throughout the State Party's territory by 14 June 2012. The national plan should build on existing structures, capacities and resources and minimize unnecessary duplication and costs.

Continuing rise of chronic diseases

The rise of chronic diseases presents a major challenge to health and health systems throughout the European Region. As an important cause of premature mortality, as well as disability, they greatly affect the number of years of life lived in good health. Modern lifestyles and behaviour (see the section above) are leading to increases in such conditions as obesity, hypertension and diabetes. This, along with ageing populations and treatment that allows individuals to survive acute events, is leading to increases in the proportion of the population living with chronic disease.

Although the term "chronic diseases" has often been used synonymously with "noncommunicable diseases", this section distinguishes them. For epidemiological purposes, the section draws on much of the data available for noncommunicable diseases, but then focuses on selected conditions of a more chronic nature.

Situation assessment

According to global burden of disease estimates for 2004 *(19)*, noncommunicable diseases caused 8.45 million deaths (87% of total deaths) in the European Region, 52% of which occurred among females. The leading causes of death, cardiovascular diseases and cancer, together caused 71% of total deaths, followed by digestive diseases and respiratory diseases (Fig. 2.26). Projections to 2030 (baseline 2004) are that the ageing of populations in low- and middle-income countries will significantly increase the total deaths caused by most noncommunicable diseases so that they will account for 90% of total deaths in the Region *(19)*.

Fig. 2.26. Projected deaths by cause, WHO European Region, 2008

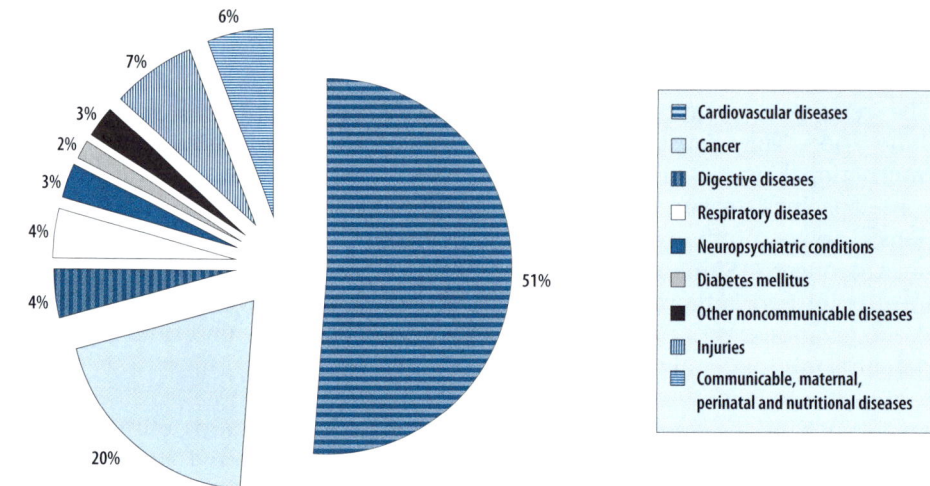

Source: The global burden of disease: 2004 update (19).

Along with injuries, cardiovascular diseases are a main contributor to the almost threefold difference in mortality between adult men and women in the Region *(1)* and the difference in life expectancy of about 15 years between the western and eastern parts of the Region. Ischaemic heart disease is the leading cardiovascular disease causing deaths, followed by cerebrovascular diseases. The average trends in ischaemic health disease mortality for Eur-A countries are declining, while the situation is more mixed for Eur-B and -C countries (Fig. 2.27). Average trends do not show improvement (stable among women, rising among men), although mortality rates have declined in some countries and risen in others for several years *(20)*.

Cancer death rates have improved somewhat in the Region (Fig. 2.28). For example, in Eur-A countries, average lung cancer mortality is relatively low in younger age groups and relatively high among the older population. The opposite tends to be true in the eastern part of the Region, while cancer mortality is high in both younger and older age groups in the central part of the Region. Mortality from lung cancer is steadily rising among women in Eur-A countries *(20)*.

Deaths from respiratory diseases are declining overall. Chronic liver disease and cirrhosis of the liver cause about half of deaths from diseases of the digestive system: mortality is steadily declining in Eur-A countries but rising in Eur-B and -C countries *(20)*.

In 2004, noncommunicable diseases caused 112.4 million DALYs lost (77.8% of the total burden of disease). The leading contributors were cardiovascular diseases (23.0%) and neuropsychiatric conditions (19.6%) followed by cancer (11.9%) and sense organ disorders (5.8%) *(19)*. Projections for the burden of disease to 2030 predict that, with an ageing population, the balance will shift to a relative increase in neuropsychiatric conditions (22.1%), cancer (13.7%) and sense organ disorders (7.3%), with cardiovascular diseases at 22.3% *(1)*.

Mental disorders are an important cause of lost years of healthy life and affect at least one in four people at some time in life *(161)*. Unipolar depressive disorder is the leading contributor

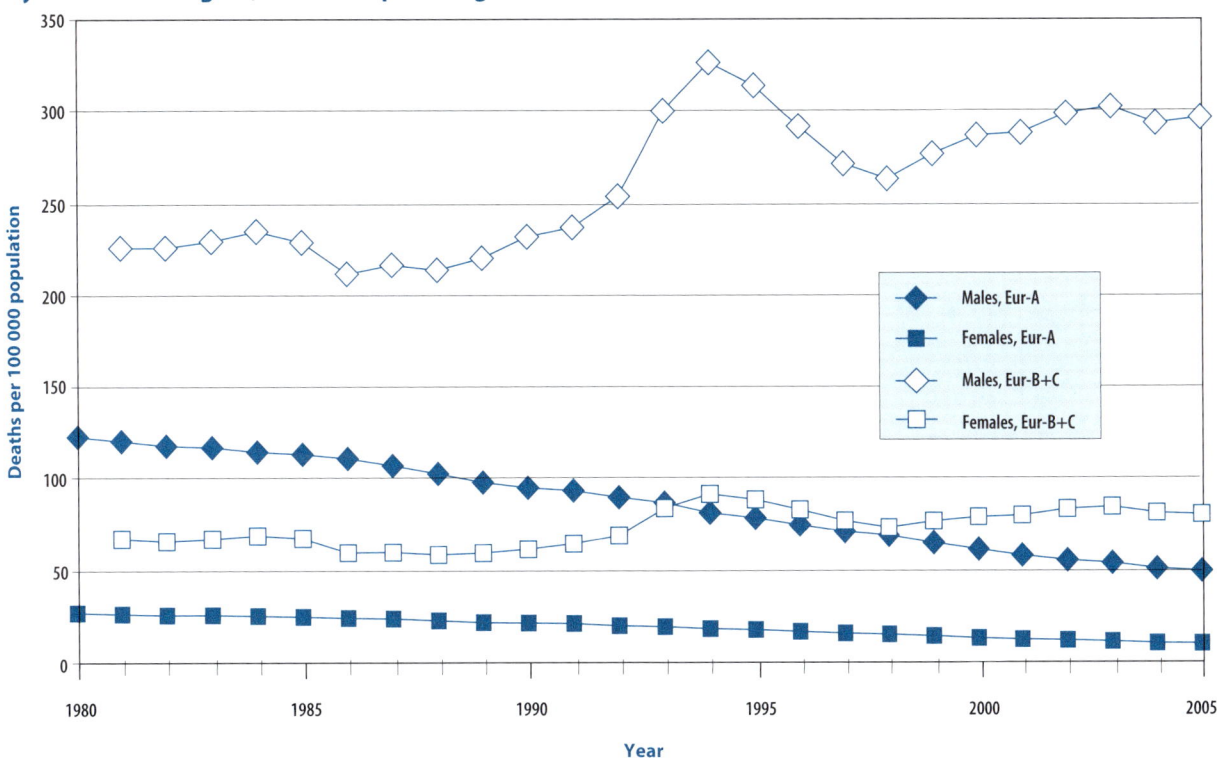

Fig. 2.27. Ischaemic heart disease among people aged 25–64 years: SDRs per 100 000 population by sex and subregion, WHO European Region, 1980–2005

Source: Atlas of health in Europe (20).

to the burden of disease among women aged 15–44 years in countries at all levels of income in the European Region and contributes 5.8% of the total burden (third leading cause) in the Region (18). Depression is frequently underdiagnosed and a major cause of suicide. Mental disorders increasingly affect children and adolescents in Europe (about 2 million): the risk of suicide among adolescents appears to be increasing in western Europe (Fig. 2.29) (161).

The incidence of noncommunicable diseases has been difficult to determine due to long incubation periods and limited country routine surveillance. Nevertheless, the global burden of disease computations for 2004 (19) made some estimates. For example, the conditions with the highest incidence in Europe were malignant neoplasms (3.1 million events; 353 per 100 000 population), strokes (2.0 million events; 228 per 100 000 population) and congestive heart failure (rheumatic fever, heart disease, hypertensive heart disease, ischaemic heart disease or inflammatory heart disease: 1.3 million events; 148 per 100 000 population). Cancer incidence by site was highest for the colon and rectum, lung, breast, stomach and prostate; these accounted for nearly half of cancer events. Appropriate and timely health care can reduce the mortality and disability impact of most of these types of cancer.

Disease prevalence indicates the number of people living with a condition and the resulting conditions at a given time, but not severity and impairment, which may vary significantly among disease conditions. The prevalence of the most frequent conditions by broad group in the European Region includes:

Fig. 2.28. Lung cancer among people aged 25–64 and ≥ 65 years: SDRs per 100 000 population by sex and subregion, WHO European Region, 1980–2005

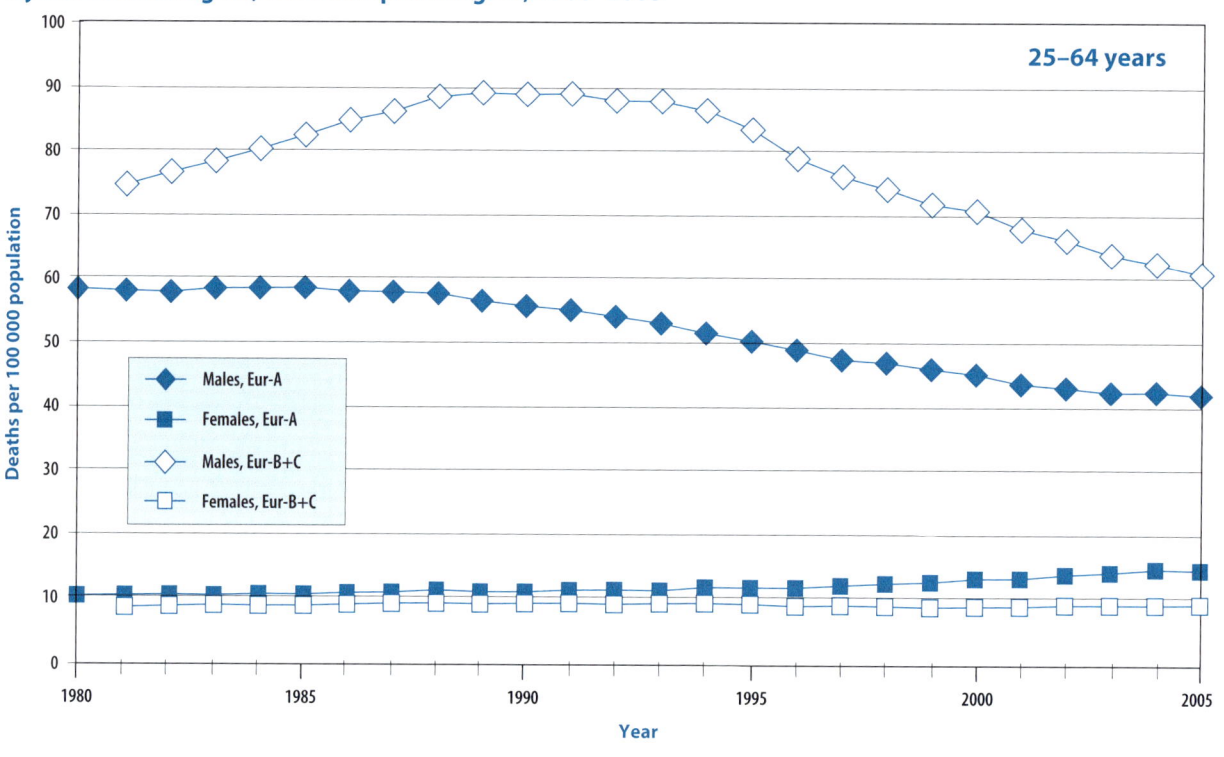

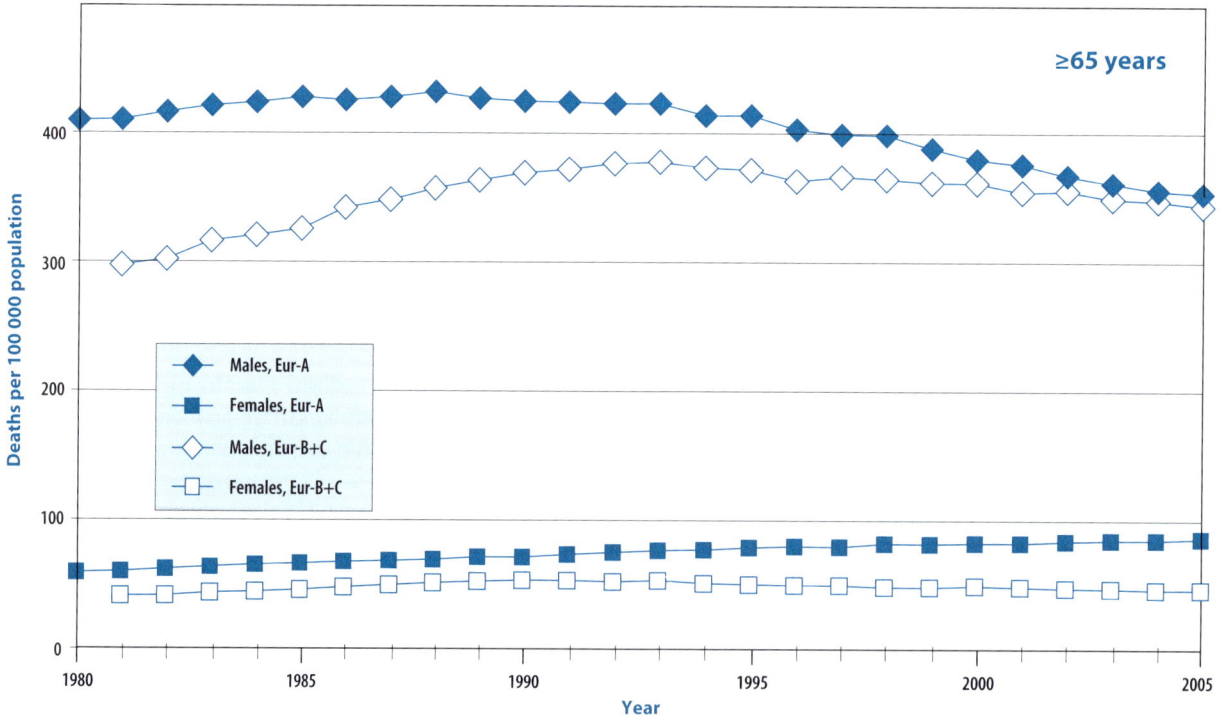

Source: Atlas of health in Europe (20).

Fig. 2.29. Suicide: SDRs per 100 000 population by sex, WHO European Region, 2006 or latest available year

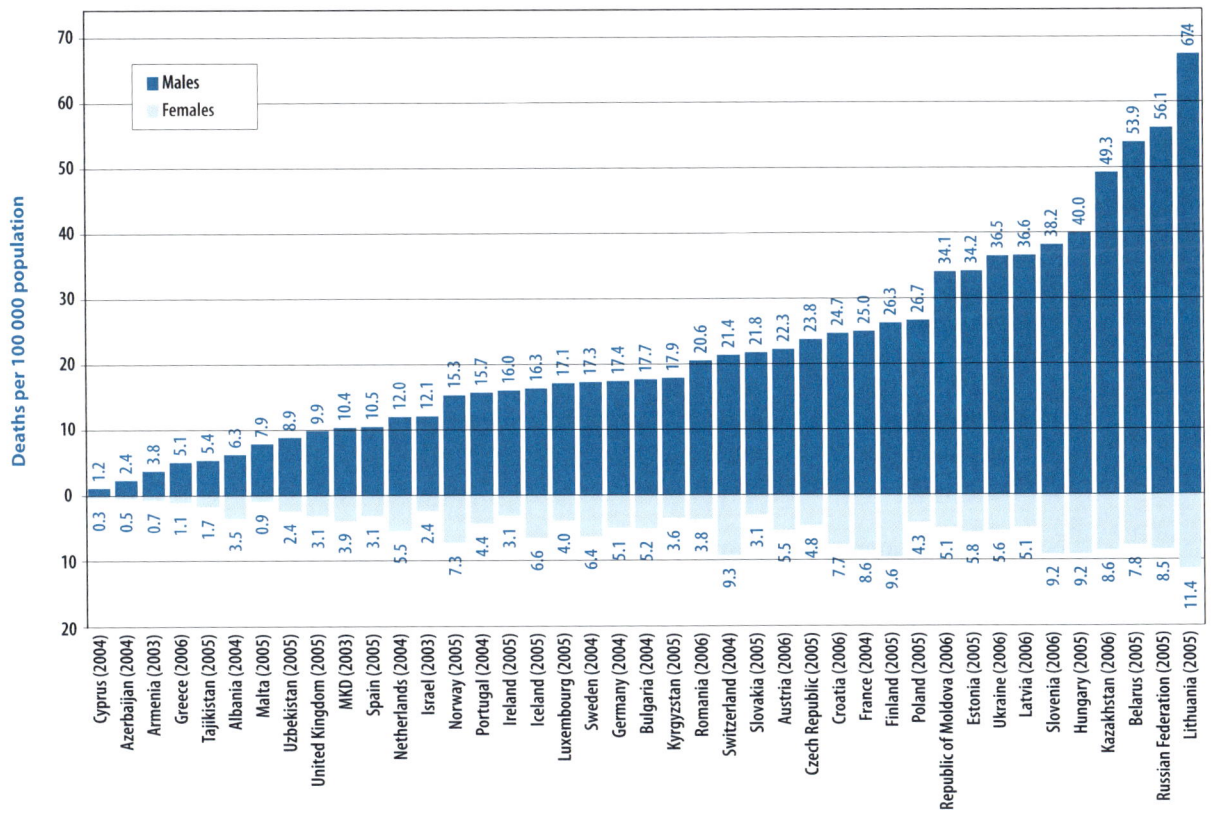

Note. MKD is the International Organization for Standardization (ISO) abbreviation for the former Yugoslav Republic of Macedonia.
Source: Atlas of health in Europe (20).

- 71.6 million people for neuropsychiatric conditions (unipolar depressive disorders, bipolar affective disorder, schizophrenia, epilepsy, alcohol use disorders, Alzheimer and other types of dementia and Parkinson's disease);
- 26.8 million for cardiovascular diseases (including angina pectoris and stroke);
- 40.1 million for respiratory diseases (chronic obstructive pulmonary disease and asthma);
- 44.5 million for hearing loss (moderate and severe);
- 46.4 million for inflammatory disorders (rheumatoid arthritis and osteoarthritis); and
- 45.4 million for diabetes (moderate to severe), the most frequent single condition.

The prevalence of diabetes in the Region ranges from 0.1 (Turkmenistan) to 7.6 (Malta) per 100 population (20). The International Diabetes Federation argues that the regional prevalence may be higher and projects that it will rise to 9.8% by 2025, partly as a result of rising obesity levels, with relatively large increases expected in countries undergoing economic and nutritional transition such as Belarus, Poland, Slovakia and Turkey (162). Diabetes adversely affects the circulatory system, eyes, kidneys and nerves, and increasing prevalence is therefore likely to increase death and disability from other conditions.

The coexistence of health conditions needs to be recognized, especially in the shift from disease-focused to person-centred care. Depression, for example, is more common among people with physical illness than the physically healthy. The prevalence of major depression in the Region includes 33% of people with cancer, 29% of those with hypertension and 27% of those with diabetes. As people age, the number of coexisting health conditions increases, especially among women *(67)*.

Finally, although estimates of disability specific to the Region are lacking by age group and sex, global figures have suggested that disability for several neuropsychiatric conditions – such as alcohol dependence and problem use, depression, schizophrenia, bipolar disorder and drug dependence use – is 20–80 times more frequent before than after the age of 60 years in countries at all income levels, but is higher in low- and middle-income countries *(19)*. Neuropsychiatric conditions tend to have higher prevalence in men; those related to alcohol and drug dependence and problem use comprise up to one third of the total burden of neuropsychiatric conditions among men. In contrast, other inflammatory and degenerative conditions (cataracts, osteoarthritis, macular degeneration, glaucoma and Alzheimer and other types of dementia) have a higher prevalence among people older than 60 years in countries at all levels of income, and among women.

Issues, challenges and responses

Burden on individuals, families and society

Focusing on epidemiological facts and figures risks missing the broader social and economic effects of chronic diseases. Much evidence suggests that these diseases impose substantial costs on society *(163)*. Cost-of-illness studies, for example, have estimated that the cost of chronic diseases and their risk factors ranges from 0.02% to 6.77% of GDP in various countries *(164)*: for the United Kingdom, cardiovascular diseases alone account for an estimated 18% of total health care expenditure *(142)*. The direct, indirect and intangible costs of illness burden individuals and their families, and include treatment costs, reduced income, early retirement and increased reliance on welfare support for ill people and/or their carers. Employers and wider society carry a burden of absenteeism, reduced productivity and employee turnover. Some chronic diseases predominate. Musculoskeletal disorders are second to respiratory disorders as a cause of short-term sickness absence and are the most common health-related cause for long-term absence *(165)*. The proportion of people on sick leave due to mental disorders is 35% in Sweden, and the proportion receiving social welfare benefits or pensions because of disability due to mental health problems varies from 44% in Denmark to 8% in the Russian Federation *(166)*.

Social exclusion can exacerbate the problems associated with poor mental health and some chronic diseases. Too often the associated stigma and discrimination can limit people's ability to obtain or return to work and to obtain housing. The Mental Health Action Plan for Europe *(161,167)* outlines action to combat stigma and discrimination, including the promotion of human rights, policies and programmes for social inclusion, legal protection against discrimination and means to support employment, such as vocational training, adaptation of workplaces and return-to-work policies.

Many people with chronic diseases need lifelong medication, and the out-of-pocket cost relative to income may place enormous strain on families and on adherence. For example, low- and middle-income families who have to choose may purchase health care focused on immediate life-threatening complications in diabetes rather than preventing cardiovascular disease, the main cause of death in diabetes. To prevent this, models of health care funding could be used to reduce financial barriers to care and to ensure universal access to a basic package of effective prevention and treatment measures *(67)*.

Disease prevention throughout life
The European Strategy for the Prevention and Control of Noncommunicable Diseases *(67)* promotes a comprehensive approach on three levels: population-level health promotion and disease prevention, identification and targeting of people at high risk and effective care of people who have noncommunicable diseases.

The onset of noncommunicable diseases needs to be prevented by changing lifestyle behaviour, developing health-promoting environments and taking action on the socioeconomic determinants of health. Once disease is established, such interventions, alongside effective and timely treatment and rehabilitation, are also important throughout the course to prevent conditions from becoming chronic and the development of disability. Physical activity, for example, can positively affect multiple chronic conditions: for example, reducing the risks of cardiovascular diseases, improving musculoskeletal health and reducing the symptoms of depression *(73)*. Stopping smoking can have substantial effects: quitting before middle age avoids more than 90% of the lung cancer risk attributable to tobacco *(78)*. Combining behavioural interventions – including smoking cessation, increased physical activity and dietary change that promotes weight loss – may reduce the risk of cardiovascular diseases by more than 60% among people with established heart disease and contribute to good blood glucose control among people with diabetes *(168)*. For people with established cardiovascular diseases, pharmaceutical interventions can further significantly reduce the risk of recurrent myocardial infarction *(169)*.

Mental well-being is increasingly recognized as fundamental to the quality of life *(161)*. Exposure to harmful stress can lead to an increase in anxiety and depression, alcohol and other substance use disorders, violence and suicidal behaviour. Promoting mental health can have benefits not only in improving well-being and preventing mental health problems but also in achieving better physical health and improving recovery from illness. Mental health is a fundamental part of the resilience and health assets that enable people to cope with adversity. In the United Kingdom, the 20–25% of people who are obese or smoke are concentrated among the 26% of the population living in poverty, who also have the highest prevalence of anxiety and depression *(39)*.

Reorienting systems of care
Health services are frequently oriented towards care rather than prevention and acute rather than chronic models of care (Table 2.17). People with mental health problems and chronic disease may require lifelong support and long-term disease management, much of which can be delivered through self-management and community-based care, but many services still focus on hospital-based specialist care *(170)*.

Even when the effectiveness of primary care has been demonstrated, the treatment provided in this setting may be limited. A WHO survey found that 31 countries in the Region limited GP care for people with mental disorders by, for example, limiting the right to prescribe medication or to perform certain tasks *(166)*.

Patients' active participation in their treatment can minimize the impact of chronic disease on physical and mental health status and functioning *(171)*. Therapeutic patient education, skills development and shared decision-making require shifting the role of health care professionals from authority to empowerment and facilitative changes in health systems *(172)*. Models of

Table 2.17. Requirements for and access to mental health home treatment by country group, WHO European Region

Home treatment	EU		EU15		EU12		Israel, Norway and Switzerland		South-eastern Europe		CIS		Total	
	No.	%	No.	%	No.	%	No.	%	No.	%	No.	%	No.	%
Required in policies, plans or legislation														
Yes	21	78	14	93	7	58	3	100	6	86	3	60	33	79
No	6	22	1	7	5	42	0	0	0	0	2	40	8	19
Information not available	0	0	0	0	0	0	0	0	1	14	0	0	1	2
People with mental disorders who have access														
All or almost all (81–100%)	3	11	3	20	0	0	0	0	0	0	0	0	3	7
Majority (51–80%)	1	4	1	7	0	0	1	33	0	0	1	20	3	7
Some (21–50%)	5	19	4	27	1	8	2	67	3	43	1	20	11	26
A few (1–20%)	6	22	3	20	3	25	0	0	2	29	1	20	9	21
None	5	19	0	0	5	42	0	0	1	14	2	40	8	19
Information not available	7	26	4	27	3	25	0	0	1	14	0	0	8	19

Source: Policies and practices for mental health in Europe – meeting the challenges (166).

care for chronic conditions have been proposed to facilitate disease management across health care boundaries, such as the chronic care model (173–175).

Further, involving patients and their families in designing care can be beneficial. Many countries in the Region entitle associations of service users and carers to be members of committees planning mental health services (166). Users and carers are also involved in training health care professionals and supporting patients in self-managing chronic diseases in some countries (176).

Rising health care costs

Policy-makers are concerned that health care costs have risen more rapidly than national income. As a proportion of GDP, average health expenditure in the European Region rose from 7.3% in 1998 to 7.7% in 2005 (Table 2.18). The public sector has borne most of this recent rise. The proportion of total spending deriving from public funding such as taxation and social insurance has increased in the past decade, and health care has consumed an increased share of total government expenditure. There are some exceptions to these general trends, such as the decline in health expenditure in the CIS countries and in Albania, Croatia, Estonia, Finland and Lithuania, and the fall in the relative role of public-sector funding in some countries, such as Bulgaria, the Czech Republic, Estonia, Lithuania and Slovenia. Overall, however, the picture shows continued growth in health care spending across the European Region.

Although estimates of future costs depend on the underlying assumptions on the relative role of the main cost drivers, health care costs are projected to increase even further in the future. The future level of public expenditure on health care is very uncertain but is projected to increase by 1–2 or 2–4 percentage points of GDP by 2050 (177,178). When the costs of long-term care are included, the projected increase is 1–4 or 3–6 percentage points of GDP (178). Non-demographic factors – such as the effects of new technology, rising unit costs and changes in health and disability and the associated changes in utilization – are assumed to be the main determinants of future growth. The fact that most of these factors are amenable to policy action should reassure policy-makers.

Table 2.18. Total health expenditure as a percentage of GDP and public-sector expenditure as a percentage of total health expenditure by country group, WHO European Region, 1998–2005 (estimates)

Country groups and expenditure	1998	2000	2002	2004	2005	Index, 2005 (%) (1998 = 100%)	Percentage-point change, 1998–2005
European Region							
Total health expenditure (%)	7.43	7.15	7.56	7.61	7.74	104.2	0.31
Public-sector health expenditure (%)	68.07	66.86	67.36	67.89	68.48	100.6	0.41
EU							
Total health expenditure (%)	7.87	8.07	8.42	8.78	8.92	113.3	1.05
Public-sector health expenditure (%)	74.45	74.91	75.47	75.25	75.54	101.5	1.09
EU15							
Total health expenditure (%)	8.47	8.66	9.00	9.42	9.57	113.0	1.10
Public-sector health expenditure (%)	75.66	75.53	76.20	76.43	76.78	101.5	1.12
EU12							
Total health expenditure (%)	5.75	5.70	6.33	6.40	6.49	112.9	0.74
Public-sector health expenditure (%)	70.15	72.68	72.81	70.88	70.92	101.1	0.77
CIS							
Total health expenditure (%)	6.55	5.51	5.88	5.38	5.51	84.1	−1.04
Public-sector health expenditure (%)	57.47	53.13	53.31	55.04	56.18	97.8	−1.29

Source: European Health for All database (4).

Factors driving costs

Health care costs can be understood as a simple function of price and the quantity used: costs increase if either or both of these parameters increase. Much empirical research in Europe and beyond has addressed the questions of what drives price and volume increases and their relative role in explaining past and future growth in health care costs. The cost drivers that receive the most attention are associated with the increasing volume of services used. These include population ageing and broader demographic changes (see the section above on changing demographic patterns in the Region), rising income and expectations, advances in technology and the associated changing patterns of use. Increasing relative prices of health care, especially given constrained labour markets, also drive costs.

Ageing and demographic changes

The demographic trends in Europe have increased the proportion of people aged 65 and more. These trends include fertility rates' falling below the natural replacement rate (see the section above on changing demographic patterns in the Region), rising life expectancy (with exceptions, as in some CIS countries) and an increase in internal migration within entities such as the EU. These trends have fuelled concerns about the future health and long-term care costs of caring for an ageing population. Older people's health continues to improve, however: most measures of morbidity have declined among them since the 1990s, which suggests either compression of morbidity (179) or a dynamic equilibrium of increasing longevity alongside consistent improvements in health (180).

Further, although older people have much higher health expenditure per person at a given time, the ageing of the population appears to be a relatively minor determinant of the annual growth in health care expenditure. Health care costs are concentrated in the period before death, such that the costs in old age are greater than those in youth, primarily because chronic disease is a greater burden. This needs to be accounted for to measure the relationship between age and expenditure. Actual health-related costs appear to decline with age and, over time, health care costs have risen more slowly for those who are near death than for others. The trends towards increasing life expectancy, declining mortality (which implies a reduction in costs since fewer people are dying), and reductions in morbidity among older people (which may or may not reduce the use of health services) all therefore indicate a relatively minor role of population ageing on future health care expenditure *(181)*. Analyses of patterns of health expenditure in past decades indicate that population ageing explains less than one tenth of the growth in health care costs *(178)*.

Population ageing is therefore estimated to be a minor cost driver in projections of future health care costs but a much more important one for the costs of long-term care. Nevertheless, policy-makers must consider how patterns of health care use will change over time and particularly how to promote healthy ageing and ensure the appropriate adoption of technology based on value for money.

Technological change and health care use

Technological change plays a complex role in increasing health care costs. New technologies can reduce costs by improving efficiency or health, thereby reducing the need for further care that may be more costly. Nevertheless, new technologies can lead to increased use of health care, and therefore costs, because they extend the scope and range of the treatments available and can extend treatment to a wider set of indications that may or may not contribute to overall health gain in society.

The uptake and use of new technology, and thus their potential to increase costs, depend on the incentives given to providers in the system *(182)*. Estimates of the effects of technological change on expenditure in Europe suggest that the impact of adopting technical and medical developments serves to increase use and thus costs *(177)*. Based on expenditure data for Switzerland for 1970–1995, one study has estimated an expenditure growth factor of 1% per year due to technological change *(183)*. Applying this estimate to projections of health expenditure suggests such changes in technology and its use will account for 77% of the growth in health care costs by 2050. Ensuring the use of health technology assessment to support the introduction of new technologies that offer real benefits and to discourage those that are less cost effective is an important challenge for policy-makers, given rising health care costs *(184)*.

Rising income, expectations and unit prices

Health care costs' associations with ageing and with technological advances are complex, but the other factors believed to drive up costs – such as rising income, higher expectations of health systems and unit prices – are even less measurable and well understood. Health care expenditure is closely related to national income: estimates suggest that health spending tends to rise relatively proportionately with economic growth. Thus, health care appears to be a normal good with an income elasticity that is close to one. Some studies have estimated higher income elasticity, implying that health care is a luxury good and that, as income increases, health care expenditure will increase even more. This could arise from failure to control for the relative prices of the key components of health care, however, such as wages, capital investment and drug prices. For example, one study found that health care expenditure is driven by wage increases that exceed productivity growth in the general economy in 19 OECD countries *(185)*.

On an individual level, rising incomes may also lead to increased expectations for newer and more expensive health technologies. Whether expectations are increasing and whether these may increase health care costs remain untested empirically. Providers have an important role in determining the uptake and use of health technologies. The incentives in place, in addition to providers' role in managing patients' expectations, will therefore be increasingly important in managing health expenditure in the context of an ever more educated population with a wealth of information (and, importantly, advertising) that is available through the Internet and elsewhere.

Health systems' role in improving population health

As the trends in health status and patterns in life expectancy and morbidity highlighted in the section above on key health status indicators suggest, health systems can play a major role in improving the health status of populations across the European Region. Nevertheless, although the assumption that the health system – and health-related activities and services[5] – can benefit overall population health status may be generally accepted, the extent of its contribution is less well accepted, as other factors also play significant roles to differing degrees in different contexts. These include local dietary habits, geography, social determinants of health and the effects of other sectors' policies, which may not be directed at improving health but influence it *(6,186)*. The challenge is therefore whether and how to attribute indicators of population health or specific outcomes to health service interventions.

Although recent research suggests that health systems have varying success in improving health *(187)* (see the section below on improving health outcomes), it also makes clear that health services can provide considerable potential gains. Health systems can play an important role in improving overall population health through the four functions of health systems:

- service provision: delivering personal health care services and, just as important, preventing disease and promoting healthy lifestyles;
- financing: collecting, pooling and allocating funds to providers in a manner that promotes equity and transparency, protects the population from the out-of-pocket costs of using health care and provides incentives for efficient and high-quality service provision;
- resource generation: investing in the appropriate mix of the necessary human and material resources (including facilities, technologies and pharmaceuticals) to secure good results; and
- stewardship: policies (including those that influence the determinants of health), regulatory mechanisms and implementation arrangements and tools, including systems for transparent monitoring and evaluation, to ensure guidance and accountability.

As the WHO framework for action on health systems denotes, a health system includes population and individual health services, with both public and personal aims and outcomes[6] *(188)*. The stewardship role of the government, health ministry and other key health institutions and actors is a vital part of this, embedding health aims within other policies and developing intersectoral activities to improve health (see the section on stewardship for healthy public policies in Part 3).

---

[5] For the purposes of this discussion, the terms "health services", "health care" and "health care activities" are interchangeable.
[6] Population health services – including health protection activities, disease prevention services, health promotion activities (including those outside health care settings) and health care services and interventions – underpin the health of populations and individuals and contribute to health outcomes. In addition to those that treat and cure disease, illness and injury (delivered through health care services), some services act upstream, protecting health, preventing disease and promoting health improvement (broadly regarded as public health activities). Activities that are focused on or overtly related to health, but that may not be within the health sector, are important for all these inputs into health. The performance of the whole health system, and the intersectoral activities directed at improving health, therefore contribute to the health of a population.

Despite this, policy-makers across the Region often have problems in getting drugs, vaccines, information and other forms of disease prevention, care or treatment – on time, reliably, in sufficient quantity and at reasonable cost – to those who need them *(188)*. In many countries, the people who most need care often simply do not receive it because pharmaceutical products and treatments, money, information and even health workers are not available or are ineffectively deployed. Thus, despite massive investment, health systems (especially in low- and middle-income countries) struggle to deliver priority health interventions, ensure effective services to lower-income people and find a balance between acute and long-term care. This can undermine health systems' contribution to overall population health. Further, poorly functioning health systems are becoming a major obstacle to some European countries' efforts to achieve the MDGs *(17,189)*.

To address the multiplicity of health challenges to countries across the Region, the WHO Regional Office for Europe focuses much of its efforts on helping countries to improve the performance and capacity of their health systems. Strengthening the health system is the most strategic way of meeting health needs on a long-term basis and avoiding the fragmentation, variable capacity and lack of comprehensiveness, universality and flexibility that often characterize health resources, especially in low- and middle-income countries. The effort to strengthen health systems stems from the conviction that health is a human right, from a willingness to share for reasons of solidarity, from an understanding that people's participation improves health outcomes and from an ethical standpoint on all issues related to health. Ideally, stronger health systems will improve health equitably, achieve a fairer distribution of financial contributions, respect the rights of patients and sustainably and efficiently use human, financial and other resources *(190)*. The next section thus considers how health system interventions have had and can have positive effects in the Region, thereby highlighting why governments should continue to invest adequately in them, especially in the current economic and fiscal climate.

Improving health outcomes

Addressing the burden of disease in the European Region involves many activities across and beyond the health system, aimed at both individuals and the population as a whole. Recognition is growing that effectively addressing the growing burden of noncommunicable and chronic diseases and the remaining challenges of communicable diseases means making disease prevention and health promotion a greater focus of coherent strategies and policy. This requires improving all four health system functions.

Amenable and avoidable mortality

Recent research has demonstrated that effective health services can considerably influence health outcomes. In particular, Nolte & McKee *(25)* have sought to apply the concept of avoidable mortality to assess the performance of health systems, providing evidence that improved access to effective and timely health care, combined with other factors, clearly reduced mortality in many countries in the European Region during the 1980s and 1990s. Among people under the age of 75, the reduction was up to 23% of total mortality among males and 32% among females in countries with the highest levels of avoidable mortality, including Finland, Ireland, Portugal and the United Kingdom *(25)*. This was achieved mainly by reducing mortality from diseases amenable to health care in several age groups. The largest contribution was from declining infant mortality, but mortality was also reduced among middle-aged adults in Denmark, France, the Netherlands, Sweden and the United Kingdom.

As noted in previous sections, noncommunicable diseases dominate the overall burden of disease in all Member States. As Table 2.19 shows, they account for 77% of the total burden of disease with sex differences across the various causes, such as neuropsychiatric conditions, which represent 17.5% of the total burden among males and 22.5% among women. Noncommunicable diseases account for most mortality and morbidity that is amenable to intervention of some sort, especially disease prevention. Cardiovascular diseases are the biggest killer in the European Region; in the Netherlands, for instance, 46% of the decline in mortality from heart disease between 1978 and 1985 has been attributed to treatment in coronary care units, postinfarction treatment and coronary bypass grafting. A further 44% of the decline in mortality over the same period is credited to primary prevention efforts: smoking-cessation campaigns, change in serum cholesterol and treatment of hypertension *(191)*. For more detailed breakdowns of the data in Table 2.19, see the section above on key health status indicators and the Annex to this report. These overall figures mask a disparity in the Region: countries in the eastern part have much higher rates of injuries and communicable diseases *(192)*.

Table 2.19. Burden of disease and deaths from selected leading noncommunicable diseases in the WHO European Region, by cause, 2005 estimates

Group of causes	Burden of disease		Deaths	
	DALYs lost (thousands)	Percentage of all causes	Number (thousands)	Percentage of all causes
Cardiovascular diseases	34 421	23	5 067	52
Neuropsychiatric conditions	29 370	20	264	3
Cancer (malignant neoplasms)	17 025	11	1 855	19
Digestive diseases	7 117	5	391	4
Respiratory diseases	6 835	5	420	4
Sense organ diseases	6 339	4	0	0
Musculoskeletal diseases	5 745	4	26	0
Diabetes mellitus	2 319	2	153	2
Oral conditions	1 018	1	0	2
All noncommunicable diseases	115 339	77	8 210	86
All causes	150 322	100	9 564	100

Source: *Gaining health: the European Strategy for the Prevention and Control of Noncommunicable Diseases (67)*.

Nevertheless, improving health outcomes requires health systems to address not only conditions but also their causes. This includes acting on socioeconomic factors and inequality (see the next two sections), smoking, alcohol misuse, poor diet, sedentary lifestyles and obesity, as well as ensuring efficient and effective protection from health threats. Access to health services, especially disease prevention services, and their quality and effectiveness are also important factors. Indeed, policies, programmes, strategies, activities and services across the European Region seek to meet these challenges and improve health. This element of disease prevention and preventable causes implies those outside the usual direct control of health services and differentiates the concepts of avoidable (through prevention and care) and preventable mortality *(133)*. A study of the 27 countries that are now EU members found that rates of both avoidable and preventable mortality declined substantially between 1990 and 2002 *(193)*. It also revealed significant disparities between the eastern and western parts of the Region: amenable mortality ranged from 13% in the Netherlands to 30% in Bulgaria for males aged 0–74 years, and from 26% in Sweden to 44% in Romania for females aged 0–74. The proportions of preventable mortality ranged from 10% in Sweden to 21% in Italy among males and from 4% in Bulgaria to 10% in Hungary among females. These figures illustrate the potential of health services to affect health but also highlight the influence of other parts of the health system and other sectors.

Disease prevention and health promotion

Disease prevention and health promotion activities are fundamental to improving overall health in the European Region by tackling both communicable and noncommunicable diseases. They seek to engage sectors beyond health, requiring strong execution of the stewardship function of the health system. Preventive public health interventions can substantially reduce mortality and morbidity. This applies to measures delivered through individual health care services, such as vaccination, post-exposure prophylaxis to people exposed to a communicable disease or controlling hypertension, especially when combined with population-based actions. Vaccination remains the main method of preventing disease in many countries, where comprehensive programmes are firmly established. Nevertheless, disease prevention activities can also include providing information on behavioural and health risks and advice on how to reduce them, and a strong role for primary care. Secondary prevention includes activities such as evidence-based screening programmes for early disease detection. Thus, acting upstream to prevent illness and promote health improvement requires the development of strategies that are cost-effective, engender widespread support and can be implemented. These go beyond actions with health as their primary goal (downstream measures) to those that indirectly affect health by other means, such as fiscal policy or social services and benefits, that are usually funded and delivered outside the health sector.

Health promotion activities are part of a broader process of enabling people to increase their control over their health and its determinants and thereby improve it. Health promotion includes:

- promoting changes in lifestyle and environmental conditions to develop a culture of health;
- carrying out educational and social communication activities to promote healthy conditions, lifestyles, behaviour and environments;
- reorienting health services to develop models of care that encourage health promotion;
- strengthening intersectoral partnerships for more effective health promotion activities; and
- assessing the effects of public policies on health.

Services can be focused on the general population or groups at increased risk of poor health outcomes in such areas as: sexual and mental health, health behaviour related to HIV transmission, reducing drug abuse, tobacco use and alcohol consumption, increasing physical activity, preventing obesity and promoting a healthy diet, reducing work-related health hazards, preventing injury, and promoting occupational and environmental health. Health systems have a major role in changing people's behaviour in relation to many specific risk factors *(194)*. The broader role of health promotion includes advising policy-makers on health risks, status and needs and designing strategies for various settings.

Tobacco

Tobacco use is a very straightforward public health problem and risk factor, and accounts for about 25% of mortality and 17% of DALYs lost *(132)*. In recognition of this, most countries of the Region have signed the WHO Framework Convention on Tobacco Control *(79)*, the first globally binding public health treaty, adopted in 2003. The Framework Convention requires signatories to enact a range of measures to reduce smoking. Smoking laws, which are recommended by the European Strategy for Tobacco Control *(195)* and developed within the framework of the Convention, are now in place in many countries across the Region. Beginning with Ireland and Norway, Estonia, Finland, Denmark, France, Italy, Malta, Slovenia, Sweden, Spain, Turkey and the United Kingdom, many countries are banning smoking in all public places, including bars, pubs and restaurants. Restrictions on smoking on public transport have also been introduced, with most countries in the Region now banning it in buses and taxis and more than half the countries, on trains *(69)*. Most countries have reinforced their legislation restricting advertising, promotion and sponsorship since 2002.

Research within and outside the European Region has shown that multipronged approaches that extend beyond the health sector are likely to be the most effective. The European Strategy for Tobacco Control *(195)* thus recommends strategic national action to maintain high prices and taxes for all tobacco products, in addition to bans, product labelling and warnings and other measures. For instance, a price increase of 10% leads to an estimated decline of 3–5% in consumption *(196)*. The tobacco industry has counteracted rising taxes by reducing pre-tax prices in some cases, causing prices to rise by less than the taxes imposed. In some countries, the real prices of tobacco products have declined in recent years, including Albania, Denmark, Finland, Kyrgyzstan and the Russian Federation (Table 2.20) *(69)*.

A comprehensive and intersectoral approach can produce successful outcomes. In Australia, rates of lung cancer dropped and deaths from coronary heart disease declined by 59% among men and 55% among women between 1980 and 2000. A comprehensive approach would include measures such as: pricing, pack warnings, advertising bans, national tobacco control campaigns, quitline services for smokers, extensive advocacy programmes, smoking bans, adoption of smoke-free homes and litigation by smokers and passive smokers against tobacco companies *(197)*. Within the European Region, Turkey is a front-runner in adopting comprehensive and intersectoral measures under the leadership of the Ministry of Health and specifically referring to the WHO Framework Convention on Tobacco Control (Box 2.4).

Smoking-cessation services have been an important setting for tobacco control. By 2007, 21 Member States had introduced national programmes for prevention, diagnosis and treatment as part of primary care services, and 10 additional countries implement such services at the regional level *(198)*. There are, however, no common standards for such services. Table 2.21 broadly outlines how tobacco policies and interventions cut across the four functions of the health system.

Table 2.20. Annual price variation (%) of tobacco products in real terms (adjusted for inflation), selected countries in the WHO European Region, 31 December 1997 – 31 December 2001 and 31 December 2001 – 31 December 2005

Country	Price variation (%)	
	1997–2001	2001–2005
Albania	−2.1	−0.4
Armenia	+14.0	−5.4
Austria	+1.5	+2.4
Azerbaijan	−8.9	−2.4
Belgium	+1.6	+3.5
Bulgaria	−2.1	+21.0
Croatia	–	+1.4
Cyprus	+5.8	+14.8
Czech Republic	0.0	0.0
Denmark	−1.1	−3.2
Estonia	+5.3	+5.5
Finland	+0.7	−1.1
France	+3.8	+13.1
Germany	+1.6	+11.0
Greece	+3.1	+1.5
Hungary	+0.5	+11.8
Iceland	+4.8	+5.7
Ireland	+3.2	+4.1
Israel	+4.1	+5.2
Italy	+0.9	+6.1
Kyrgyzstan	−0.2	−2.6
Latvia	+1.9	+5.3
Lithuania	–	+7.9
Luxembourg	+1.6	+1.8
Malta	–	+7.9
Netherlands	+2.6	+6.3
Norway	+7.3	+7.6
Poland	+4.3	+1.9
Portugal	+1.8	+2.8
Republic of Moldova	+3.5	−3.8
Romania	–	+2.9
Russian Federation	–	−6.2
Slovakia	+1.6	+10.7
Slovenia	0	+9.3
Spain	+4.7	+2.3
Sweden	+2.9	+0.7

Source: The European tobacco control report 2007 (69).

Box 2.4. Political commitment to and leadership of tobacco control in Turkey

Turkey is a major tobacco producer, with 280 000 local growers, and one of the top 10 consuming countries, with 20 million smokers. Nevertheless, it has come a long way in its efforts to stem the tobacco epidemic. This is largely due to the high level of leadership and political commitment. When the first tobacco control law was enacted in 1996, banning advertising and smoking in public places, many complained that it was contrary to Turkish culture and could never be enforced. There were some setbacks to full enforcement of the smoking ban at the time, but the law not only remained unadulterated, despite many attempts by various pro-tobacco lobbyists but was strengthened in 2008. This was largely a result of Turkey's ratification of the WHO Framework Convention on Tobacco Control *(79)* in 2004, which allowed policy-makers to further pursue the issue.

The commitment and leadership of the Ministry of Health has been crucial throughout. First, a special unit was established in 2006 devoted exclusively to tobacco control. Second, a National Tobacco Control Committee was created, with high-level representation of key ministries and civil-society organizations, as stipulated by the Framework Convention. Third, in 2007 the Prime Minister launched the first five-year National Tobacco Control Programme and Action Plan, prepared by the National Tobacco Control Committee. Fourth, the Government continually increased taxation on tobacco products to reach a compound tax rate of 73–87%, depending on the brand, one of the highest rates in the world. Finally, the amended law in 2008 expanded smoke-free environments to cover all indoor areas. This includes the hospitality and tourism sector – a major source of foreign exchange – which was given an eighteen-month transition period. When the law entered into force for this sector on 19 July 2009, Turkey became the sixth country globally with national smoke-free laws containing no exemptions: no provisions for designated smoking rooms in public places.

The new law and the political commitment that supports it are an example of best practice from which other countries can learn. The law was judiciously rendered free of loopholes or ambiguities that could be abused. For instance, the previous law required 90 minutes of air time for information, education and communication for tobacco control on broadcast mass media, but the amended law specifies that 30 of the 90 minutes must be during prime time, for greater exposure to achieve the objective of creating an antismoking culture among 90% of the population by 2012. In addition, tobacco products may not be displayed in television programmes, films, music videos and advertisements, and all smoking scenes are blurred. Enforcement is taken very seriously, as all broadcast mass media stations are required to use a set of messages approved by the Ministry of Health for information, education and communication, and to prepare a compact disc of their advertisements every month for review by the Higher Radio and Television Council. This is a major undertaking in a country in which the penetration of broadcast mass media is almost universal, with some 1400 national, regional and local television and radio stations.

Despite the initial objections on cultural grounds, recent polls show that more than 85% of the population now favours the smoke-free legislation. Attitudes and awareness have changed to such an extent that the Prime Minister has publicly mentioned the fight against tobacco in relation to the fight against terrorism (personal communication from the Ministry of Health, Turkey, June 2009).

Table 2.21. Examples of action on tobacco control by health system function

Function	Action
Service delivery	Smoking-cessation services given opportunistically by GPs
	Anti-tobacco health promotion activities in schools
	Tobacco-free environments
Financing	Specified funds for smoking-cessation services in primary care
	Ring-fenced funding for health promotion in schools
Resource generation	Ensuring that relevant expertise is available in the community to conduct smoking-cessation counselling
Stewardship	Taxation and revenue policy – excise duties on tobacco products
	Intersectoral coordination to implement tobacco-related health promotion in settings, especially schools and workplaces
	Enacting and enforcing comprehensive public smoking bans

Diet and physical activity

As highlighted above, poor diet and insufficient physical activity, leading in particular to overweight and obesity, are significant problems across the European Region. Energy-dense, nutrient-poor foods are a key target of action in this respect, as are sedentary lifestyles, since two thirds of adults in the EU are insufficiently active for optimal health *(199)*. Many countries have unwillingly enabled obesogenic (obesity-causing) environments to develop. Obesity is related to many growing health challenges, such as type 2 diabetes, cardiovascular diseases, joint problems and other musculoskeletal conditions associated with excess weight *(200)*. Illness related to obesity is an economic as well as a health issue. For example, the health care costs associated with obesity account for an estimated 4.6% of the total in the United Kingdom *(192)*. The WHO Global Strategy on Diet, Physical Activity and Health *(201)*, which the World Health Assembly endorsed in 2004, sets out goals and actions for improving diet and physical activity across all countries.

Available data show that fruit and vegetable consumption is low in western, northern and central Europe and saturated fat consumption is high in north-western Europe *(33)*. In addition, countries in the Region differ widely in consumption of sugar-rich beverages. Consumption of soft drinks in 11 western countries in 1999 ranged from less than 50 ml in Italy to 200 ml per day in the United Kingdom *(199)*. Nevertheless, dietary patterns in the Region are converging; for example, fat consumption in southern, central and eastern Europe is rising from historically low levels and fruit and vegetable intake has increased in many countries in northern and western Europe *(33)*.

Many recognized downstream interventions can deal with obesity, including long-term lifestyle changes involving diet and physical activity, behavioural therapy, surgery and drug treatment *(199)*. Broader population-level activities are also becoming more prominent and being recognized as crucial for effective long-term solutions. These include intersectoral activities targeting lifestyles and behaviour that create health-supporting environments. A project in Norway addressing physical activity and nutrition in schools, for instance, focused not only on providing healthier meals and snacks but also on changing schools' physical environments and altering class timetables to accommodate more physical activity. This resulted in improved classroom concentration among students (70% in primary school and 50% in junior high school), an improved school environment and one in three students reporting less victimization and bullying (personal communication, Ministry of Health, Norway, 2008). A review of economic studies of obesity *(202)* found that investing in programmes that promote physical activity and healthy eating is highly cost-effective.

Reducing obesity and the associated morbidity and mortality requires multisectoral activity. In particular, tackling the obesogenic environments in many countries requires cooperation across a range of sectors including public health professionals, the food industry, urban planners and education authorities. This is therefore a task of the whole health system (Table 2.22) to be pursued via the stewardship role of health ministries in building intersectoral cooperation.

Table 2.22. Examples of action on diet and physical activity by health system function

Function	Action
Service delivery	Advice on diet and physical activity given by GPs Opportunistically identifying patients at risk in all parts of the health system, such as in health-promoting hospitals Health sector advice to schools about meals and sport Family-friendly leisure environments
Financing	Specified funds for action related to diet and physical activity in primary care, such as targeting high-risk people, measuring BMI and serum cholesterol, etc. Ring-fenced funding for health promotion in schools
Resource generation	Ensuring that relevant expertise is available in primary and secondary care to target people at increased risk of noncommunicable diseases from unhealthy diet and physical inactivity Ensuring that relevant expertise is available in various settings such as schools Funding designated to local authorities for community-level actions and facilities, such as sports facilities, public spaces and bicycle lanes
Stewardship	Coordinating health promotion functions across the health system Making laws, regulations, codes of conduct and agreements with retailers on food labelling Restricting sales of some goods in some places, such as vending machines in schools Restricting advertising Intersectoral coordination on health-promoting environments

Alcohol

Alcohol consumption is an issue of increasing importance. Some countries are showing clear increases in alcohol-related disease. For example, the prevalence of chronic liver disease is rising in the United Kingdom, albeit from a low base, and in countries in south-eastern Europe, where it is significantly higher than in the EU15 *(203)*. About 8% of mortality and 14% of DALYs lost can be attributed to alcohol consumption *(133)* despite declining overall recorded consumption in many countries. Nevertheless, two factors are important: the quantity of unrecorded alcohol consumption, often of homemade products, and the rise of binge drinking, which is especially damaging to health. Further, overall recorded alcohol consumption has risen significantly in many countries.

Countries are using a range of activities to tackle alcohol misuse, reflecting their circumstances and the nature of the problem. For instance, upstream interventions, such as taxation, may work in high-income countries. In Sweden, a combination of legislation, taxes and certification programmes for businesses involved in alcohol reduced health gaps due to alcohol, at least until Sweden joined the EU in 1995 *(204)*. Downstream activities such as improved control of liquids containing alcohol may be more successful in low- and middle-income countries. This applies especially to the CIS and Baltic countries. Research on the Russian Federation has shown that alcohol accounts for 40% of deaths among working-age men *(205)*. The EU has an alcohol strategy that monitors good practice across a range of actions in countries *(206)*. This shows that many countries have taken actions in a variety of fields to address alcohol misuse, including mass-media campaigns, stakeholder intervention, education programmes and legal provisions on sales, purchases, drink–driving and police powers. The EU12 have been at least as active as and often more active than the EU15. Poland and the Baltic countries, for example, have undertaken comprehensive approaches to controlling alcohol, as Norway and Sweden are already renowned for having done. Table 2.23 highlights examples of alcohol control policy across the four functions of the health system.

Table 2.23. Examples of action on alcohol control by health system function

Function	Action
Service delivery	Advice on alcohol consumption given by GPs Availability of specialist counselling services for people with alcohol-related problems Alcohol-related health promotion activities in schools Family-friendly leisure environments
Financing	Specified funds for alcohol control services in primary care Ring-fenced funding for health promotion in schools
Resource generation	Ensuring that relevant expertise is available in general practice and secondary care opportunistically to identify alcohol-related problems Ensuring that relevant expertise is available in relevant settings, including among police officers, teachers, etc. Funding designated to local authorities for community-level actions
Stewardship	Taxation and revenue policy, raising excise duties on alcohol products to reduce consumption Licensing and other restrictions on sales Restrictions on advertising Intersectoral coordination to implement alcohol-related health promotion in various settings

Conclusion

The role of sectors other than health is key to effective long-term action for healthy diets, increased physical activity and alcohol and tobacco control, and positive outcomes are most likely to arise from combining intersectoral action in both population-based and individual services. Most activities to ameliorate – and specifically to prevent – the greatest burdens of disease in the European Region can therefore benefit from comprehensive and strategic intersectoral activity: a health-in-all-policies approach. Many such activities exist in the

Region. A central aspect of the stewardship function of the health system is to influence policies and actions in all the sectors that may affect population health, including actions beyond the health system. This is a key role for the government as a whole, and the health ministry as its health agency in particular (see the section on stewardship for healthy public policies in Part 3). Australia's approach to tobacco and nonsmoking provides a good example.

Health impact assessment of all policy decisions can support or implement a health-in-all-policies approach to health. It supports decision-making with evidence about the likely effects on health of given and alternative decisions, both to help in decision-making and to enable action to ameliorate any negative effects of the decisions made. Health impact assessment is mostly carried out in western European countries, especially in Finland, the Netherlands and the United Kingdom *(207)*. Among the EU12, Slovenia has used it the most. Health impact assessment demonstrates its ability to inform decision-making mainly on a case-by-case basis, although research suggests that it can be both effective as a decision support tool and cost-effective *(207)*.

The purpose of policy and action across the health sector is to improve health outcomes in the European Region. Health policy-makers and health professionals can make the greatest contributions to reducing the burden of disease by focusing on the major determinants of ill health. Progress has been made in each of these areas across all countries. The role of the health system is key, not only in terms of its own actions but also through the intersectoral action it is primarily responsible for overseeing, based on the stewardship function of health ministries.

In addition, health systems globally face new challenges from lifestyle-related illness, disease and causes of premature morbidity and mortality, and established and novel communicable diseases that require comprehensive national action and international cooperation. Recent strategies to strengthen health systems in Europe in order to attain better population health have therefore ranged from broadly changing the organization and/or financing of the health sector to making more discrete efforts focusing on specific elements of the health system. Countries have developed health sector strategies, approaches for assessing the performance of health systems, priority-setting mechanisms to decide on the interventions with the greatest impact on population health at an affordable cost (such as WHO's CHOICE tool *(208)*) and medium-term expenditure frameworks. Other countries have adopted disease- or service-specific strategies to address specific causes of ill health or intersectoral strategies to address inequality in health. These types of approaches and measures are crucial if policy-makers are to ensure that they are targeting and spending their limited resources effectively. In addition, outcomes need to demonstrate both cost–effectiveness and positive health effects to make the continued case for sustained health system investment.

Increasing coverage and financial protection

As a policy objective, coverage involves both access to care and protection from the out-of-pocket costs of using health care services. The goal of universal coverage means ensuring that all in the population can use the services they need and that this does not impose out-of-pocket expenses high enough to impoverish them or their families. This section focuses first on the financial protection aspect of coverage in the European Region and then addresses issues related to access to care. Closely linked to the goal of financial protection is the goal of equity in finance, which means that people with lower incomes should not pay more as a percentage of income for health services than people with higher incomes.

Financial protection and equity in financing

A fundamental goal of a health system is to ensure that no one becomes poor as a result of using health services and that people should not be forced to choose between their health (both physical and mental) and their economic well-being when they become sick *(36,209)*. This reflects one of the most direct associations between health and welfare: the extent to which out-of-pocket health expenditure impoverishes people or, conversely, the effectiveness of the health financing system in protecting people from becoming poor while enabling them to use services. Two widely used measures of this objective can be produced for any country that has reliable household survey data:

- the percentage of households experiencing catastrophic out-of-pocket health expenses; and
- impoverishing expenditure, measured as the impact of health spending on the poverty headcount (the number or percentage of households that fall below the nationally defined poverty line as a result of their health spending) or poverty gap (the extent to which households fall below the poverty line as a result of their health spending).

Catastrophic health expenditure is health spending that exceeds a certain threshold percentage of either total or non-subsistence household spending. The choice of a threshold may vary. This report chooses a threshold of 40% of household non-subsistence income: the income available after basic needs, such as food, have been met. Once out-of-pocket spending exceeds this level for a given period of time, it is considered to be catastrophic for the household.

Even without an in-depth analysis of survey data to determine catastrophic and impoverishing effects, international evidence strongly suggests that high levels of out-of-pocket spending should cause concern. A WHO analysis of data from nearly 80 countries reveals a strong correlation between the share of out-of-pocket payments in total health spending and the percentage of families that face catastrophic health spending *(210)*. One clear message from such findings is that catastrophic payments all but disappear once out-of-pocket payments fall below 15% of total health spending.

Based on this relationship, there is certainly cause for concern that many people in the European Region risk incurring catastrophic levels of out-of-pocket health spending. As shown in Fig. 2.30, out-of-pocket payment as a proportion of total health expenditure exceeds 15% in most countries, 30% in many and 50% in some. The risk of catastrophic levels of spending is great at these very high levels. These data suggest that the risk of incurring catastrophic expenditure is greater in the Caucasus and central Asian countries, but other countries, including such EU countries as Bulgaria, Cyprus, Greece and Latvia, also have high levels of out-of-pocket payments and may need to examine options to address this.

What explains this variation in dependence on out-of-pocket spending – and hence variation in financial protection and equity – across the Region? Most low- and middle-income countries require more out-of-pocket spending, but there are several exceptions.

The relationship between public and private spending can partly explain these patterns. Public spending on health is determined by both the overall size of the public sector in the economy (total government spending as a percentage of GDP) and the relative priority governments give to health in allocating resources (health as a percentage of total government spending). Fig. 2.31 and 2.32 summarize data on each of these for the Region and reflect the substantial variation across the Region in both. The product of these indicators of fiscal capacity and public

Fig. 2.30. Out-of-pocket payment on health as a percentage of total health expenditure, 2006

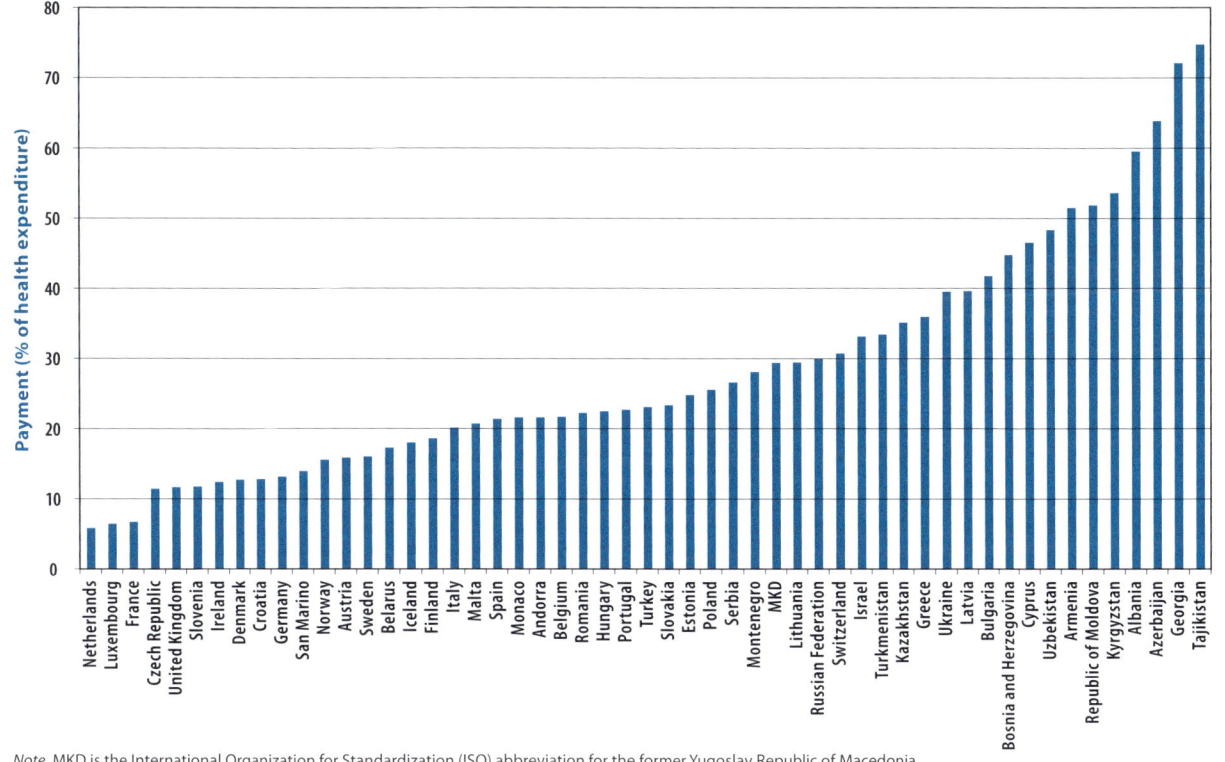

Note. MKD is the International Organization for Standardization (ISO) abbreviation for the former Yugoslav Republic of Macedonia.
Source: National health accounts. Country information [web site] (211).

sector priority for health is government health spending as a percentage of GDP. As shown in Fig. 2.33, this varies considerably across the Region and has a strong inverse correlation with country health systems' dependence on out-of-pocket spending and hence the extent to which financial protection is or is not likely to be a problem.

The association between levels of public spending and health systems' dependence on out-of-pocket payments is strong, but there is substantial variation around the trend shown in Fig. 2.33. For example, the governments of 12 countries had health expenditure of about 6% of GDP in 2006. Of these, out-of-pocket payment as a proportion of total health expenditure ranged from 11% in the Czech Republic to 36% in Greece. Hence the data suggest that both fiscal context and public-sector priorities are important determinants of financial protection in European countries, but the variation also suggests that how health care is funded – health financing policy – matters as well. Although this overall relation between government health spending, out-of-pocket payment and catastrophic expenditure gives a broad picture, understanding the situation in any country requires in-depth analysis of household survey data. A few country examples illustrate this.

In Fig. 2.33, Estonia is a positive outlier, with a relatively low level of out-of-pocket payment for its level of public spending on health. In-depth analysis of Estonia's data reveals how patterns of impoverishing out-of-pocket payments have changed over time. The data (Fig. 2.34) indicate that these payments have been a particular burden for poor and near-poor people, suggesting the need to protect this part of the population from out-of-pocket

Fig. 2.31. Fiscal capacity: total government expenditure as a percentage of GDP, WHO European Region, 2006

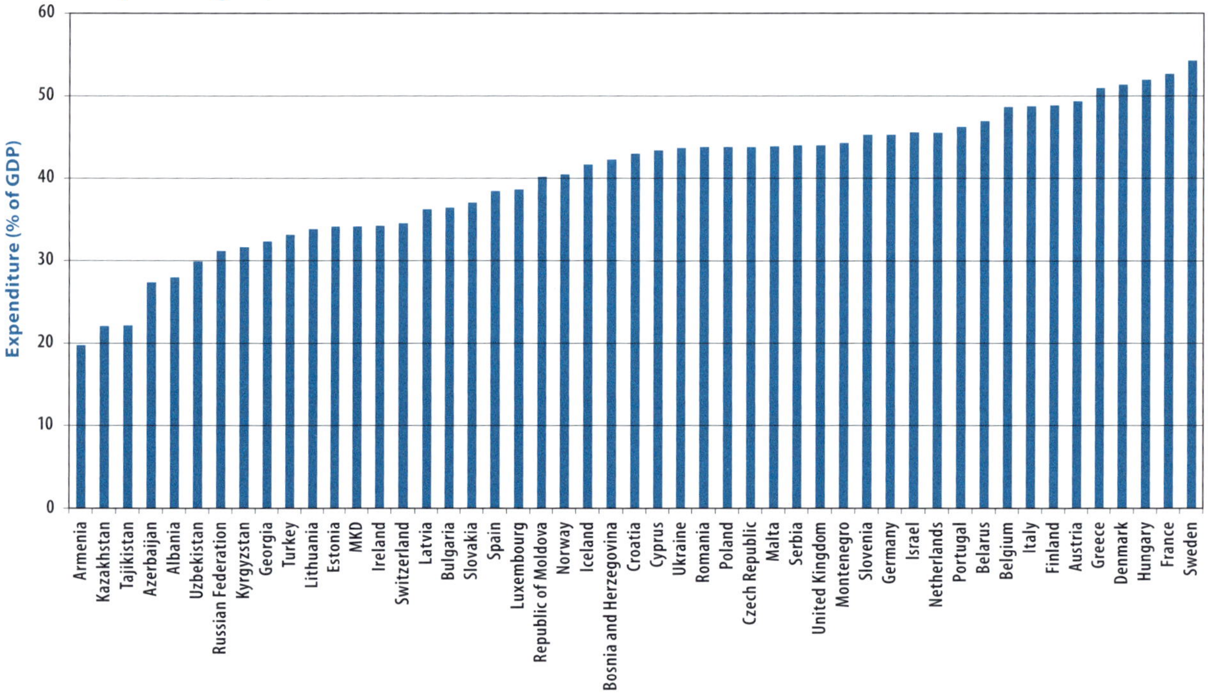

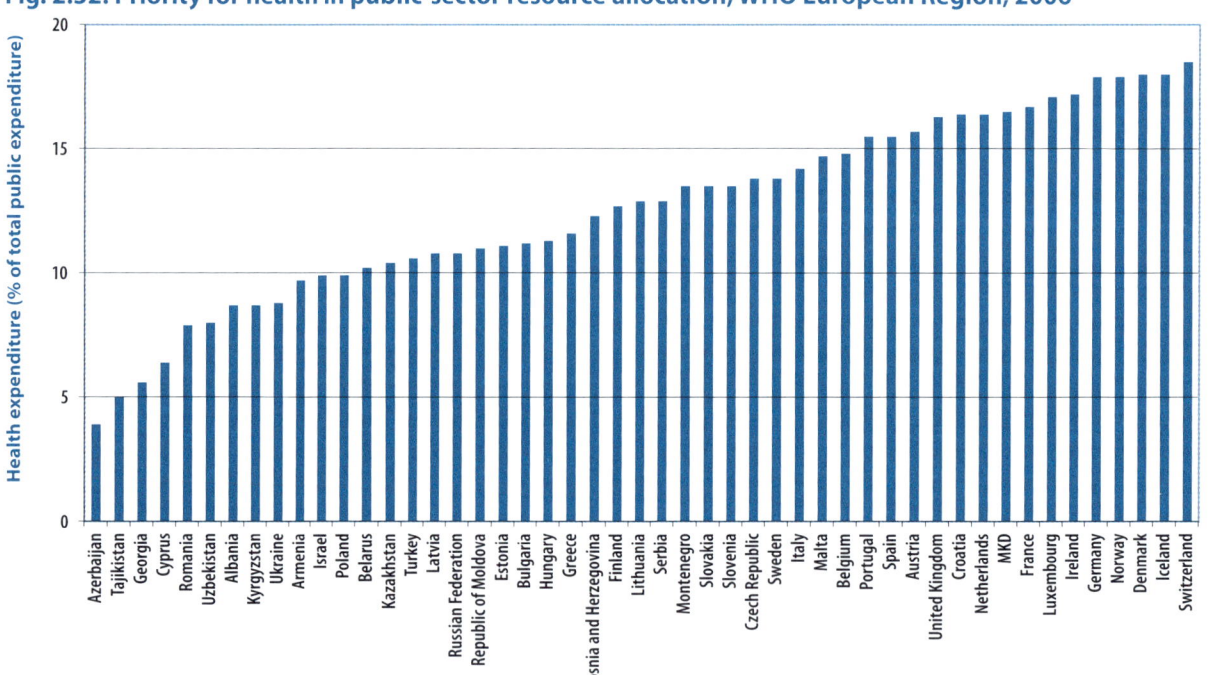

Note. MKD is the International Organization for Standardization (ISO) abbreviation for the former Yugoslav Republic of Macedonia.
Source: National health accounts. Country information [web site] (211).

Fig. 2.32. Priority for health in public-sector resource allocation, WHO European Region, 2006

Note. MKD is the International Organization for Standardization (ISO) abbreviation for the former Yugoslav Republic of Macedonia.
Source: National health accounts. Country information [web site] (211).

Fig. 2.33. Relationship between the level of government health spending and the share of total health expenditure from out-of-pocket payments, WHO European Region, 2006

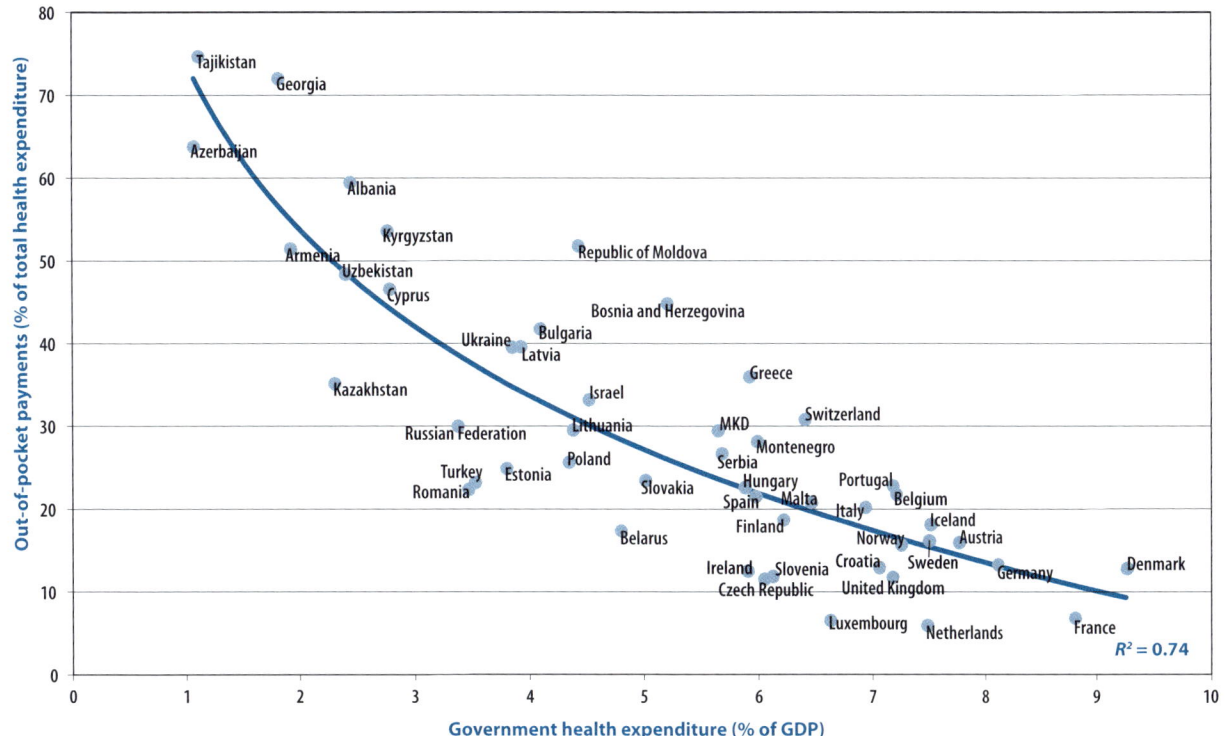

Note. MKD is the International Organization for Standardization (ISO) abbreviation for the former Yugoslav Republic of Macedonia.
Source: National health accounts. Country information [web site] (211).

payments to avoid pushing them more deeply into poverty (212). Thus, although Estonia appears to be doing well in financial protection – based on its overall proportion of out-of-pocket spending in total health spending, especially relative to most other countries at its level of public spending on health – the analysis reveals that improving financial protection for the people most at risk needs to remain on the policy agenda.

In Latvia, concerns about financial protection are driven by its relatively high proportion of out-of-pocket payment in total health expenditure: about 40%, which is among the highest in the EU and high relative to its level of government health spending (Fig. 2.35) (213). According to 2006 survey data, 3.2% of households in Latvia experienced an illness that forced them into catastrophic levels of health spending. In addition, a further 8.2% of households paid 20–40% of non-subsistence expenditure on health care (214). As shown in Fig. 2.35, catastrophic expenditure was closely linked with high expenditure on pharmaceuticals, especially for the 40% of the population with the lowest incomes (213).

Unfortunately, some households do not seek health services at all when their members feel ill because they expect to incur high out-of-pocket payments. In such cases, private spending by the household is zero, and this analysis does not capture this very important effect. In Latvia, 30% of the population reported not using health services when feeling ill for precisely this reason, with the figure even higher among poorer households.

Fig. 2.34. Proportion of households impoverished by out-of-pocket payments, Estonia, 2000–2007

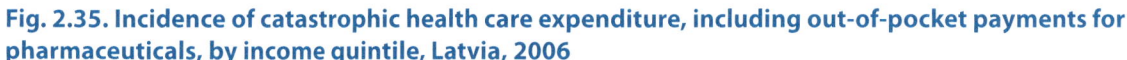

Source: Võrk (212).

Fig. 2.35. Incidence of catastrophic health care expenditure, including out-of-pocket payments for pharmaceuticals, by income quintile, Latvia, 2006

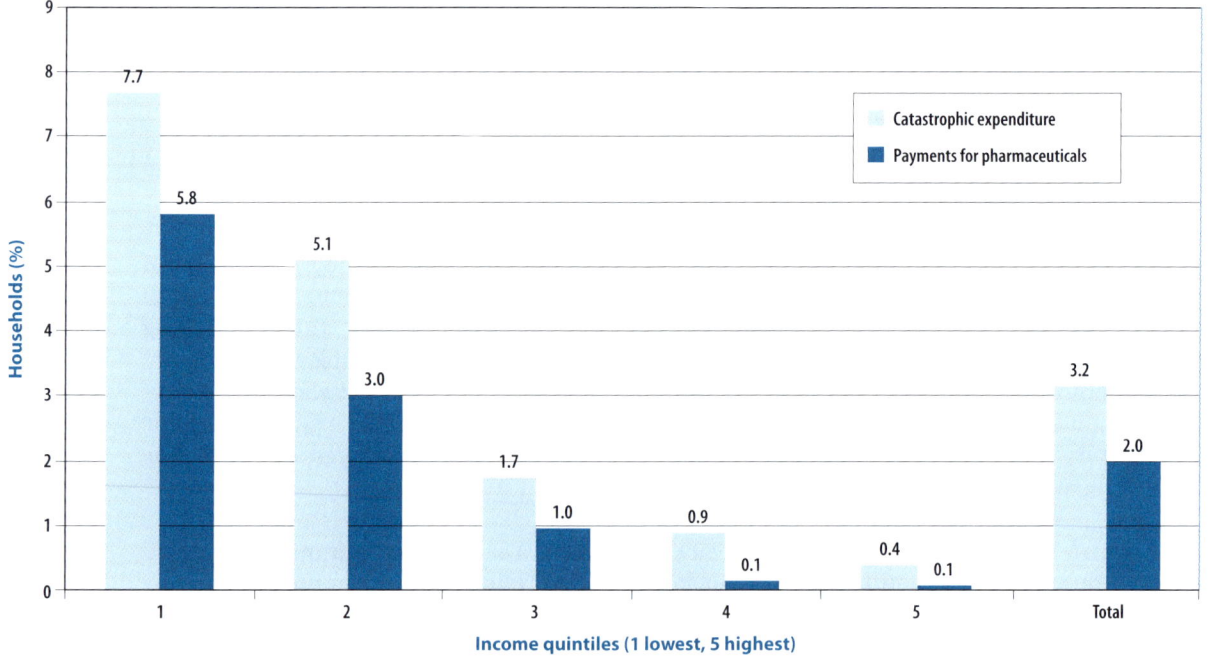

Source: Xu et al. (213).

This type of analysis can be useful to inform policy or to monitor the effects of reforms over time. Using an indicator of equity in financing, household survey data in Kyrgyzstan show that the financial burden for the 40% of the population with the lowest income declined significantly between 2003 and 2006 (Fig. 2.36) *(215,216)*. This calculation of out-of-pocket payments covers all household payments for health, including: fees for outpatient visits and medicine, co-payments for hospitalization, other official fees for laboratory tests and diagnostics, and informal payments to providers for medicine and supplies. Use of services among the 40% of the population with the lowest income increased, again suggesting that coverage – both access and risk protection – improved during this period *(215)*.

Fig. 2.36. Mean out-of-pocket payments for health care as a proportion of total household consumption by income quintile, Kyrgyzstan, 2003 and 2006

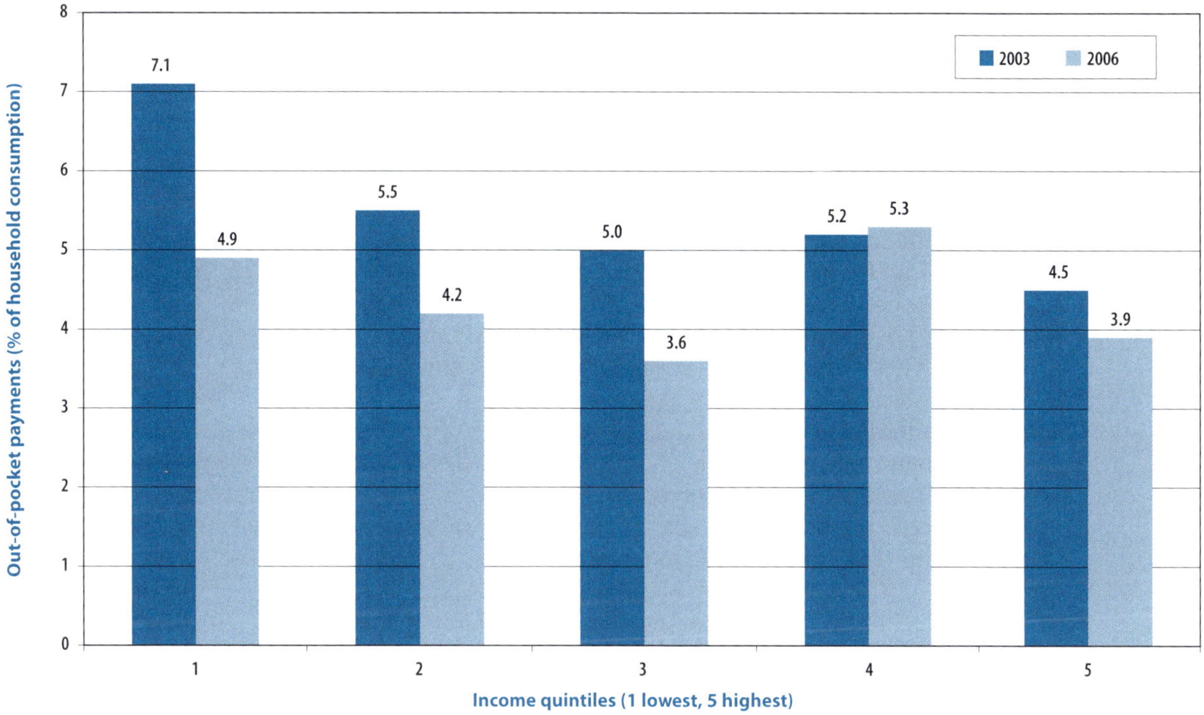

Income quintile	2003	2006
1	7.1	4.9
2	5.5	4.2
3	5.0	3.6
4	5.2	5.3
5	4.5	3.9

Source: Mid-term review report: Manas Taalimi Health Sector Strategy (215).

The overall pattern of health expenditure in the Region suggests that financial protection remains a concern. In general, the more affluent countries tend to have a larger public sector and give higher priority to health in allocating public resources, leading to higher government health expenditure and hence lower out-of-pocket payments and risk of catastrophic household expenditure. There are numerous exceptions, however, and the need to ensure financial protection thus remains a concern throughout the Region, not solely in lower-income countries. Further, the cross-country variation in out-of-pocket payments at any given level of government health expenditure indicates that health financing policy decisions matter as well. Part 3 reviews recent trends in health financing policy.

Reducing inequity in health and access to health care

The previous section presented the relationship between the social determinants of health and inequity in health *(84)* and highlighted the rising inequity in health in both high-income and low- and middle-income countries in the European Region *(9,92)*. The global economic downturn gives greater urgency to identifying options for action: what can be done and what works.

Leveraging the health system

Health systems are a vital determinant of health, and unequal distribution of care is a social determinant of health *(6)*. Health systems are responsible for ensuring that their policies and interventions do not unintentionally increase socioeconomic and health inequity. In addition, they can directly address the effects of socially determined inequity in health through health services and act on the social determinants of health outside the health sector *(6,217)*. The scope for health-sector action goes beyond health care services to other health system functions, especially stewardship.

Three types of action by health systems can help to reduce inequity in health:

- putting its own house in order by addressing the types of inequity in health services that contribute to inequity in health status;
- preventing or addressing the harm to health caused by living in disadvantaged circumstances; and
- tackling poverty and other wider social determinants of health more directly, including advocacy with other sectors for change, through stewardship *(218)*.

Action to put the health system's house in order ranges from providing services that counteract the principle that the availability of high-quality health care tends to vary inversely with the need of the population group served (inverse care law), to matching resource allocation to increased need, maintaining a set of comprehensive universal services and/or preventing health systems from contributing to poverty.

An example is Poland's strengthening its national health insurance system through legislative and regulatory mechanisms to improve the access of vulnerable groups to universal health care services. Five legislative and/or regulatory solutions were introduced to ensure that people with low incomes have better access to health care, ranging from free access to publicly financed health services for uninsured people to protecting the access of insured people to dental care. The changes emerged from monitoring the introduction of the new universal health insurance system: all information on unintentional exclusion was analysed to identify new or excluded social groups so that they could be included in the legislation to ensure equity of access to health services. Post-implementation monitoring identified a lower-than-expected number of intended beneficiaries and lower total expenditure. Further analysis, however, identified that the uptake was greatest in the administrative divisions that included major or capital cities (such as Warsaw) because more population groups who are likely to be uninsured and have low incomes (such as homeless people) live in major cities, and/or that had promoted the new rights where uninsured low-income people live *(219)*.

Another example is the resource allocation formula that the Department of Health in England uses to allocate funding to primary care trusts. The funding formula is weighted to allow for extra health needs that primary care trusts need to meet by working in disadvantaged areas *(220,221)*.

Action to prevent or address the harm to health caused by living in disadvantaged circumstances takes the form of providing extra support services to cater for increased need. These include boosting sensitive or selective disease prevention and health promotion services and intersectoral or multisectoral work to address the harmful effects of living in disadvantaged circumstances. Box 2.5 provides two examples *(222–224)*.

Box 2.5. Addressing the harmful effects of living in disadvantaged circumstances

Prison health reform in England and Wales

Prisoners often come from the poor, deprived and marginalized groups in any society, which are particularly vulnerable to communicable diseases such as HIV, other sexually transmitted infections and TB. The Department of Health is responsible for the health of prisoners but has an equal partnership with H.M. Prison Service, which aims to provide improved health services for prisoners. As part of the North West Health Service (England) initiative, Target: Wellbeing, additional funding has been provided to promote healthy eating, exercise and positive mental health among inmates in 17 prisons. The longer-term goal is to enhance the employment opportunities for prisoners through specific health promotion resources and to improve the health literacy of prisoners' families. This initiative involves many partners and stakeholders from other agencies, including nongovernmental organizations *(222,223)*.

Romania: a community approach to TB

TB is a resurging and growing public health threat in Romania, and disproportionately affects the Roma population. Poverty and marginalization of the Roma has led to higher TB mortality, treatment default and failure rates. Using a knowledge, attitudes and practices survey and other data, the Ministry of Health and HealthRight International developed a community-based information, education and communication campaign to expand knowledge about TB in vulnerable groups and Roma in selected counties, to reduce the stigma of and negative attitudes towards TB within these groups and to increase the detection of cases and adherence to treatment for TB *(224)*. Evaluation revealed that the exposed respondents were better informed than the unexposed respondents about treatment for and the transmission of TB. At the end of the project, the Ministry of Health hired some peer health educators as Roma health mediators. At the level of policy-making and stewardship, the project provided important feedback and input for adapting the National Tuberculosis Control Programme.

Addressing poverty and the wider determinants of health directly includes health system actions such as working intersectorally and making health impact assessments of national and/or subnational policies within and outside the health sector. For example, equity-focused health impact assessment of regional development plans can identify their potential effects on equity in health and recommend how they can be strengthened to maximize and distribute potential health gains more equitably. It also includes the health system in its role as a major employer at the national and subnational levels. Box 2.6 provides an example from Norway *(225,226)*.

Box 2.6. Norway: working intersectorally to tackle the social gradient

Norway's national strategy to reduce social inequalities in health *(225)* – along with the reports to the Storting on employment, welfare and inclusion and on early intervention for lifelong learning – form part of the Government's comprehensive policy for reducing social inequity, promoting inclusion and combating poverty. This is one of the first national policies explicitly to tackle the social gradient in health.

The national strategy sets out guidelines for the efforts of the Government and ministries to reduce social inequality in health during the next decade. Its primary objective is to reduce social inequality in health by levelling up. The strategy responds to health intelligence demonstrating that social inequality in health affects all population groups in Norway *(226)*. The four priority areas include:

- reducing social inequality that contributes to inequality in health by such means as creating safe childhood conditions and inclusive working life and healthy working environments;
- reducing inequality in health in health-related behaviour and use of the health services by such means as reducing the second upper limit for user charges and working intersectorally to develop systematic programmes for physical activity, dietary guidance and smoking cessation;
- using targeted initiatives to promote social inclusion by such means as creating better living conditions for the most disadvantaged people; and
- developing knowledge and intersectoral tools to help increase knowledge about causes and effective measures.

Another example of the health system acting with others to directly tackle wider social determinants of health is the use of cash benefit programmes. These are incentive-based approaches for individuals, with cash benefits provided on the fulfilment of particular conditions, such as children receiving health services and attending school, expectant mothers receiving antenatal care and unemployed young people accepting job counselling and support *(227)*.

A recent review of the global evidence on social exclusion found that: "… conditional transfer programmes are associated with a range of positive outcomes in the short to medium term including modest but important health status outcomes" *(227)*. Nevertheless, it noted that such programmes pose challenges in low-income settings. The changes recommended to maximize potential health and equity benefits included using conditionality solely when it is necessary to achieve the intended outcome and providing higher levels of cash transfers and/or quality of services *(227)*. The recent additions to the cash transfer programme in Kyrgyzstan (Box 2.7) *(228)* provide an example of how this type of programme can be tailored for greater equity in health. Cash transfer programmes are increasingly part of poverty reduction strategies and initiatives to reduce social exclusion.

Box 2.7. Additions to the cash transfer programme in Kyrgyzstan

In 2008, the World Bank approved an additional US$ 10 million as part of the cash transfer programme in Kyrgyzstan in response to soaring food prices, such as the tripling of bread prices, which meant that some families might not be able to buy enough food for their children *(228)*. The 450 000 people who were already receiving the cash transfer would receive an additional 10%. This included a strategy to reduce the exclusionary error: the people who were eligible to receive the transfer but did not. To address this, social workers are interviewing families to raise awareness of the initiative and ensure that everyone who is eligible receives the cash transfer to purchase food.

Linking to health system functions

All three categories outlined above include action across one or more of the functions of health systems *(190)*. Table 2.24 uses examples of health system action to highlight how these functions are important for reducing inequity in health. The four features of health systems that are critical in promoting equity *(217,218)* are:

- leveraging of intersectoral action across government departments to promote population health;
- organizational arrangements and practices that involve population groups and civil-society organizations;
- progressive universalism: health care funding and provision arrangements that aim at universal coverage with particular benefits for socially disadvantaged and marginalized groups; and
- revitalization of the comprehensive primary health care approach.

These features therefore comprise an important foundation for developing and assessing health systems' action on health inequities.

Changing the design and delivery of public health programmes

Increasing and emerging evidence indicates how to design and deliver public health programmes (for communicable and noncommunicable conditions) for improved health equity as well as improved coverage. The Priority Public Health Conditions Knowledge Network *(231)* looked at 14 noncommunicable and communicable conditions and related

Table 2.24. Cross-cutting the functions of the health system with three types of action to address socially determined inequity in health

Function	Health system action: example		
	Health system putting its own house in order: Inequalities Sensitive Practice Initiative, National Health Service, Greater Glasgow and Clyde, and addressing discrimination, Scotland, United Kingdom (229)	Health services preventing or ameliorating the harm to health caused by living in disadvantaged circumstances: Liverpool Healthy Homes initiative, England, United Kingdom (230)	Health services preventing or ameliorating the harm to health caused by living in disadvantaged circumstances: a community approach to controlling TB among the Roma in Romania (224)
Service delivery	Gender-sensitive smoking cessation in maternity services to build capacity to support pregnant women to quit smoking. Housebound service to enable delivery of primary care to hard-to-reach group	Health needs assessment and referrals to relevant health services, including health trainers, health visitors and lifestyle advisers where appropriate	Facilitation of Roma's access to and use of existing diagnosis and treatment services by providing training to specialized TB health service providers (doctors and nurses) and local doctors. More client-oriented approach resulting in better use of health services
Financing	Funding available to support participation by disabled people in developing new services. Resource allocation plan for community health and care partnerships for children's and older people's services using deprivation as an indicator	Health service financing and resource allocation structures for local health authorities enable the pooling of funds for a partnership and intersectoral initiative between the health sector and others, such as the local council	Services funded through National Tuberculosis Control Programme. Additional funding from nongovernmental organizations (United States Agency for International Development and the Open Society Institute) for the targeted health education components of the project and recruitment of peer health educators and community nurses. The Ministry of Health now also responsible for financing and management of the targeted/selective health education components of the project
Resource generation	Direct access hubs planned to increase access of people in disadvantaged areas to health and social care services. Training of practitioners and National Health Service staff to raise awareness of inequality and how it affects health and well-being	Partnership initiative involving the local primary care trust: 27 staff from the participating National Health Service and local government services over three years, at a total cost of £4 million, in addition to capital investment of £4.7 million	Peer health educators selected from the Roma community and trained to communicate a health message on TB. Over half the educators hired by the Ministry of Health when the project ended to continue working with the Roma community, medical staff and public health authorities
Stewardship	Improved health intelligence: increasing collection and disaggregation of patient information by sex, race, disability and sexual orientation	Improvements to the worst private rented homes – such as removing serious health hazards identified by environmental health inspection – to control their most significant and life-threatening hazards, especially to vulnerable people	Health intelligence and oversight improved by a baseline survey to identify knowledge, attitudes and practices about TB among Roma in three counties. Policy guidance enhanced by using survey to inform training of peer health educators and development of appropriate information, education and communication materials for Roma about TB; and by using results of project to revise National Tuberculosis Control Programme. Baseline survey used to evaluate the impact and outcomes of the project. Coalitions between the Ministry of Health and nongovernmental organizations strengthened

issues, including violence and injury, TB, malaria, neglected tropical diseases, alcohol-related disorders, children's health, cardiovascular diseases, diabetes, food safety, HIV, maternal health, mental health, nutrition, oral health, sexual and reproductive health and tobacco and health. The Network's final report is not yet publicly available, but preliminary results have been made available within WHO and demonstrate how programmes can be made more effective and equitable.

According to Blas et al., "… ample opportunities exist to adjust the design and coordinated implementation of these initiatives to enhance health equity when a social determinants of health approach is adopted" (232). This can be accomplished by identifying barriers to and facilitators of access to public health programmes, including analysing the social determinants of health that affect the accessibility, acceptability and appropriateness of programmes (233) and thus reduce effective coverage or increase inequity in health (231). A recent study (234) found that successfully implementing current best practice interventions on four classical risk factors to reduce coronary heart disease in groups with both high and low socioeconomic status could reduce most of the inequity in mortality from this cause.

Using this approach, public health programmes may take action individually or collectively to achieve more equitable health outcomes, especially when different health conditions, such as TB, HIV infection and poor nutrition, have common social determinants. Achieving greater equity in health might therefore not only involve new sets of interventions but also probably require modifying the organization and operation of public health programmes, including involving sectors other than health as the norm rather than the exception (Box 2.8) *(231)*.

Box 2.8. Incorporating a focus on social determinants of health into a national programme to stop TB

TB remains an increasing public health threat in Tajikistan. The country is one of the 18 high-priority countries for implementing the updated Stop TB Strategy *(144)*. A social gradient for TB exists in all countries: the risk of TB is much higher among people with low socioeconomic status. A global WHO network, as part of the Priority Public Health Conditions Knowledge Network of the Commission on Social Determinants of Health, examined the role of TB risk factors and the social determinants of health, especially how to combine the current approaches, such as the Stop TB Strategy, with preventive action, including reducing people's vulnerability to developing TB by addressing such determinants as migration.

Given the high level of labour migration and TB incidence in Tajikistan, the Ministry of Health is conducting a knowledge, attitudes and practices survey on TB among migrant labourers to better understand how this affects the treatment of TB and to improve programme coverage and outcomes. WHO and the International Organization for Migration are supporting the Ministry of Health in improving health intelligence on labour migration as a social determinant of health and its effects on TB *(235)*.

Developing a systematic approach to measuring and evaluating action by health systems

This section has given a brief overview of the types of action health systems are taking across the European Region to reduce socially determined inequity in health. This action reflects countries' increased acceptance of the need to develop and implement policy-level responses in health systems to reduce inequity, as reflected in the Tallinn Charter *(36)*. This has accompanied a demand for greater specificity in health intelligence about how such action affects inequity in terms of: measuring the relative, absolute and/or scale or magnitude of inequity, making relevant data available and identifying which actions or policies are most effective. Countries including Lithuania, Norway, Slovakia, Slovenia and the United Kingdom have invested significantly in improving the assessment of policies to reduce socially determined inequity in health.

These challenges suggest that information about health systems' actions to address inequity in health needs to be collected more systematically, to provide better support to policy-makers and policy development in this area, especially regarding the transferability of action across countries in the Region. This is consistent with the recommendations of other major initiatives in this field, such as the Eurothine project on socially determined inequity in health, which recommended establishing a databank and a European clearinghouse for initiatives on equity *(92)*.

Finally, all the actions outlined require changing the approach to designing, delivering and evaluating health services. In turn, this has implications for human resources and requires changing methods of education and training for all who work in the health system, so that they are more aware not only of the effects of social determinants on health outcomes but also of how to respond appropriately and not worsen existing inequity in health.

Contributing to health and societal well-being

Health care costs continue to rise faster than national income. In recent decades, this trend has focused policy attention on cost-containment initiatives. Nevertheless, the growing understanding of the interdependence of health and wealth, the value that citizens and societies place on health and health systems' role in improving health provide strong arguments for re-examining this long-standing focus *(133)*. Instead of concentrating solely on reducing health care costs, policy-makers could view increased spending on effective health care as contributing to a more productive economy and a way of improving health and well-being. Strengthening health systems, based on sound evidence of cost–effectiveness and performance assessment, can thus potentially improve health, increase wealth and enhance societal well-being.

The intricate linkage between health systems, health and well-being can be conceptualized in a triangle that outlines the causal, direct and indirect relationships between these three dimensions (Fig. 2.37). The WHO European Ministerial Conference on Health Systems: "Health Systems, Health and Wealth", held in June 2008 in Tallinn, Estonia, examined how the relationships between these three dimensions play out at the practical and policy levels in the European Region. The Tallinn Charter, which resulted from the Conference, is thus based on a shared commitment to optimize outcomes within this constellation of health systems, health and wealth *(36,37)*.

Fig. 2.37. Interrelationships between health systems, health, wealth and societal well-being

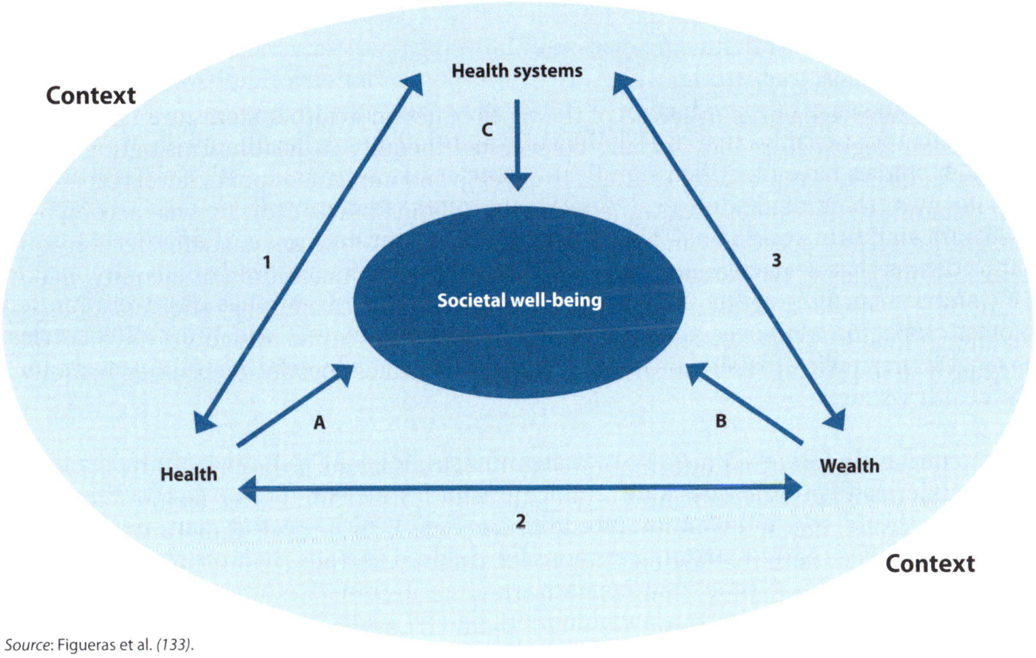

Source: Figueras et al. *(133)*.

Societal well-being can be understood as the total well-being of the entire society: it encompasses happiness and quality of life, in addition to broader elements of the environmental, social and spiritual aspects of life. As the conceptual triangle illustrates, health systems contribute to broader societal well-being in three main ways. They:

1. contribute to health and well-being both directly and by affecting the creation of wealth;
2. contribute to economic growth; and
3. directly increase societal well-being because societies value and derive satisfaction from the existence and accessibility of health services.

Health systems improve health and well-being

Policy-makers across the European Region give priority to health systems' improving population health (see the section above on improving health outcomes). The combined functions of health systems aim to improve health by: delivering effective and high-quality services in a manner that is equitable and responds to patients' needs; funding health care fairly, separating payment from receiving services; investing in a skilled and flexible workforce and innovative technologies; and regulation and stewardship, ensuring that all functions are aligned with the broader objectives of the health system.

The existence and accessibility of health systems directly improve not only health but also societal well-being and social cohesion. The European Member States of WHO have explicitly recognized the value societies place on health, declaring their commitment to health protection, equity and solidarity (36). Further, health improvement, as measured by healthy life-years, is an indicator of progress towards increasing economic competitiveness and social cohesion as part of the EU Lisbon Strategy for Growth and Jobs.

The function of health systems in improving health has been empirically assessed and debated for decades. Some studies have taken an inventory approach to examining how individual health services affect the burden of disease. These types of study have demonstrated a positive effect on health in terms of reducing disease or mortality, although the findings assume that health gains in clinical trial settings will translate into population-level improvements in health (187). Other studies take a production–function approach, identifying the health input and other explanatory variables that are significantly associated with health outcomes. Although many such studies have identified significant associations between health care expenditure and outcomes, their methodological limitations, often stemming from data availability, prevent drawing firm conclusions about the causal relationship. A third approach aims to monitor deaths that are amenable to health care. These avoidable deaths have declined in most countries since the 1980s, suggesting that improved health care has positively affected outcomes (186,236). Moreover, the rates of avoidable mortality vary widely across countries. This suggests that policy-makers can improve population health by enhancing the performance of the health system.

Beyond acute health care, evidence also indicates how public health initiatives affect population health. Public health programmes may produce greater health gain for a given cost than some types of acute health care intervention. In addition to their health benefits, many public health programmes, such as early-years interventions for children and healthy workplace initiatives, can also have significant economic benefits, such as improved educational performance among children and job performance among working-age adults (237).

As highlighted in the section above on the social determinants of health, social inequality in health is widespread in the European Region. Nevertheless, growing evidence indicates the causes of inequality and the potential mechanisms for reducing it through the health care system or broader social policy (238). Reducing inequality by improving the health of relatively disadvantaged people would not only improve overall population health but can also potentially increase societal well-being because it is more equitable. Policy-makers in Europe recognize that both health and equity in health are important components of societal welfare and indicate social progress *(133)*.

Health systems have an important role in reducing inequality in health through health care and public health initiatives that improve health but also through their organizational features, which affect the patterns of service use across social groups. Despite having better health on average, people with higher socioeconomic status in most countries use more specialized and preventive health services than those with lower socioeconomic status. Along with cultural and geographical factors, the methods used to fund health care affect the patterns of service use. Out-of-pocket payments have been shown to reduce the use of necessary services, especially among people with lower income. Higher socioeconomic groups have more private insurance, and such coverage may enable more rapid access to needed services or reduce the out-of-pocket payments for public services *(239)*. Reducing inequality in health therefore requires policy-makers to consider the multiple factors that affect inequality, to offer targeted services to people with lower socioeconomic status and to work across sectoral boundaries *(238)*.

Health contributes to wealth and well-being

Health contributes to well-being both directly and indirectly. The direct contribution is widely known: health is a critical dimension of well-being, and international conventions and national legislation therefore recognize it as a human right. Nevertheless, health also affects well-being indirectly through its role in increasing economic productivity and wealth at the individual and societal levels. Estimating the value societies place on health in monetary terms is complex, but studies suggest that this value is very high. One analysis of western European countries suggests that the increases in life expectancy in the past three decades have been associated with welfare gains totalling about one third of GDP *(240)*.

Health will lead to economic growth if it affects a component of the economy. GDP is the most common measure of the size of the economy; its components include physical capital and labour, both of which could be affected by health. For instance, healthier people are likely to contribute more productively to the workforce and to have higher earnings. Moreover, they have greater economic incentives to invest in education and training, which then stimulates greater labour productivity. Research and development in health and health care also stimulate broader economic growth.

There is some empirical support for these theoretical associations. Although the evidence on how health affects wealth macroeconomically is mixed, studies from the EU15, the countries of central and eastern Europe and the CIS countries (including a study of the Russian Federation) have shown that improving health leads to enhanced economic productivity *(240)*. Countries with poorer initial health are likely to have greater economic gains. For instance, in some countries in the eastern part of the Region, small reductions in mortality could result in GDP growth in the range of 20–40% in the next 25 years. Moreover, numerous single-country and cross-country studies support the theory that, on an individual level, physical and mental health affects labour force participation, earnings and retirement decisions *(240)*.

The relationship between health and wealth is also bidirectional: wealth is an important social determinant of health. On both the collective and individual levels, wealth significantly affects health, both directly through the material conditions that wealth creates and indirectly through its social and psychological effects. Studies therefore require longitudinal data and methodological tools to identify the direction of the causal effect. Many studies have used such methods, mostly on the individual level, and have found evidence for both income affecting health and health affecting wealth.

Health systems contribute to wealth

Health systems contribute to economic development since they are often the largest employer in a country and play a significant role in driving and consuming technological innovation, research and development. Nevertheless, this direct wealth-creating effect of health systems is not straightforward, and investment in other sectors may yield greater economic returns. Moreover, not only do health systems contribute to economic growth, but expenditure on health care rises as national incomes rise.

The links between health systems, health, wealth and societal well-being provide a framework for policy-makers to balance the key elements in decision-making and to highlight the importance of looking beyond cost-containment for health reform. This also emphasizes the need for measuring, assessing and monitoring health systems' performance to maximize improvements in health and societal well-being. Not all investment in health systems will lead to health and economic benefits. Continuing to monitor how health systems and health reform initiatives affect population health improvement and health inequality is therefore vital.

References

1. Nolte E, McKee M, Gilmore A. Morbidity and mortality in the transition countries of Europe. In: Macura M, MacDonald AL, Haug W, eds. *The new demographic regime. Population challenges and policy responses*. New York, United Nations, 2005 (http://www.unece.org/pau/_docs/pau/PAU_2005_Publ_NDRCh09.pdf, accessed 28 June 2009).
2. Smits J, Monden C. Length of life inequality around the globe. *Social Science and Medicine*, 2009, 68:1114–1123.
3. Mackenbach JP. Politics is nothing but medicine at a larger scale: reflections on public health's biggest idea. *Journal of Epidemiology and Community Health*, 2009, 63:181–184.
4. European Health for All database [online database]. Copenhagen, WHO Regional Office for Europe, 2009 (http://www.euro.who.int/hfadb, accessed 28 June 2009).
5. Zaridze D et al. Alcohol poisoning is a main determinant of recent mortality trends in the Russian Federation: evidence from a detailed analysis of mortality statistics and autopsies. *International Journal of Epidemiology*, 2009, 38:143–153.
6. Commission on Social Determinants of Health. *Closing the gap in a generation: health equity through action on the social determinants of health*. Geneva, World Health Organization, 2008 (http://www.who.int/social_determinants/en, accessed 28 June 2009).
7. Marmot M, Bell R. Action on health disparities in the United States. *Journal of the American Medical Association*, 2009, 301:1169–1171.
8. Marmot M. Achieving health equity: from root causes to fair outcomes. *Lancet*, 2007, 370:1153–1163.
9. *Tackling health inequalities in Europe: an integrated approach*. Rotterdam, Erasmus University Medical Centre, 2007 (EUROTHINE Final Report; http://survey.erasmusmc.nl/eurothine, accessed 28 June 2009).

10. *Report on health systems: health creates welfare – The role of the health system in Norwegian society, 2008*. Oslo, Norwegian Directorate of Health, 2008 (http://www.helsedirektoratet.no/vp/multimedia/archive/00062/Health_creates_welfa_62299a.pdf, accessed 28 June 2009).
11. *The world health report 2004. Changing history*. Geneva, World Health Organization, 2004 (http://www.who.int/whr/2004/en, accessed 28 June 2009).
12. *World health statistics 2009*. Geneva, World Health Organization, 2009 (http://www.who.int/whosis/whostat/2009/en/index.html, accessed 28 June 2009).
13. *The European health report 2005. Public health action for healthier children and populations*. Copenhagen, WHO Regional Office for Europe, 2005 (http://www.euro.who.int/ehr2005, accessed 28 June 2009).
14. Fogel RW. *Forecasting the cost of U.S. health care in 2040*. Cambridge, MA, National Bureau of Economic Research, 2008 (NBER Working Paper 14361; http://www.nber.org/papers/w14361, accessed 28 June 2009).
15. European mortality database [online database]. Copenhagen, WHO Regional Office for Europe, 2009 (http://data.euro.who.int/hfamdb, accessed 28 June 2009).
16. Shkolnikov V, McKee, Leon DA. Changes in life expectancy in the Russian Federation in the mid-1990s. *Lancet*, 2001, 357:917–921.
17. Health in the Millennium Development Goals [web site]. Geneva, World Health Organization, 2004 (http://www.who.int/mdg/goals/en, accessed 28 June 2009).
18. OECD, World Bank. *OECD reviews of health systems – Turkey*. Paris, Organisation for Economic Co-operation and Development, 2008.
19. *The global burden of disease: 2004 update*. Geneva, World Health Organization, 2004 (http://www.who.int/healthinfo/global_burden_disease/2004_report_update/en/index.html, accessed 28 June 2009).
20. *Atlas of health in Europe*, 2nd ed. Copenhagen, WHO Regional Office for Europe, 2008 (http://www.euro.who.int/InformationSources/Publications/Catalogue/20080905_1, accessed 28 June 2009).
21. Hirte L et al. The changing regional pattern of ischaemic heart disease mortality in southern Europe: still healthy but uneven progress. *Journal of Epidemiology and Community Health*, 2008, 62:e4.
22. Stuckler D, King L, McKee M. Mass privatization and the post-communist mortality crisis: a cross-national analysis. *Lancet*, 2009, 373:399–407.
23. Bobak M, Marmot M. Societal transition and health. *Lancet*, 2009, 373:360–363.
24. Rutstein D et al. Measuring the quality of medical care. *New England Journal of Medicine*, 1976, 294:582–588.
25. Nolte E, McKee M. *Does health care save lives? Avoidable mortality revisited*. London, Nuffield Trust, 2004 (http://www.nuffieldtrust.org.uk/ecomm/files/21404avoidablemortality2.pdf, accessed 28 June 2009).
26. Johnston SC, Mendis S, Mathers CD. Global variation in stroke burden and mortality: estimates from monitoring, surveillance, and modelling. *Lancet Neurology*, 2009; 8:345–354.
27. Nolte E, Bains C, McKee M. Diabetes as a tracer condition in international benchmarking of health systems. *Diabetes Care*, 2006, 29:1007–1011.
28. Mackenbach JP et al. Socioeconomic inequalities in cardiovascular disease mortality: an international study. *European Heart Journal*, 2000, 21:1141–1151.
29. Moon L, Waters A-M. *Socioeconomic inequalities in cardiovascular disease in Australia: current picture and trends since the 1990s*. Canberra, Australian Institute for Health and Welfare, 2006 (Bulletin No. 37).

30. Ezzati M et al., eds. *Comparative quantification of health risks*. Geneva, World Health Organization, 2004 (http://www.who.int/healthinfo/global_burden_disease/cra/en, accessed 28 June 2009).
31. Kjellstrom T et al. Comparative assessment of transport risks: how it can contribute to health impact assessment of transport policies. *Bulletin of the World Health Organization*, 2003, 81:451–457.
32. *The world health report 2002. Reducing risks, promoting healthy life*. Geneva, World Health Organization, 2002 (http://www.who.int/whr/2002/en, accessed 28 June 2009).
33. Allender S et al. *European cardiovascular disease statistics 2008*. Oxford, European Heart Network, 2008.
34. McKee M, Nolte E. Health sector reforms in central and eastern Europe: how well are health services responding to changing patterns of health? *Demographic Research*, 2004, Special collection 2, Article 7: 163–181.
35. *The European health report 2002*. Copenhagen, WHO Regional Office for Europe, 2002 (http://www.euro.who.int/InformationSources/Publications/Catalogue/20020913_1, accessed 28 June 2009).
36. *The Tallinn Charter: Health Systems for Health and Wealth*. Copenhagen, WHO Regional Office for Europe, 2008 (http://www.euro.who.int/document/e91438.pdf, accessed 28 June 2009).
37. *WHO European Ministerial Conference on Health Systems: "Health Systems, Health and Wealth", Tallinn, Estonia, 25–27 June 2008. Report*. Copenhagen, WHO Regional Office for Europe, 2009 (http://www.euro.who.int/InformationSources/Publications/Catalogue/20090122_1, accessed 28 June 2009).
38. Mackenbach JP. *Health inequalities: Europe in profile*. London, Department of Health, 2005.
39. Friedl L. *Mental health, resilience and inequalities*. Copenhagen, WHO Regional Office for Europe, 2009 (http://www.euro.who.int/mentalhealth/topics/20090309_1, accessed 28 June 2009).
40. Environmental burden of disease: country profiles [web site]. Geneva, World Health Organization, 2007 (http://www.who.int/quantifying_ehimpacts/countryprofiles/en, accessed 28 June 2009).
41. *Preventable environmental impact on mortality and morbidity in countries of the WHO European Region (2007)*. Copenhagen, WHO Regional Office for Europe, 2007 (http://www.euro.who.int/envhealth/data/20070831_4, accessed 28 June 2009).
42. Deaths and DALYs attributable to three environmental risk factors [online database]. Geneva, World Health Organization, 2007 (http://www.who.int/entity/quantifying_ehimpacts/countryprofilesbd.xls, accessed 28 June 2009).
43. Valent F et al. Burden of disease attributable to selected environmental factors and injury among children and adolescents in Europe. *Lancet*, 2004, 363:2032–2039.
44. Joint Monitoring Programme for Water Supply and Sanitation [web site]. Geneva, World Health Organization and New York, United Nations Children's Fund, 2009 (http://www.wssinfo.org/en, accessed 28 June 2009).
45. *Protocol on Water and Health to the 1992 Convention on the Protection and Use of Transboundary Watercourses and International Lakes*. Geneva, United Nations Economic Commission for Europe and Copenhagen, WHO Regional Office for Europe, 2006 (http://www.euro.who.int/Document/Peh-ehp/ProtocolWater.pdf, accessed 28 June 2009).

46. *Air quality guidelines. Global update 2005. Particulate matter, ozone, nitrogen dioxide and sulfur dioxide.* Copenhagen, WHO Regional Office for Europe, 2006 (http://www.euro.who.int/Document/E90038.pdf, accessed 28 June 2009).
47. *Health risks of heavy metals from long-range transboundary air pollution.* Copenhagen, WHO Regional Office for Europe, 2007 (http://www.euro.who.int/document/E91044.pdf, accessed 28 June 2009).
48. *Persistent organic pollutants (POPs) in human milk.* Bilthoven, National Institute for Public Health and the Environment, 2007 (http://www.enhis.org/object_document/04733n27532.html, accessed 28 June 2009).
49. *World Health Assembly resolution WHA60.26. Workers' health: global plan of action.* Geneva, World Health Organization, 2007 (http://www.who.int/gb/ebwha/pdf_files/WHA60/A60_R26-en.pdf, accessed 28 June 2009).
50. Pruss-Ustin A, Corvalan C. *Preventing disease through healthy environments – Toward an estimation of the environmental burden of disease.* Geneva, World Health Organization, 2006 (http://www.who.int/quantifying_ehimpacts/publications/preventingdisease.pdf, accessed 28 June 2009).
51. Sethi D et al. *Injuries and violence in Europe. Why they matter and what can be done.* Copenhagen, WHO Regional Office for Europe, 2006 (http://www.euro.who.int/document/E88037.pdf, accessed 28 June 2009).
52. *WHO Regional Committee for Europe resolution EUR/RC55/R9 on prevention of injuries in the WHO European Region.* Copenhagen, WHO Regional Office for Europe, 2005 (http://www.euro.who.int/eprise/main/WHO/AboutWHO/Governance/resolutions/2005/20050922_1, accessed 28 June 2009).
53. Confalonieri U et al. Human health. In: Parry ML et al., eds. *Climate change 2007: impacts, adaptation and vulnerability. Contribution of Working Group II to the Fourth Assessment Report of the Intergovernmental Panel on Climate Change.* Cambridge, Cambridge University Press, 2007:391–431 (http://www.ipcc-wg2.org, accessed 28 June 2009).
54. Robine JM et al. Death toll exceeded 70 000 in Europe during the summer of 2003. *Comptes Rendus Biologies*, 2008, 331:171–178.
55. The PESETA project: impacts of climate change in Europe [web site]. Brussels, European Commission Joint Research Centre, 2009 (http://peseta.jrc.ec.europa.eu/index.html, accessed 28 June 2009).
56. Menne B et al., eds. *Protecting health in Europe from climate change.* Copenhagen, WHO Regional Office for Europe, 2008 (http://www.euro.who.int/Document/E91865.pdf, accessed 28 June 2009).
57. *World Health Assembly resolution WHA61.19 on climate change and health.* Geneva, World Health Organization, 2008 (http://www.who.int/gb/ebwha/pdf_files/A61/A61_R19-en.pdf, accessed 28 June 2009).
58. Kovats RS, Ebi K, Menne B. *Methods of assessing human health vulnerability and public health adaptation to climate change.* Copenhagen, WHO Regional Office for Europe, 2003 (Health and Global Environmental Change Series, No. 1; http://www.euro.who.int/globalchange/Publications/20031125_1, accessed 28 June 2009).
59. Kovats S, ed. *Health effects of climate change in the United Kingdom 2008. An update of the Department of Health report 2001/2002.* London, Health Protection Agency, Department of Health, 2008.
60. Mitis F, Martuzzi M, eds. *Population health and waste management: scientific data and available options. Report of a WHO workshop, Rome, Italy, 29–30 March 2007.* Copenhagen, WHO Regional Office for Europe, 2007 (http://www.euro.who.int/document/E91021.pdf, accessed 28 June 2009).

61. Martuzzi M et al. Cancer mortality and congenital anomalies in a region of Italy with intense environmental pressure due to waste. *Occupational and Environmental Medicine* (in press; doi:10.1136/oem.2008.044115).
62. *WHO European Action Plan for Food and Nutrition Policy 2007–2012*. Copenhagen, WHO Regional Office for Europe, 2008 (http://www.euro.who.int/nutrition/actionplan/20070620_3, accessed 28 June 2009).
63. International Public Health Symposium on Environment and Health Research: Science for policy, policy for science: bridging the gap, Madrid, Spain, 20–22 October 2008 [web site]. Copenhagen, WHO Regional Office for Europe, 2009 (http://www.euro.who.int/symposium2008, accessed 28 June 2009).
64. Stahl T et al., eds. *Health in all policies: prospects and potentials*. Helsinki, Ministry of Social Affairs and Health, 2006.
65. *Amsterdam Declaration – Making THE Link: transport choices for our health, environment and prosperity*. Geneva, Transport, Health and Environment Pan-European Programme, 2009 (http://www.euro.who.int/document/E92356.pdf, accessed 28 June 2009).
66. Fifth Ministerial Conference on Environment and Health [web site]. Copenhagen, WHO Regional Office for Europe, 2009 (http://www.euro.who.int/parma2010, accessed 28 June 2009).
67. *Gaining health: the European Strategy for the Prevention and Control of Noncommunicable Diseases*. Copenhagen, WHO Regional Office for Europe, 2006 (http://www.euro.who.int/InformationSources/Publications/Catalogue/20061003_1, accessed 23 September 2009).
68. *Report on alcohol in the WHO European Region. Background paper for the Framework for alcohol policy in the WHO European Region*. Copenhagen, WHO Regional Office for Europe, 2005 (EUR/RC55/BD/1; http://www.euro.who.int/Document/RC55/ebd01.pdf, accessed 28 June 2009).
69. *The European tobacco control report 2007*. Copenhagen, WHO Regional Office for Europe, 2007 (http://www.euro.who.int/InformationSources/Publications/Catalogue/20070226_1, accessed 28 June 2009).
70. *WHO report on the tobacco epidemic, 2008 – the MPOWER package*. Geneva, World Health Organization, 2008 (http://www.who.int/tobacco/mpower/en, accessed 28 June 2009).
71. Hibell B et al. *The 2007 ESPAD report: substance use among students in 35 European countries*. Stockholm, European School Survey Project on Alcohol and Other Drugs, 2007 (http://www.espad.org/espad-reports, accessed 28 June 2009).
72. *The challenge of obesity in the WHO European Region and the strategies for response. Summary*. Copenhagen, WHO Regional Office for Europe, 2007 (http://www.euro.who.int/InformationSources/Publications/Catalogue/20070220_1, accessed 28 June 2009).
73. Cavill N, Kahlmeier S, Racioppi F, eds. *Physical activity and health in Europe: evidence for action*. Copenhagen, WHO Regional Office for Europe, 2006 (http://www.euro.who.int/InformationSources/Publications/Catalogue/20061115_2, accessed 28 June 2009).
74. *Steps to health: a European framework to promote physical activity for health*. Copenhagen, WHO Regional Office for Europe, 2007 (http://www.euro.who.int/hepa/publications/publications, accessed 28 June 2009).
75. Edwards P, Tsouros A, eds. *Promoting physical activity and active living in urban environments. The role of local governments. The solid facts*. Copenhagen, WHO Regional Office for Europe, 2006 (http://www.euro.who.int/InformationSources/Publications/Catalogue/20061115_1, accessed 28 June 2009).

76. *European Charter on Counteracting Obesity*. Copenhagen, WHO Regional Office for Europe, 2006 (http://www.euro.who.int/obesity/conference2006, accessed 28 June 2009).
77. *Framework for alcohol policy in the WHO European Region*. Copenhagen, WHO Regional Office for Europe, 2005 (http://www.euro.who.int/InformationSources/Publications/Catalogue/20060403_1, accessed 28 June 2009).
78. *Disease control priorities in developing countries*, 2nd ed. Washington, DC, World Bank, 2006.
79. *WHO Framework Convention on Tobacco Control*. Geneva, World Health Organization, 2003 (http://www.who.int/fctc/en, accessed 28 June 2009).
80. Transport, Health and Environment Pan-European Programme (THE PEP) [web site]. Geneva, Transport, Health and Environment Pan-European Programme, 2009 (http://www.thepep.org/en/welcome.htm, accessed 28 June 2009).
81. Healthy Cities and urban governance [web site]. Copenhagen, WHO Regional Office for Europe, 2005 (http://www.euro.who.int/healthy-cities, accessed 28 June 2009).
82. European network for the promotion of health-enhancing physical activity (HEPA Europe) [web site]. Copenhagen, WHO Regional Office for Europe, 2009 (http://www.euro.who.int/hepa, accessed 28 June 2009).
83. Tarlov A. Social determinants of health: the sociobiological translation. In: Blane D, Brunner E, Wilkinson R, eds. *Health and social organization*. London, Routledge, 1996:71–93.
84. Equity [web site]. Geneva, World Health Organization, 2009 (http://www.who.int/healthsystems/topics/equity/en, accessed 28 June 2009).
85. *Economic crisis gives Europe, central Asia chance to reach for social goals*. New York, United Nations News Centre, 2009 (http://www.un.org/apps/news/story.asp?NewsID=29868&Cr=international+labour+organization&Cr1=, accessed 28 June 2009).
86. *May 2009: euro area unemployment up to 9.5%; EU27 up to 8.9%*. Brussels, EUROSTAT, 2009.
87. Irwin A et al. Commission on Social Determinants of Health: tackling the social roots of health inequities. *PLoS Medicine*, 2006, 3(6):e106.
88. Constitution of the World Health Organization. In: *Basic documents, Forty-fifth ed. Supplement, October 2006*. Geneva, World Health Organization, 2006 (http://www.who.int/governance/eb/who_constitution_en.pdf, accessed 28 June 2009).
89. Waters S, Suhrcke M. *Socioeconomic inequalities in health and health care access in central and eastern Europe and the CIS: a review of the recent literature*. Copenhagen, WHO Regional Office for Europe, 2005 (Working Paper 2005/1; http://www.euro.who.int/socialdeterminants/develop/20050929_1, accessed 28 June 2009).
90. Jagger C et al. Inequalities in healthy life years in the 25 countries of the European Union in 2005: a cross-national meta-regression analysis. *Lancet*, 2008, 372:2124–2131.
91. Suhrcke M, Rocco L, McKee M. *Health: a vital investment for economic development in eastern Europe and central Asia*. Copenhagen, WHO Regional Office for Europe on behalf of the European Observatory on Health Systems and Policies, 2007 (http://www.euro.who.int/observatory/Publications/20070618_1, accessed 28 June 2009).
92. Mackenbach J et al. Strategies to reduce socio-economic inequalities in health in Europe: lessons from the Eurothine Project. In: *Tackling health inequalities in Europe: an integrated approach*. Rotterdam, Erasmus University Medical Centre, 2007 (EUROTHINE Final Report; http://survey.erasmusmc.nl/eurothine, accessed 28 June 2009).

93. *The Millennium Development Goals report*. New York, United Nations, 2008 (http://www.un.org/millenniumgoals/pdf/The%20Millennium%20Development%20Goals%20Report%202008.pdf, accessed 28 June 2009).
94. *Millennium Development Goals: progress and prospects in Europe and central Asia*. Washington, DC, World Bank, 2005 (http://siteresources.worldbank.org/INTECA/Resources/ECA-MDG-full.pdf, accessed 28 June 2009).
95. *Millennium Development Goals in the WHO European Region: health systems and health of mothers and children – lessons learned*. Copenhagen, WHO Regional Office for Europe, 2008 (Document EUR/RC57/8; http://www.euro.who.int/document/rc57/edoc08.pdf, accessed 28 June 2009).
96. Alam A et al. *Growth, poverty and inequality: eastern Europe and the former Soviet Union*. Washington, DC, World Bank, 2005 (http://siteresources.worldbank.org/INTECA/Resources/complete-eca-poverty.pdf, accessed 28 June 2009).
97. Johansson B. Sweden: FRISK – Addressing underemployment and sick leave. In: *Poverty and social exclusion in the European Region: health systems respond*. Copenhagen, WHO Regional Office for Europe (in press).
98. Kopp M et al. Psychosocial determinants of premature cardiovascular mortality differences within Hungary. *Journal of Epidemiology and Community Health*, 2006, 60:782–788.
99. Artacoz L et al. Social inequalities in the impact of flexible employment on different domains of psychosocial health. *Journal of Epidemiology and Community Health*, 2005, 59:761–767.
100. Seguino S. Emerging issue: the gender perspectives of the financial crisis. *Expert panel on the gender perspectives of the financial crisis, United Nations Commission on the Status of Women, Fifty-third Session, New York, 2–13 March 2009*.
101. Gushulak B, Pace P, Weekers J. Migration and health of migrants. In: *Poverty and social exclusion in the European Region: health systems respond*. Copenhagen, WHO Regional Office for Europe (in press).
102. United Nations Economic and Social Council. *World demographic trends*. New York, United Nations, 2009 (United Nations document E/CN/2009/6).
103. *Council of Europe Parliamentary Assembly recommendation 1503 (2001) on health conditions of migrants and refugees in Europe*. Strasbourg, Council of Europe, 2001 (http://assembly.coe.int/main.asp?Link=/documents/adoptedtext/ta01/erec1503.htm, accessed 28 June 2009).
104. Measuring inequality: Gender-related Development Index (GDI) and Gender Empowerment Measure (GEM) [web site]. New York, United Nations Development Programme, 2008 (http://hdr.undp.org/en/statistics/indices/gdi_gem, accessed 28 June 2009).
105. Decision-making in national parliaments [web site]. Brussels, European Commission, 2008 (http://ec.europa.eu/employment_social/women_men_stats/out/en010.htm, accessed 28 June 2009).
106. Saurel-Cubizolles MJ et al. Social inequalities in mortality by cause among men and women in France. *Journal of Epidemiology and Community Health*, 2009, 63:197–202.
107. Östlin P. *Equity in access to health care and treatment – A global view*. Stockholm, Karolinska Institute and National Institute of Public Health, 2007 (http://www.gesundheit-nds.de/downloads/05.10.07.berlin.oestlin.pdf, accessed 28 June 2009).

108. National Health Survey 2006 [web site]. Madrid, National Statistics Institute, 2008 (http://www.ine.es/jaxi/menu.do?type=pcaxis&path=%2Ft15/p419&file=inebase&L=1, accessed 28 June 2009).
109. Mackenbach J et al. Socioeconomic inequalities in health in 22 European countries. *New England Journal of Medicine*, 2008, 358:2468–2481.
110. Rueda S, Artazcoz L, Navarro V. Health inequalities among the elderly in western Europe. *Journal of Epidemiology and Community Health*, 2008, 62:492–498.
111. Graham H. Building an inter-disciplinary science of health inequalities: the example of lifecourse research. *Social Science and Medicine*, 2002, 55:2005–2016.
112. Graham H. *Unequal lives: health and socioeconomic inequalities*. Maidenhead, Open University Press, 2007.
113. Power C, Manor O, Matthews S. The duration and timing of exposure: effects of socioeconomic environment on adult health. *American Journal of Public Health*, 1999, 89:1059–1065.
114. Siddiqi A, Irwin L, Hertzman C. *Total environment assessment model for early child development. Evidence report for the World Health Organization's Commission on Social Determinants of Health*. Geneva, World Health Organization, 2007 (http://www.who.int/social_determinants/resources/ecd_kn_evidence_report_2007.pdf, accessed 28 June 2009).
115. Irwin L, Siddiqi A, Hertzman C. *Early childhood development: a powerful equalizer. Final report of the Early Childhood Development Knowledge Network of the Commission on the Social Determinants of Health*. Geneva, World Health Organization, 2007 (http://www.who.int/social_determinants/resources/ecd_kn_final_report_072007.pdf, accessed 28 June 2009).
116. Grantham-McGregor S et al. Development potential in the first 5 years for children in developing countries. The International Child Development Steering Group. *Lancet*, 2007, 369:60–67.
117. Walker S et al. Child development: risk factors for adverse outcomes in developing countries. *Lancet*, 2007, 369:145–157.
118. *Thematic study on policy measures concerning child poverty*. Brussels, European Commission, 2008 (http://ec.europa.eu/employment_social/spsi/docs/social_inclusion/2008/child_poverty_leaflet_en.pdf, accessed 28 June 2009).
119. Engle P et al. Strategies to avoid the loss of development potential in more than 200 million children in the developing world. *Lancet*, 2007, 369:229–242.
120. Mercy J, Saul J. Creating a healthier future through early interventions for children. *Journal of the American Medical Association*, 2009, 301:2262–2264.
121. Wilkinson R, Marmot M, eds. *Social determinants of health: the solid facts*, 2nd ed. Copenhagen, WHO Regional Office for Europe, 2003 (http://www.euro.who.int/InformationSources/Publications/Catalogue/20020808_2, accessed 28 June 2009).
122. Social inclusion [web site]. Brussels, European Commission, 2009 (http://ec.europa.eu/employment_social/spsi/poverty_social_exclusion_en.htm, accessed 28 June 2009).
123. Suhrcke M et al. *Socioeconomic differences in health, health behaviour and access to health care in Armenia, Belarus, Georgia, Kazakhstan, Kyrgyzstan, the Republic of Moldova, the Russian Federation and Ukraine*. Copenhagen, WHO Regional Office for Europe, 2008 (http://www.euro.who.int/InformationSources/Publications/Catalogue/20081027_1, accessed 28 June 2009).

124. Farrell C et al. *Tackling health inequalities – An all-Ireland approach to social determinants*. Dublin, Combat Poverty Agency and Institute of Public Health in Ireland, 2008.
125. Kelly M et al. *The social determinants of health: developing an evidence base for political action. Final report to World Health Organization Commission on Social Determinants of Health from Measurement and Evidence Knowledge Network*. Geneva, World Health Organization, 2007 (http://www.who.int/social_determinants/publications/measurementandevidence/en/index.html, accessed 28 June 2009).
126. *Economic implications of socio-economic inequalities in health in the European Union*. Brussels, European Commission, 2007 (http://ec.europa.eu/health/ph_determinants/socio_economics/documents/socioeco_inequalities_en.pdf, accessed 28 June 2009).
127. *Reducing health inequities through action on the social determinants of health*. Geneva, World Health Organization, 2009 (EB124.R6; http://www.who.int/gb/ebwha/pdf_files/EB124/B124_R6-en.pdf, accessed 28 June 2009).
128. *Health in times of global economic crisis: implications for the WHO European Region, Oslo, Norway, 1–2 April 2009. Meeting report*. Copenhagen, WHO Regional Office for Europe, 2009 (http://www.euro.who.int/document/HSM/Oslo_report.pdf, accessed 28 June 2009).
129. United Nations Population Division. World population prospects: the 2008 revision population database [online database]. New York, United Nations, 2008 (http://esa.un.org/unpp/index.asp?panel=2, accessed 28 June 2009).
130. United Nations Population Division. World urbanization prospects: the 2007 revision population database [online database]. New York, United Nations, 2007 (http://esa.un.org/unup, accessed 28 June 2009).
131. *The status of health in the European Union: towards a healthier Europe*. Rome, EUGLOREH Project, Ministry of Health, 2009 (http://www.eugloreh.it/ActionPagina_993.do, accessed 28 June 2009).
132. Coleman D. Facing the 21st century: new developments, continuing problems. In: Macura M, MacDonald AL, Haug W, eds. *The new demographic regime. Population challenges and policy responses*. New York, United Nations, 2005 (http://www.unece.org/pau/_docs/pau/PAU_2005_Publ_NDRCh09.pdf, accessed 28 June 2009).
133. Figueras J et al. Health systems, health, wealth and societal well-being: an introduction. In: Figueras J et al., eds. *Health systems, health and wealth: assessing the case for investing in health systems*. Copenhagen, WHO Regional Office for Europe, 2008 (http://www.euro.who.int/document/hsm/3_hsc08_eBD3.pdf, accessed 28 June 2009).
134. Rechel B et al. *How can health systems respond to population ageing?* Copenhagen, WHO Regional Office for Europe, 2009 (http://www.euro.who.int/HEN/policybriefs/20090519_1, accessed 28 June 2009).
135. Wait S, Harding E. *The state of ageing and health in Europe*. London, International Longevity Centre – United Kingdom and the Merck Co. Foundation, 2006.
136. Fogel R. *Forecasting the costs of U.S. health care in 2040*. Cambridge, National Bureau of Economic Research, 2008 (Working Paper 14361).
137. Poisal J et al. Health spending projections through 2016: modest changes obscure Part D's impact. *Health Affairs*, 2007, 26:w242–w253.
138. Brockman H. Why is less money spent on health care for the elderly than the rest of the population? Health care rationing in German hospitals. *Social Science and Medicine*, 2002, 55:593–608.

139. Vignon J. Responses to the new demographics: present and future strategies for the European Region. In: Macura M, MacDonald AL, Haug W, eds. *The new demographic regime. Population challenges and policy responses.* New York, United Nations, 2005 (http://www.unece.org/pau/_docs/pau/PAU_2005_Publ_NDRCh09.pdf, accessed 28 June 2009).
140. Bogaert H. *Long-term population projections in Europe: how they influence policies and accelerate reforms.* Brussels, Federal Planning Bureau, 2008 (Working Paper 2–08).
141. *European Population Conference 2005. Demographic challenges for social cohesion. Proceedings of the Council of Europe Conference, Strasbourg, 7–8 April 2005.* Strasbourg, Council of Europe, 2005.
142. Suhrcke M, Fahey DK, McKee M. Economic aspects of chronic disease and chronic disease management. In: Nolte E, McKee M, eds. *Caring for people for chronic conditions. A health system perspective.* Maidenhead, Open University Press, 2008 (http://www.euro.who.int/InformationSources/Publications/Catalogue/20081027_2, accessed 28 June 2009).
143. *Plan to Stop TB in 18 High-priority Countries in the WHO European Region, 2007–2015.* Copenhagen, WHO Regional Office for Europe, 2007 (http://www.euro.who.int/InformationSources/Publications/Catalogue/20071221_1, accessed 28 June 2009).
144. *WHO report 2009: global tuberculosis control: epidemiology, strategy, financing.* Geneva, World Health Organization, 2009 (http://www.who.int/entity/tb/publications/global_report/2009/pdf/full_report.pdf, accessed 28 June 2009).
145. *The Beijing "Call for Action" on Tuberculosis Control and Patient Care: Together Addressing the Global M/XDR-TB Epidemic.* Geneva, World Health Organization, 2009 (http://www.who.int/tb_bejingmeeting/en, accessed 28 June 2009).
146. *WHO European Ministerial Forum "All against Tuberculosis".* Copenhagen, WHO Regional Office for Europe, 2007 (http://www.euro.who.int/Document/E91369.pdf, accessed 28 June 2009).
147. *The Stop TB Strategy.* Geneva, World Health Organization, 2006 (WHO/HTM/TB/2006.368; http://www.stoptb.org/resource_center/assets/documents/The_Stop_TB_Strategy_Final.pdf, accessed 28 June 2009).
148. European Centre for Disease Prevention and Control, WHO Regional Office for Europe. *HIV/AIDS surveillance in Europe 2007.* Stockholm, European Centre for Disease Prevention and Control, 2008.
149. Matic S et al., eds. *Progress on implementing the Dublin Declaration on Partnership to Fight HIV/AIDS in Europe and Central Asia.* Copenhagen, WHO Regional Office for Europe, 2008 (http://www.euro.who.int/document/e92606.pdf, accessed 28 June 2009).
150. WHO, UNODC, UNAIDS. *Technical guide for countries to set targets for universal access to HIV prevention, treatment and care for injecting drug users (IDUs).* Geneva, World Health Organization, 2009 (http://www.who.int/hiv/pub/idu/targetsetting/en/index.html, accessed 28 June 2009).
151. *HIV and other STIs among MSM in the European Region.* Copenhagen, WHO Regional Office for Europe, 2008 (http://www.euro.who.int/document/SHA/bled_report.pdf, accessed 28 June 2009).
152. 4th European Immunization Week 2009: 20–26 April 2009 [web site]. Copenhagen, WHO Regional Office for Europe, 2009 (http://www.euro.who.int/vaccine/eiw/20081205_33, accessed 28 June 2009).

153. *WHO vaccine-preventable diseases: monitoring system – 2008 global summary.* Geneva, World Health Organization, 2008 (http://www.who.int/immunization_monitoring/data/en, accessed 28 June 2009).
154. Centralized information system for infectious diseases (CISID) [online database]. Copenhagen, WHO Regional Office for Europe, 2009 (http://data.euro.who.int/cisid, accessed 28 June 2009).
155. *WHO Regional Committee for Europe resolution EUR/RC55/R7 on strengthening national immunization systems through measles and rubella elimination and prevention of congenital rubella infection in WHO's European Region.* Copenhagen, WHO Regional Office for Europe, 2005 (http://www.euro.who.int/Governance/resolutions/2005/20050920_3, accessed 28 June 2009).
156. European Influenza Surveillance Scheme [web site]. Stockholm, European Centre for Disease Prevention and Control, 2009 (http://www.eiss.org, accessed 28 June 2009).
157. Global Health Atlas [online database]. Geneva, World Health Organization, 2007 (http://www.who.int/globalatlas/dataQuery/default.asp, accessed 28 June 2009).
158. *Tashkent Declaration: "the Move from Malaria Control to Elimination" in the WHO European Region.* Copenhagen, WHO Regional Office for Europe, 2009 (http://www.euro.who.int/Document/E89355.pdf, accessed 28 June 2009).
159. Pandemic (H1N1) 2009 [web site]. Copenhagen, WHO Regional Office for Europe, 2009 (http://www.euro.who.int/influenza/ah1n1, accessed 20 July 2009).
160. WHO/Europe influenza surveillance [web site]. Copenhagen, WHO Regional Office for Europe, 2009 (http: //www.euroflu.org/index.php, accessed 23 September 2009).
161. *Mental health: facing the challenges, building solutions.* Copenhagen, WHO Regional Office for Europe, 2005 (http://www.euro.who.int/InformationSources/Publications/Catalogue/20050912_1, accessed 28 June 2009).
162. *Diabetes atlas*, 3rd ed. Brussels, International Diabetes Federation, 2007 (http://www.eatlas.idf.org, accessed 28 June 2009).
163. Suhrcke M et al. *Chronic disease: an economic perspective.* Oxford, Oxford Health Alliance, 2006.
164. Petersen S, Peto V, Rayner M. *European cardiovascular disease statistics.* London, British Heart Foundation, 2005.
165. Woolf AD. Musculoskeletal conditions. In: *Major and chronic diseases – Report 2007.* Brussels, European Commission, 2008 (http://ec.europa.eu/health/ph_threats/non_com/docs/mcd_report_en.pdf, accessed 23 September 2009).
166. *Policies and practices for mental health in Europe – Meeting the challenges.* Copenhagen, WHO Regional Office for Europe, 2008 (http://www.euro.who.int/InformationSources/Publications/Catalogue/20081009_1, accessed 28 June 2009).
167. *Mental Health Action Plan for Europe – Facing the challenges, building solutions.* Copenhagen, WHO Regional Office for Europe, 2005 (http://www.euro.who.int/Document/MNH/edoc07.pdf, accessed 24 September 2009).
168. *Preventing chronic diseases: a vital investment.* Geneva, World Health Organization, 2005 (http://www.who.int/chp/chronic_disease_report/contents/en/index.html, accessed 28 June 2009).
169. *Prevention of recurrent heart attacks and strokes in low and middle income populations. Evidence-based recommendations for policy-makers and health professionals.* Geneva, World Health Organization, 2003.
170. *The world health report 2008. Primary health care – Now more than ever.* Geneva, World Health Organization, 2008 (http://www.who.int/whr/2008/en, accessed 28 June 2009).

171. Coulter A, Parsons S, Askham J. *Where are the patients in decision-making about their own care?* Copenhagen, WHO Regional Office for Europe, 2008 (http://www.euro.who.int/healthsystems/Conference/Documents/20080620_34, accessed 28 June 2009).
172. *Therapeutic education of patients with coronary heart disease: training guide for general practitioners.* Copenhagen, WHO Regional Office for Europe, 2006 (http://www.euro.who.int/noncommunicable/publications/20050628_1, accessed 28 June 2009).
173. *Innovative care for chronic conditions: building blocks for action.* Geneva, World Health Organization, 2002 (http://www.who.int/diabetesactiononline/about/icccreport/en/index.html, accessed 28 June 2009).
174. Singh D. *How can chronic disease management programmes operate across care settings and providers?* Copenhagen, WHO Regional Office for Europe, 2008 (http://www.euro.who.int/document/hsm/6_hsc08_ePB_9.pdf, accessed 28 June 2009).
175. Bodenheimer T, Wagner EH, Grumbach K. Improving primary care for patients with chronic illness: the chronic care model. Part 2. *Journal of the American Medical Association*, 2002, 288:1909–1914.
176. Rijken M et al. Supporting self-management. In: Nolte E, McKee M, eds. *Caring for people with chronic conditions. A health system perspective.* Maidenhead, Open University Press, 2008 (http://www.euro.who.int/InformationSources/Publications/Catalogue/20081027_2, accessed 28 June 2009).
177. Economic Policy Committee and European Commission. *The impact of ageing on public expenditure: projections for the EU25 Member States on pensions, health care, long-term care, education and unemployment transfers (2004–2050).* Brussels, European Commission, 2006 (http://ec.europa.eu/economy_finance/publications/publication6654_en.pdf, accessed 23 September 2009).
178. *Projecting OECD health and long-term care expenditures: what are the main drivers?* Paris, Organisation for Economic Co-operation and Development, 2006 (Economics Department Working Papers No. 477).
179. Fries JF. Aging, natural death, and the compression of morbidity. *New England Journal of Medicine*, 1980, 303:130–135.
180. Manton KG. Changing concepts of morbidity and mortality in the elderly population. *Milbank Memorial Fund Quarterly*, 1982, 60:183–244.
181. Payne G et al. Counting backward to health care's future: using time-to-death modeling to identify changes in end-of-life morbidity and the impact of aging on health care expenditures. *Milbank Quarterly*, 2007, 85:213–257.
182. Evans RG. *Economic myths and political realities: the inequality agenda and the sustainability of Medicare.* Vancouver, Centre for Health Services and Policy Research, University of British Columbia, 2007.
183. Breyer F, Felder S. Life expectancy and health care expenditures: a new calculation for Germany using the costs of dying. *Health Policy*, 2006, 75:178–186.
184. Sorenson C et al. *How can the impact of health technology assessments be enhanced?* Copenhagen, WHO Regional Office for Europe, 2008 (http://www.euro.who.int/document/hsm/2_hsc08_ePB_5.pdf, accessed 28 June 2009).
185. Hartwig J. What drives health care expenditure? Baumol's model of "unbalanced growth" revisited. *Journal of Health Economics*, 2008, 27:603–623.
186. Nolte E, McKee M. Measuring the health of nations: analysis of mortality amenable to health care. *British Medical Journal*, 2003, 327:1129.

187. Nolte E, McKee M, Evans D. Saving lives? The contribution of health care to population health. In: Figueras J et al., eds. *Health systems, health and wealth: assessing the case for investing in health systems.* Copenhagen, WHO Regional Office for Europe, 2008 (http://www.euro.who.int/document/hsm/3_hsc08_eBD3.pdf, accessed 28 June 2009).
188. *Everybody's business: strengthening health systems to improve health outcomes. WHO's framework for action.* Geneva, World Health Organization, 2007 (http://www.who.int/healthsystems/strategy/en, accessed 28 June 2009).
189. Travis P et al. Overcoming health-systems constraints to achieve the Millennium Development Goals. *Lancet*, 2004, 364:900–906.
190. *Strengthened health systems save more lives: an insight into WHO's European health systems strategy.* Copenhagen, WHO Regional Office for Europe, 2005 (http://www.euro.who.int/financing, accessed 28 June 2009).
191. Bots ML, Grobbee DE. Decline of coronary heart disease mortality in the Netherlands from 1978 to 1985: contribution of medical care and changes over time in presence of major cardiovascular risk factors. *Journal of Cardiovascular Risk*, 1996, 3:271–276.
192. McDaid D, Drummond M, Suhrcke M. *How can European health systems support investment in and the implementation of population health strategies?* Copenhagen, WHO Regional Office for Europe, 2008 (http://www.euro.who.int/document/hsm/1_hsc08_ePB_2.pdf, accessed 28 June 2009).
193. Newey C et al. *Avoidable mortality in the enlarged European Union.* Paris, Institut des Sciences de la Santé, 2004.
194. *Behaviour change strategies and health: the role of health systems.* Copenhagen, WHO Regional Office for Europe, 2008 (EUR/RC58/10; http://www.euro.who.int/document/rc58/rc58_edoc10.pdf, accessed 28 June 2009).
195. *European Strategy for Tobacco Control.* Copenhagen, WHO Regional Office for Europe, 2002 (http://www.euro.who.int/tobaccofree/Policy/20030826_3, accessed 28 June 2009).
196. Chaloupka F, Warner W. The economics of smoking. In: Culyer A, Newhouse J, eds. *Handbook of health economics.* Amsterdam, Elsevier Science, 2000, Volume 18: 1539–1627.
197. Chapman S. Reducing tobacco consumption. *NSW Public Health Bulletin*, 2003, 14:46–48.
198. Framework Convention Alliance [web site]. Geneva, Framework Convention Alliance, 2009 (http://www.fctc.org, accessed 28 June 2009).
199. Branca F, Nikogosian H, Lobstein T, eds. *The challenge of obesity in the European Region and the strategies for response.* Copenhagen, WHO Regional Office for Europe, 2007 (http://www.euro.who.int/eprise/main/who/progs/obe/home, accessed 28 June 2009).
200. Anandacoomarasamy A, Fransen M, March L. Obesity and the musculoskeletal system. *Current Opinion in Rheumatology*, 2009, 21:71–77.
201. *WHO Global Strategy on Diet, Physical Activity and Health.* Geneva, World Health Organization, 2004 (http://www.who.int/dietphysicalactivity/strategy/eb11344/en/index.html, accessed 28 June 2009).
202. *Ökonomische Beurteilung von Gesundheitsförderung und Prävention.* Winterthur, Winterthurer Institut für Gesundheitsökonomie, 2004.
203. *Health and economic development in south-eastern Europe.* Copenhagen, WHO Regional Office for Europe, Paris, Council of Europe Development Bank, 2006 (http://www.euro.who.int/InformationSources/Publications/Catalogue/20061009_1, accessed 28 June 2009).

204. European Directory of Good Practices to Reduce Health Inequalities [online database]. Cologne, DETERMINE (European Consortium for Action on the Socioeconomic Determinants for Health), Federal Centre for Health Education, 2008 (http://www.health-inequalities.eu/?uid=651e4e7cbe2af9488f7809341e36d69a&id=main2, accessed 28 June 2009).
205. Leon DA et al. Hazardous alcohol drinking and premature mortality in the Russian Federation (the Izhevsk Family Study): a population based case-control study. *Lancet*, 2007, 369:2001–2009.
206. Alcohol [web site]. Brussels, European Commission, 2009 (http://ec.europa.eu/health/ph_determinants/life_style/alcohol/alcohol_en.htm, accessed 28 June 2009).
207. Wismar M et al. *The effectiveness of health impact assessment: scope and limitations of supporting decision-making in Europe*. Copenhagen, WHO Regional Office for Europe on behalf of the European Observatory on Health Systems and Policies, 2007 (http://www.euro.who.int/observatory/Publications/2007/20071016_1, accessed 28 June 2009).
208. WHO-CHOICE [web site]. Geneva, World Health Organization, 2009 (http://www.who.int/choice/en, accessed 28 June 2009).
209. *The world health report 2000. Health systems: improving performance*. Geneva, World Health Organization, 2000 (http://www.who.int/whr/2000/en, accessed 28 June 2009).
210. Xu K. *Designing health financing systems to reduce catastrophic health expenditure*. Geneva, World Health Organization, 2005 (Technical Briefs for Policy-Makers Number 2/2005; http://www.who.int/health_financing/documents/cov-pb_e_05_2-cata_sys/en, accessed 28 June 2009).
211. National health accounts. Country information [web site]. Geneva, World Health Organization, 2009 (http://www.who.int/nha/country/en, accessed 28 June 2009).
212. Võrk A. *Household catastrophic expenditures on health care and distribution of taxation burden to households in Estonia 2000–2006*. Copenhagen, WHO Regional Office for Europe (in press).
213. Xu K et al. *Access to health care and the financial burden of out-of-pocket health payments in Latvia*. Geneva, World Health Organization, 2009 (Technical Briefs for Policy-Makers, Number 1/2009; http://www.who.int/health_financing/documents/cov-pb_e_09_01-oopslat/en/index.html, accessed 28 June 2009).
214. *Out-of-pocket health payments in households of Latvia and their impact on the capacity to pay*. Riga, Central Statistical Bureau of Latvia, 2008.
215. *Mid-term review report: Manas Taalimi Health Sector Strategy*. Bishkek, Ministry of Health of the Kyrgyz Republic, 2008.
216. Falkingham J, Akkazieva B, Baschieri A. *Health, health seeking behavior and out of pocket expenditures in Kyrgyzstan, 2007*. Bishkek, Republican Center for Health System Development and Information Technologies, 2007 (Policy Research Paper 46, MANAS Health Policy Analysis Project; http://chsd.studionew.com/images//prp46khhs.pdf, accessed 28 June 2009).
217. Gilson L et al. *Challenging inequity through health systems: final report of Knowledge Network on Health Systems*. Geneva, World Health Organization, 2007 (http://www.who.int/social_determinants/resources/csdh_media/hskn_final_2007_en.pdf, accessed 28 June 2009).
218. Dahlgren G, Whitehead M. *European strategies for tackling social inequities in health: levelling up part 2*. Copenhagen, WHO Regional Office for Europe, 2006 (http://www.euro.who.int/socialdeterminants/publications/publications, accessed 28 June 2009).

219. Marek M. Poland: poverty and health. In: *Poverty and social exclusion in the European Region: health systems respond*. Copenhagen, WHO Regional Office for Europe (in press).
220. House of Commons Health Committee. *Health inequities*. London, The Stationery Office, 2009 (Third Report of Session 2008–09. Volume I; http://www.publications.parliament.uk/pa/cm200809/cmselect/cmhealth/286/28602.htm, accessed 28 June 2009).
221. Diderichsen F, Varde E, Whitehead M. Resource allocation to health authorities: the quest for an equitable formula in Britain and Sweden. *British Medical Journal*, 1997, 315:875–878.
222. Hayton P, Boyington J. Prison and health reforms in England and Wales. *American Journal of Public Health*, 2006, 96:1730–1733.
223. Pan-regional prisons programme: health, inclusion and citizenship [web site]. Lancashire, University of Central Lancashire, 2009 (http://www.uclan.ac.uk/health/schools/sphcs/hsdu_pan_regional_prisons_programme.php, accessed 28 June 2009).
224. Berger D et al. Romania: controlling TB among the Roma – A community approach. In: *Poverty and social exclusion in the European Region: health systems respond*. Copenhagen, WHO Regional Office for Europe (in press).
225. *National strategy to reduce social inequalities in health*. Oslo, Ministry of Health and Care Services, 2007 (Report No. 20 (2006–2007) to the Storting; http://ec.europa.eu/health/ph_determinants/socio_economics/documents/Norway_rd01_en.pdf, accessed 28 June 2009).
226. Dahl E. Health inequalities and health policy: the Norwegian case. *Norsk Epidemiologi*, 2002, 12:69–75.
227. Popay J et al. *Understanding and tackling social exclusion. Final report to the WHO Commission on Social Determinants of Health by the Social Exclusion Knowledge Network*. Geneva, World Health Organization, 2008 (http://www.who.int/social_determinants/knowledge_networks/final_reports/sekn_final%20report_042008.pdf, accessed 28 June 2009).
228. Food crisis in Kyrgyz Republic [web site]. Washington, DC, World Bank, 2008 (http://go.worldbank.org/7VIFYUOKJ0, accessed 28 June 2009).
229. Equalities in Health [web site]. Glasgow, National Health Service Greater Glasgow and Clyde, 2009 (http://www.equalitiesinhealth.org/, accessed 20 November 2009).
230. Healthy Homes Programme [web site]. Liverpool, Liverpool City Council, 2009 (http://www.liverpool.gov.uk/Environment/Environmental_health/healthyhomes/index.asp, accessed 23 November 2009).
231. Priority public health conditions [web site]. Geneva, World Health Organization, 2009 (http://www.who.int/social_determinants/themes/prioritypublichealthconditions/background/en/index.html, accessed 28 June 2009).
232. Blas E et al. Addressing social determinants of health inequities: what can the state and civil society do? *Lancet*, 2008, 372:1684–1689.
233. Tanahashi T. Health service coverage and its evaluation. *Bulletin of the World Health Organization*, 1978, 56:295–303.
234. Kivimaki M et al. Best-practice interventions to reduce socioeconomic inequities of coronary heart disease mortality in the United Kingdom: a prospective occupational cohort study. *Lancet*, 2008, 372:1648–1654.

235. Gilpin C. *Research proposal: to explore the TB related knowledge, attitude, practice and behaviour among migrant labour workers in Tajikistan*. Geneva, International Organization for Migration, 2009.
236. Nolte E, McKee M, eds. *Caring for people with chronic conditions. A health system perspective*. Maidenhead, Open University Press, 2008 (http://www.euro.who.int/InformationSources/Publications/Catalogue/20081027_2, accessed 28 June 2009).
237. McDaid D, Suhrcke M. The contribution of public health interventions: an economic perspective. In: Figueras J et al., eds. *Health systems, health and wealth: assessing the case for investing in health systems*. Copenhagen, WHO Regional Office for Europe, 2008 (http://www.euro.who.int/document/hsm/3_hsc08_eBD3.pdf, accessed 28 June 2009).
238. Mackenbach JP, Kunst AE. Evidence for strategies to reduce socioeconomic inequalities in health in Europe. In: Figueras J et al., eds. *Health systems, health and wealth: assessing the case for investing in health systems*. Copenhagen, WHO Regional Office for Europe, 2008 (http://www.euro.who.int/document/hsm/3_hsc08_eBD3.pdf, accessed 28 June 2009).
239. Mossialos E, Thomson S. *Voluntary health insurance in the European Union*. Copenhagen, WHO Regional Office for Europe on behalf of the European Observatory on Health Systems and Policies, 2004 (http://www.euro.who.int/observatory/Publications/20041014_3, accessed 28 June 2009).
240. Suhrcke M et al. Economic costs of ill health in the European Region. In: Figueras J et al., eds. *Health systems, health and wealth: assessing the case for investing in health systems*. Copenhagen, WHO Regional Office for Europe, 2008 (http://www.euro.who.int/document/hsm/3_hsc08_eBD3.pdf, accessed 28 June 2009).

Part 3.
Strengthening health systems

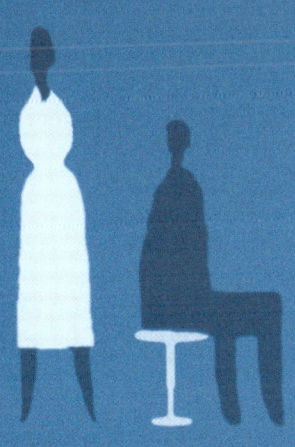

Investing in health systems

A process of wide-ranging reform across the European Region in the past decade has sought to invest in and improve the performance of health systems. Current health system reform in Europe is broadly consistent with the type of reforms called for at the time of the 1996 WHO Conference on European Health Care Reforms in Ljubljana, Slovenia (1). The recent reforms have addressed all four of a health system's functions: service delivery, resource generation, financing and stewardship. Each is discussed below.

Delivering integrated and cost-effective services

Delivering health care services is perhaps the most widely discussed and visible function, and has received considerable attention in the past decade of health care reform. The Ljubljana Charter on Reforming Health Care (2) emphasized the need to improve the quality and cost–effectiveness of care and to move towards primary care, comprehensiveness and continuity of care. In accordance with this, many countries' reform efforts have focused on these dimensions of service delivery. The current demographic and epidemiological trends towards increasing numbers of older people with chronic and often multiple health conditions have increased the need to reconsider the models of care delivery.

Integrating and coordinating services

One reform strategy that has been adopted across Europe has been to integrate clinical services across primary (or ambulatory) and hospital care (3). Evidence indicates that strong primary care systems lead to healthier populations (4) and that putting primary care in the driver's seat (5) would improve the continuity of care for patients and exert pressure to reduce the cost of hospital care. Many tools have therefore been introduced to shift budgetary and/or decision-making power from hospital care to primary care in various countries in the European Region. The section on revitalizing primary health care discusses in detail the issues related to strengthening primary care in general and delivering people-centred care in particular.

Some countries have introduced financial incentives for providers and patients to encourage more cost-effective patterns of health care use. Primary care providers face both clinical and cost considerations when some or all of the hospital-sector budget is given to primary care holders, such as primary care trusts in England, municipal health and social boards in Finland and subcounty district health boards in Sweden. The recent introduction of practice-based commissioning in England further devolves the budget to GPs themselves (as with GP fundholding in the 1990s) to shift care out of the hospital and improve coordination, although little evidence so far indicates success (6). Countries without a tradition of physician gatekeeping (in which primary care physicians serve as gatekeepers to higher-level, specialized services through referrals), such as in France, Germany, the Netherlands and Sweden, have tried to encourage such a system with financial incentives.

Restructuring the organization of primary care has been a common reform strategy across Europe. For example, some countries have encouraged providers to group together in larger primary care centres (Denmark, Finland, the Netherlands, Sweden and parts of the United Kingdom). Germany has introduced larger centres or polyclinics that bring together primary care, diagnostic and specialty providers. This contrasts with the situation in many countries of central and eastern Europe, such as Estonia and Hungary, which have sought to transform substantial numbers of polyclinic specialists into freestanding GPs since the mid-1990s.

Evidence indicates that care is being shifted from inpatient to day-case and ambulatory settings, perhaps owing in part to such reforms in how care is organized and delivered but also to technological and clinical innovation. In particular, inpatient care has been transferred to other settings: for example, replacing high-cost inpatient care with the more cost-effective alternative of day-care surgery *(7,8)*. From 1996 to 2005, the number of hospital beds per capita visibly declined across the Region, reflecting at least two policy objectives: shifting inpatient care to ambulatory settings and shifting mental health care from institutions to the community. The decline has been most pronounced (22%) in the CIS countries, which have had an oversupply of hospitals: from 1077 hospital beds per 100 000 population in 1996 to 845 in 2007. Nevertheless, the supply is still much greater than in the EU, where beds declined 17%: from 689 to 570 per 100 000 population in the same period *(9)*.

One widespread reform to the organization of care delivery, given the rising prevalence of chronic conditions, has been the development and introduction of disease management programmes, which are now in place in some form in most countries *(10)*. Disease management has thus become a key initiative for addressing the growing burden of chronic diseases and the need for new models of care delivery. The key objective of these reforms has been to promote seamless treatment of chronically ill people in the most clinically appropriate and cost-effective setting. Evidence indicates that coordinating care across settings and providers is more effective than traditional, uncoordinated interventions *(11)*. The model that has been adopted in most countries is individualistic and delivery level, however, in contrast to system-level initiatives that not only rely on changing methods of delivery but also build on policy, structures and community resources. System-level initiatives may be more effective in achieving sustained effects on quality and health outcome *(11)*.

Countries with less of a traditional primary care focus have introduced formal disease management programmes to address the fragmentation of care *(10)*, including those initiated in Germany, followed by France and, on a smaller scale, the Netherlands. Countries with strong primary care traditions have had similar objectives of improving care coordination, albeit with different policy tools. Efforts have been made to increase the role of nurses in delivering and managing care, as in Denmark, England, the Netherlands and Sweden, and to integrate care across traditional health and social care boundaries. In Sweden, nurse-led clinics are integral to managing diabetes and hypertension, along with other chronic conditions: models that have also been adopted in Denmark, England and the Netherlands.

Making health systems more responsive to patients

The Tallinn Charter: Health Systems for Health and Wealth *(12)* recognizes the importance of making the health system more responsive to patients' needs, preferences and expectations. Responsiveness is a relatively recent concept that is closely related to satisfaction. Both measure the degree to which health care systems meet public and patient expectations, although responsiveness includes solely the expectations that can be considered legitimate and within the scope of the health system *(13)*. Numerous strategies have been adopted across countries to make the system more responsive, including *(13)*:

- defining entitlements and benefits, making benefit packages more transparent and integrating broader services into the benefit packages that address patient dignity (such as palliative care);
- reducing waiting times and lists;
- introducing patients' rights legislation and patient charters;

- incorporating patient dignity and respect into health care professional training; and
- expanding patients' choice of provider or purchaser.

To monitor responsiveness, the World Health Survey *(14)* includes all countries, with some (such as England and Sweden) also conducting regular surveys of patients, in addition to the perceived quality of care, to measure some of the dimensions of responsiveness.

Within the past decade, explicit policy efforts combining supply-side and demand-side approaches significantly reduced waiting times in Denmark, England and Spain *(13,15)*. Substantial increases in capacity, alongside waiting-time targets and combined with expanded patient choice of hospital, brought about these reductions and corresponding improvements in responsiveness.

Many countries have adopted various models of patient choice, seeking to harness patient preferences to generate greater responsiveness and satisfaction, as well as market-oriented pressures for greater fiscal efficiency. In tax-funded health systems (as in Denmark, Norway and Sweden), choice has typically been introduced among providers on the production side of the system. England has introduced patient choice of both private and public hospitals funded by the public-sector National Health Service (NHS) system and, at the first point of contact in the system, by introducing nurse-led walk-in clinics and telephone-based services (NHS Direct). In countries with health systems based on social insurance models, new choice arrangements have focused on selecting sickness funds (Germany and Switzerland) or "insurance companies" (the Czech Republic and the Netherlands). Nevertheless, these insurer choice arrangements have been introduced within a tightly regulated environment with mechanisms of risk adjustment to reduce but not eliminate the incentive for insurers to select risks. Experience with these reforms suggests that regulation by the state, providing sufficient information to patients and sufficient support for making choices, is needed to improve economic efficiency without adversely affecting solidarity.

In addition to increased choice, countries have implemented a wide range of measures to empower patients, including patients' rights legislation, requiring formal representation on the boards of purchaser and provider organizations, introducing ombudsperson services and increasing patients' participation in making decisions about their care. This is especially relevant in chronic diseases, where patients' participation and self-management have been shown to improve outcomes *(10)*. This requires the system to build health literacy, promote patients' involvement in treatment decisions and educate patients to play an active role in self-managing chronic conditions *(16)*.

Enhancing the quality of care

Improving quality has been a key feature of recent health reforms across Europe. Strategies incorporate organizational, financial and regulatory tools, with initiatives that range from the broad system level to the clinical setting. The numerous initiatives adopted include:

- national legislation and policies on the quality of care;
- comprehensive strategies to improve patient safety;
- new systems of registration and licensing for new technologies and pharmaceuticals;
- incorporating quality assurance into professional training programmes and continuous professional development;
- pursuing clinical guidelines and audit processes;
- establishing information systems and quality assurance methods at the clinical level; and

- including quality indicators in methods of paying providers (performance-based payment).

In addition, OECD, the European Commission and WHO have been influential in guiding and advising on national strategies for improving quality and patient safety *(17)*.

Many countries have established comprehensive strategies and legislation to make systematic efforts to improve quality, but the countries in the Region vary in the extent to which they have used legislation to ensure quality improvements *(17)*. Some countries use local initiatives and voluntary quality assurance mechanisms instead of national quality or safety legislation (such as Bulgaria, Cyprus, Estonia, Greece, Hungary, Latvia, Luxembourg, Malta, Poland, Portugal, Romania and Slovakia). Others have recently adopted explicit laws on the quality of care (such as the Czech Republic, Ireland, Lithuania and Slovenia). Many countries have a longer tradition of national quality measures; some are undergoing minor reform (such as Finland, France, Germany, Italy, Spain and Sweden), and others are experiencing major organizational reform with quality as a key focus (such as Austria, Belgium, Denmark, England and the Netherlands). Specific institutional structures to ensure patient safety appear to be limited to Denmark, Germany, the Netherlands, Spain and the United Kingdom *(17)*. Despite the flurry of legislative and regulatory activity in recent years across Europe to ensure the quality of health care, its effects have rarely been evaluated.

In addition to the legislative approaches to improving quality, numerous regulatory and organizational tools have been introduced across Europe. Clinical practice guidelines represent one common instrument for improving quality, reducing disparities in clinical practice and improving patient safety. Most countries have such systems in place, and others are beginning to introduce guidelines, such as Austria, Cyprus, Greece, Latvia, Poland and Romania. The ability of guidelines to improve quality, however, depends on whether they lead to changes in provider behaviour. In addition to clinical guidelines, the assurance of minimum standards of competence can be incorporated into registration and licensing approaches related to the training, certification or revalidation of professionals and provider organizations. Such approaches vary across the Region: some are self regulated and others have an external regulatory body; some are voluntary and others mandatory. Nevertheless, there is a general consensus that lifelong learning and revalidation to assess fitness to practise are useful in ensuring the quality of care and safety in delivery *(18)*.

Strengthening public health, disease prevention and health promotion

European health policy-makers have increasingly recognized the important role that public health, including disease prevention, can play in improving population health. This has led to the establishment of numerous research and advisory bodies and the development of national and international strategies related to public health.

Public health has historically addressed the broader material and social conditions that affect health, such as sanitation and standards of living, which were linked closely to the control of infectious diseases and the basis for many public health interventions. Given the increases in chronic diseases, the scope of public health has widened to include more health promotion activities, in addition to efforts to reduce the prevalence of chronic diseases by targeting the known risk factors, minimizing the risk of complications and the development of additional diseases, and prolonging life among the people affected. Reform efforts have attempted to strengthen the role of public health in health systems by using upstream measures, such as alleviating poverty and improving living and working conditions in combination with downstream measures, such as health promotion and disease prevention, that often target known high-risk behaviour and lifestyle issues such as tobacco smoking and physical inactivity (19).

The integration and coordination of care efforts in the European Region have involved efforts to strengthen the role of primary care in the health system, but integrating health promotion and disease prevention activities into primary care has also been important. GPs spend much of their working time delivering primary prevention, including health advice, screening and vaccinations (20). In this way, primary health care has taken on an increasing role in cost-effective public health interventions such as systematic screening for hypertension, high serum cholesterol and a range of types of cancer and providing health advice on risks including diet, alcohol and smoking. Other health workers at the patient's first point of contact are also important. For example, in a drive to tackle obesity in Scotland in 2008, the government sent guidance to GPs, nurses, health visitors and pharmacists in the NHS on how to advise their patients to incorporate exercise into their daily routines.

The reform of the sanitary–epidemiological services in countries in the eastern part of the European Region was motivated by the lack of adequate public health services. These services had produced tangible achievements through their vaccination and communicable disease control programmes, but largely neglected promoting health and addressing the risk factors for chronic diseases (21,22). Some countries have abolished their sanitary–epidemiological services altogether and introduced new organizational settings. For example, Kazakhstan established a National Centre for Healthy Lifestyles in 1997. The Centre monitors the implementation of the national health promotion policy, develops the regulatory framework for health promotion and is responsible for cooperating with the mass media and public organizations. By 2006, this structure had moved from the national to the oblast level. In parallel, an intersectoral health promotion council has been established (23). The National Centre for Healthy Lifestyles attracted the attention of neighbouring countries, and similar services are now established in Kyrgyzstan, Tajikistan and Uzbekistan (23,24).

Investing in human and capital resources

Policy-makers in the European Region face considerable challenges in developing appropriate plans and securing adequate investment in human and capital resources. Countries need to engage in long-term planning of and investment in the health workforce, manage challenges faced by migrating health workers and invest in research and health technology assessment. The Tallinn Charter (12) explicitly took up these challenges. This section addresses the recent reforms and current challenges in these key areas of resource generation.

Investing in the health care workforce
The changing health care needs of the population and models of service delivery require a skilled and flexible workforce. Some of the main challenges facing the health care workforce in the European Region arise from the increasing pace of change in the delivery and organization of health care, such as changing patterns of disease and demographic factors, diffusion of new and sophisticated technologies, increasingly informed and demanding patients, growing demands for evidence-based medicine and the broader economic conditions (25). The health workforce itself is also changing; for example, the growing proportion of women among physicians blurs old boundaries between categories of workers. Reflecting their divergent situations, policy-makers have sought a variety of different approaches through which to

address the efficiency and effectiveness of the development and use of resources in their health systems.

Countries face different human resources challenges and needs. The current supply and distribution of health workers vary across the European Region. Shortages of staff (especially primary care physicians and higher-level nurses) in many parts of western Europe contrast with the inherited oversupply of physicians and beds in many countries in central and eastern Europe and CIS. In 2002, the European Region had an estimated 16.6 million health workers *(26)*.

Variation in supply may reflect not only different organizational arrangements for ambulatory care, such as in the patient's first point of contact with the system, but also differences in underlying demographic and economic trends. Georgia and Greece have the highest density of physicians, with almost 5 per 1000 population. Belarus, Belgium and the Russian Federation also have high density (for example, more than 4 GPs per 1000 population), with the lowest density in Albania, Bosnia and Herzegovina, Montenegro, Romania, Tajikistan, Turkey and the United Kingdom (less than 2 GPs per 1000 population). The supply of nurses also varies widely across the Region. Some countries may have shortages: Albania, Greece, Romania and Turkey have less than 4 nurses per 1000 population. Belarus, Belgium, Ireland, the Netherlands, Norway, Sweden and Uzbekistan have many more nurses (10–15 per 1000 population) *(9)*. Some countries, such as Denmark, France, Iceland, Norway and Sweden, are concerned about the ageing nursing workforce that may lead to future shortages of nurses *(26)*. Because of the long-term implications of reducing medical school admissions in many countries, alongside the coming retirement of the cohort of physicians born after 1945, countries increasingly depend on health professionals trained in other countries (see below).

Planning the proportions of general to specialist physicians and of nurses to physicians raises particular challenges. In some countries, mainly in western Europe, the proportion of physicians who are generalists appears to be declining, reflecting not only the increasing complexity of medical treatment *(27)* but also cultural and financial factors. Many countries have therefore recently stepped up measures to train and/or retrain additional primary care physicians (the United Kingdom) and/or sought to encourage more graduating medical students to take up positions in primary care (Finland and Sweden). Countries have also accelerated efforts to train more nurses (the Netherlands), to retain nurses who are thinking about leaving and to reattract those who have already left the profession.

The public health workforce has also received much attention as a result of the increased evidence on the social determinants of health and evidence of the effectiveness and cost–effectiveness of public health interventions. Countries throughout the Region are taking different approaches to strengthen the public health workforce in terms of both numbers and qualifications.

- Hungary and Kazakhstan established new schools of public health.
- Between 1989 and 1995, Germany established several postgraduate courses.
- France reconfigured its public health training as part of its public health reform in 2004.
- Estonia introduced health promotion in the curriculum of medical and nursing training and initiated public health training for civil servants and teaching staff *(28)*.
- Croatia used a modular county training programme to compensate for a lack of competencies in public health, especially health management and strategy development but also health surveillance and disease prevention *(29)*.

- Universities and public health associations from other European countries also appear to be helpful in strengthening public health training collaboration with schools of public health *(30)*.

The migration of health care personnel is a key human resource issue in the European Region, presenting both challenges to and opportunities for the performance of health systems. Since the late 1990s, international recruitment and migration of health care personnel have grown significantly. Policy-makers have sought to plug gaps by bringing in physicians and nurses from other EU countries and beyond. Further, the process of EU enlargement has enabled greater mobility, causing some concern about the emigration of health professionals, especially from the EU12 *(26)*.

International migration of health care personnel may solve shortages, improve living conditions for migrants and address the oversupply of personnel in source countries *(26,31)*. Migration poses challenges, however, both to the countries that lose their workers and to those that rely on workers from other countries (at least in terms of language and other obstacles to integrating into the new system). Through an explicit human resources planning policy, the United Kingdom relies heavily on migrant health professionals mainly from countries outside the EU, such as India and South Africa. About one third of the 71 000 NHS hospital physicians were from other countries in 2002, and more than two thirds of the 15 000 new full registrants on the United Kingdom's medical register were from outside the country in 2003 *(31)*. Poland is one of the Region's countries experiencing the most emigration, although the level here and in other countries appears to have been less than feared at the time it joined the EU *(26)*.

There has been some progress in monitoring and measuring the migration process, but the information base still needs to be developed to monitor the relative loss of staff in source countries (and loss to other forms of employment within the country) and the inflow (both numbers and sources) to destination countries to improve the planning process. The effects of health worker emigration and the various attempts to constrain it or encourage staff retention need to be evaluated, and information is needed on why shortages arise. Policy options to address the challenges of immigration and emigration include monitoring flows and developing better information bases, or actively managing the migration process. Managed migration will gain importance owing to demographic changes and continued EU enlargement, and can take the form of introducing educational and training support, developing bilateral agreements across governments and/or employers in countries and considering the possibility of arranging compensation for source countries.

Assessing health technology

Research into health policy, health services and, more specifically, the ethical and effective use of health technology is an important component of the health system's function of creating resources. Given the considerable growth in health technology in recent years, policy-makers across the European Region have turned to health technology assessment for its effective regulation, diffusion and use. Assessments of pharmaceuticals and other medical technologies have aimed to ensure that service delivery avoids inefficacious or iatrogenic interventions and that they achieve value for money. Moreover, as pharmaceuticals now account for up to 30% of total health spending *(9)*, efforts have increased across Europe to contain costs through price regulation *(32)* and to make reimbursement decisions based on evidence of cost–effectiveness.

Health technology assessment tends to consider the criteria of safety, efficacy, cost and cost–effectiveness, as well as social, organizational, legal and ethical implications. Formal health technology assessment agencies have been established in many countries; others, especially smaller countries and those outside the EU, are currently developing or considering them *(33,34)*. Most agencies responsible for health technology assessment play an advisory or regulatory role in the decision-making process *(35)*, although all can potentially bring together commitment to quality and efficiency and enhance the sustainability of the health system. Health technology assessment programmes have generally improved transparency in decision-making processes through mechanisms such as conducting independent systematic reviews, involving stakeholders and producing guidance. Nevertheless, no country has an explicitly defined and cost-effective benefit package *(36)*.

Some barriers to the more effective use of health technology assessment include resource constraints and limited technical expertise, lack of transparency in the criteria for including or excluding interventions and a lack of political will to enforce the decisions based on assessments *(34)*. The trend, however, appears to be towards greater reliance on health technology assessment to review existing and new services, which has the potential to improve value for money and transparency in the system.

Reinvigorating primary care in Europe for people-centred services

The renewal of primary health care has been advocated in recent years. Under the banner of Health for All, the 1978 Declaration of Alma-Ata *(37)* laid the foundation for a holistic view of health that went well beyond a narrow medical model. WHO renewed this commitment on the thirtieth anniversary of the Declaration in *The world health report 2008 (38)*. The report urges countries to act on evidence demonstrating that access to primary care forms the core of an efficient health care system and, more specifically, that people-centred care implies a fundamental change in service delivery *(38)*. Modern people-centred primary care is characterized as: coordinated, integrated and providing comprehensive and continuous care that is accessible to all *(4)*.

Putting people first: the meaning of people-centred care

Accessibility means that primary care is geographically and financially accessible to the whole population. It also includes the notion of organizational access that relates, for example, to dimensions such as convenient office hours, out-of-office hours, distance consultations, short waiting times and the possibility of home visits *(39)*. Continuous care means the "follow-up from one visit to the next" *(40)*. It distinguishes between informational continuity, related to the routine keeping of medical records for each patient and visit, and longitudinal continuity, meaning that primary care is provided at a specific locus over a longer time. Most significant is the issue of interpersonal continuity, defined as a continuing personal relationship between the patient and the care provider characterized by personal trust and respect *(41)*. Coordinating primary care services is important in determining the responsiveness of health services as a whole, especially because primary care is the entry point to the health system and often serves a gatekeeping function to other levels of health care. The potential for problems in managing patients is especially evident at the interface between primary and secondary care or between curative care and other (public health) services in health promotion *(42)*. Other dimensions of coordination encompass collaboration within the primary care practice and between primary care providers (such as family doctors, nurses and physical therapists).

A further characteristic of people-centred care is a comprehensive range of curative, rehabilitative and preventive services either directly provided by a primary care physician or specifically arranged elsewhere. Comprehensiveness is also linked to practice conditions, facilities and equipment and the professional skill of the primary care provider. The community orientation of primary care workers also plays a role *(43)*. Table 3.1 briefly summarizes the key elements of people-centred care compared with more conventional approaches.

Table 3.1. Aspects that distinguish conventional health care from people-centred primary care

Conventional ambulatory health care in clinics or outpatient departments	Disease control programmes	People-centred primary care
Focus on illness and cure	Focus on priority disease	Focus on health needs
Relationship limited to the moment of consultation	Relationship limited to programme implementation	Enduring personal relationship
Episodic curative care	Programme-defined disease control interventions	Comprehensive, continuous and person-centred care
Responsibility limited to effective and safe advice to the patient at the moment of consultation	Responsibility for disease-control targets among the target population	Responsibility for the health of everyone in the community along the life cycle; responsibility for tackling the determinants of ill health
Users are consumers of the care they purchase	Population groups are targets of disease-control interventions	People are partners in managing their own health and that of their community

Source: The world health report 2008. Primary health care – Now more than ever *(38)*.

Diversity of primary care in the WHO European Region

Many countries in the European Region have implemented health reforms to strengthen primary care in recent decades. The rationale and background for such reforms vary, however, and reflect the diversity of primary care in the Region.

In western Europe, primary care was expected to address rising costs and changing demands resulting from demographic and epidemiological trends, especially ageing populations and unhealthy lifestyles and the consequent increase in chronic diseases and multiple illnesses. In general, primary care reforms have focused more on adjusting existing structures than on large-scale changes in the health sector. In contrast, countries in the eastern part of the European Region, with their legacy of the Semashko model, have given priority to more comprehensive health system reform, moving away from very narrow disease-oriented specialties and a hospital-based service delivery system. Primary care reforms were thus part of an overall health sector reform programme, aimed at changing funding, the design of education and training for health professionals and the organization and delivery of primary care. Box 3.1 gives two examples.

Achieving people-centred care in the WHO European Region

Although clear progress has been made in improving health systems, patients continue to experience shortages of primary care physicians (especially in rural areas) and longer waiting times. They are also asked to contribute more money to a system that seems insufficiently responsive, spending a vast proportion of its resources on specialized

> **Box 3.1. Aims of primary care reforms in Germany and Kyrgyzstan**
>
> **Germany**
>
> In 2006, Germany attempted to strengthen the gatekeeping role of GPs, traditionally based on private practitioners operating mainly in solo practices and competing with specialists for patients. The social health insurance system offers voluntary gatekeeping contracts to the insured population. People register with a GP of their choice and agree always to see this GP first before contacting any kind of specialist. People entering into and complying with the contract save the obligatory €10 user charge per quarter.
>
> By May 2007, 5.3 million insured people, many of them older or chronically ill, had subscribed to a gatekeeper contract. Evaluation of the effects shows that 90% of the people registered with a GP did not perceive any difference in care delivery after joining the contracting model *(44)*.
>
> **Kyrgyzstan**
>
> Primary care was one of the cornerstones of the health sector reform programme that started in 1996. The main characteristics were an organizational and financial split between primary and hospital care, with newly created family group practices as the organizational locus of primary health care. In addition to nurses and midwives, family group practices were staffed by at least one physician (family doctor), and this team approach was introduced at all service delivery levels. Previously, people had been required to register with a family doctor of their choice, but each family group practice would serve up to 2000 people. The new family doctors thus act as gatekeepers to the secondary and tertiary levels.
>
> As part of a second phase of restructuring the delivery system, traditional polyclinics were merged into comprehensive polyclinics for men and women and, from 2002, polyclinics were further reorganized and renamed as family medicine centres. They now combine primary care and secondary outpatient services, ranging from general health care to specialized care and diagnostics – the aim is to gradually decrease the number of specialists working in these centres.
>
> Evaluation has shown that health care has shifted from secondary care to primary care. Increased volume and coverage of primary health services coincide with declines in referrals and unnecessary hospitalization *(45)*.

curative services rather than preventing disease and promoting health: activities that could eliminate an estimated 70% of the global burden of disease *(38)*. Rising care costs are of particular concern in the current global economic climate, increasing the risk of more people being without access to care.

Primary care physicians face challenges as well, such as too many, often older, patients with increasingly complex chronic comorbidity that would need more time for consultation, a growing administrative burden, inability to remain up to date with new clinical innovations and in general too little time to do a good job *(46)*. This applies across the Region. For instance, a recent study in Kyrgyzstan showed that excessive reporting requirements adversely affect the quality of care by limiting the time available for patients. During an average working day, family doctors spend only 34% of the time available on direct patient care and the rest on documentation and reporting *(47)*.

Aspects of practice organization that can explain the level of organizational access vary considerably between countries. Table 3.2 shows that GPs in Finland and Sweden can dedicate more time to their patients than their colleagues in the Netherlands and the United Kingdom. Nevertheless, waiting times between the appointment and the actual consultation appear to be higher in Finland and Sweden. GP workload is another aspect that affects organizational access and patient satisfaction, and is measured here as the average number of office consultations, telephone contacts and home visits. This varies considerably between countries, with GPs in Germany and Hungary working more than 10 hours per day.

High workload in some countries might also indicate shortages or a declining workforce in primary care. For instance, in Germany the number of GPs within the overall physician workforce declined by more than 10% from 1990 to 2007, while the number of primary care physicians remained more or less constant and at a high level in France (Fig. 3.1). Finland, a frontrunner in Europe for a strong primary care system, lost 25% of its primary care

Table 3.2. Aspects of workload and practice organization in primary care in selected countries

Country	Average inhabitants per GP (list size)[a]	Number of patients treated			Average length of patient consultation (minutes)	GPs with waiting time ≥ 2 days (%)[b]
		Office consultations (per day)	Telephone contacts (per day)	Home visits (per week)		
Croatia	2010	44	6	6	12	11
Finland	1582	19	6	3	18	80
France	943	16	7	27	20	12
Germany	2110	50	11	34	13	25
Hungary	1975	48	7	27	15	0
Lithuania	NA	17	3	15	17	0
Netherlands	2310	32	12	21	10	6
Slovenia	NA	42	8	7	13	18
Spain	1970	39	4	9	10	23
Sweden	2870	16	7	2	24	91
United Kingdom	1892	34	6	19	8	31

[a] Data are from 1993.
[b] GP-reported days between appointment and consultation for non-acute problems.
NA: not available.
Source: adapted from Boerma (43).

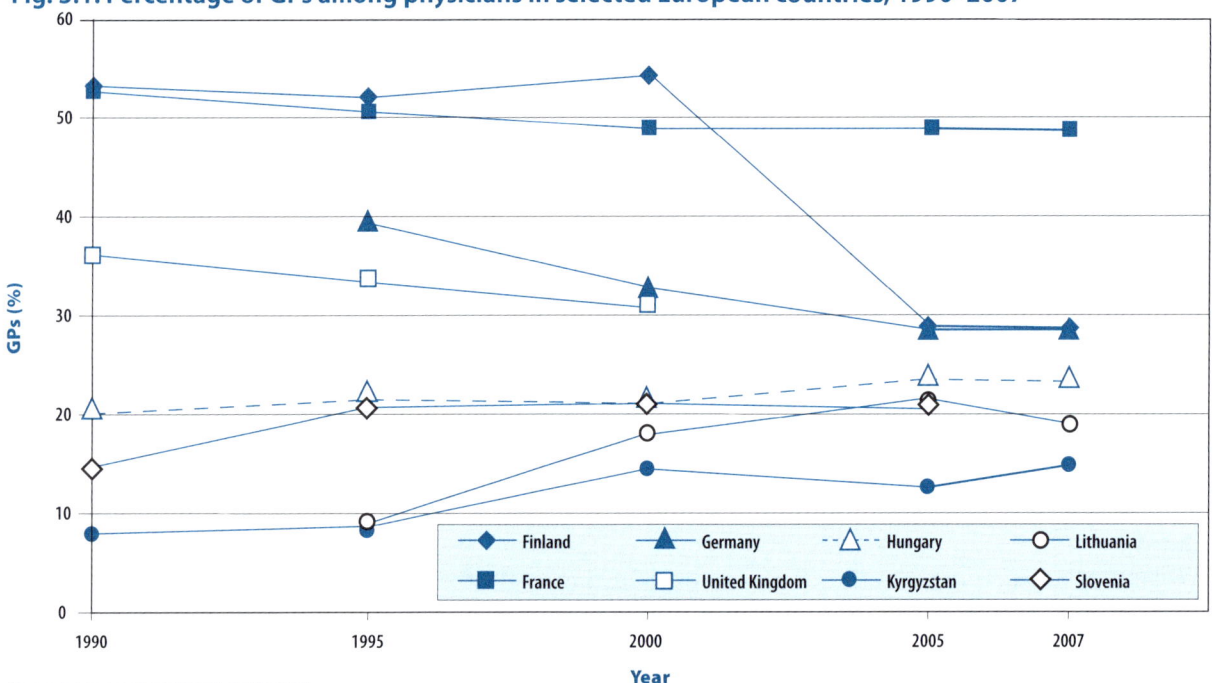

Fig. 3.1. Percentage of GPs among physicians in selected European countries, 1990–2007

Source: European Health for All database (9).

physicians between 2000 and 2005. This has been attributed to: physicians complaining about a loss of control and influence over their own work, less professional incentives in terms of support from colleagues, the sharing of on-call duties and limited opportunity for research and continuing education compared with specialists working in hospitals (48). The level of remuneration, which is relatively low compared with the Netherlands and the United Kingdom, has also contributed to opposition to primary care among GPs in Finland (49).

In central and eastern Europe and central Asia, the picture of the primary care workforce clearly differs from that in western Europe, with a much lower baseline. Nevertheless, the challenge in establishing a more people-centred system is essentially the same: human resources in primary care remain scarce. Countries such as Kyrgyzstan, Lithuania and Slovenia have increased the number of physicians working in primary care since 1990, but the percentage of 12–20% is still relatively low compared with physicians working in other sectors (Fig. 3.1). In addition, countries such as Croatia and Slovenia are struggling with the fact that many of their GPs have retired or will retire soon, and the new generation is not yet ready to replace the old one *(50)*.

Although such information on shortages in the primary care workforce is easy to find, dimensions such as coordination and integration are less demonstrable. There are no firm indicators or data, and they differ from country to country. Primary care is not a closed and controllable environment, such as a hospital, so sometimes only proxy indicators based on surveys can give some indications of existing barriers.

Turkey has embarked on large-scale reform of family medicine in primary care. A study of its effects in two provinces (Table 3.3) revealed, for example, that not all family doctors routinely kept medical records for each patient visit, a prerequisite for informational continuity. Since 2005, however, routine clinical records have been kept for all patient visits and, since May 2009, all records have been transferred to the Ministry of Health electronically. Most family doctors also had difficulty in generating a list of patients by diagnosis or health risk, which would be required to analyse the practice population and organize coherent treatment plans for individuals or groups in this population. Such data must be compiled for coordinated and integrated care. Although weaknesses in the coordination and interface between primary, secondary and tertiary care are quite common in a transitional process – Turkey is just one example – patients seem to value governments' efforts to bring services closer to them. About 95% of the patients sampled in the two provinces in Turkey declared that they were "satisfied with how my family doctor treats me" *(51)*.

Table 3.3. Availability and use of clinical information considered prerequisites for continuity and integrated care based on self-reported information from family doctors in two provinces in Turkey

Items	Bolu (N = 37)		Eskişehir (N = 41)	
	N	%	N	%
Keeping patients' medical records				
Routinely	13	35	20	49
With some reservation	24	65	21	51
Generating a list of patients by diagnosis or health risk				
Easy	10	28	11	27
Somewhat difficult	14	39	14	34
Very difficult or impossible	12	33	16	39
Using referral letters for all or most referred patients	20	56	5	12
Receiving information from medical specialist after treatment				
Usually	1	3	1	2
In a minority of cases	8	22	5	12
Seldom or never	28	75	35	86
Receiving discharge report after hospitalization				
Within 30 days	3	8	4	10
Seldom or never	30	81	30	73

Source: Kringos et al. *(51)*.

Overcoming challenges to people-centred care: European examples

Pursuing people-centred care is a major challenge, and countries across the European Region continue to struggle to achieve it. This ultimately requires a paradigm shift; rather than spending all day in traditional 10–15-minute patient visits, primary care physicians and teams would analyse the health needs of their registered population and manage them accordingly, either with individual case strategies or in groups according to health risks *(46)*. Country strategies and options to achieve this appear to follow two main trends:

- experimenting with new provider qualifications and practice organizations; or
- implementing integrated care schemes along with disease management programmes.

Transforming practice and provider qualifications

Given the restrictions on human resources outlined above, solutions for more people-centred primary care are limited. One option is gradually to transform practice settings and organizations and to introduce new provider qualifications based primarily on teamwork and networking. Some countries have changed the roles of and introduced new qualifications for nurses and other health care staff to manage select tasks that primary care physicians would otherwise carry out. For example, nurse practitioners have been established in the Netherlands and the United Kingdom. These university-trained professionals carry out regular nursing duties but also assume traditional physicians' tasks such as prescribing drugs and giving uncomplicated treatment. Germany has recently created community nurses who, while executing tasks similar to those of nurse practitioners, focus on providing home care for chronically ill people in rural areas *(52)*. Similarly, the primary care trusts in the United Kingdom have started to employ case managers to coordinate services for people with long-term conditions or with complex social and health needs. The managers' tasks include analysing the registry to assess people's needs, developing care plans and organizing services accordingly and monitoring the quality of care. In addition, England changed the roles of pharmacists by enabling them to provide repeat prescriptions, review medication and provide smoking-cessation services *(53)*.

In 2003, the region of Castilla y León, Spain embarked on a programme to improve efficiency in providing care for people that have both social and health needs, such as those with chronic diseases. The authorities quickly realized that shifting tasks from physicians to nurses and other new social care providers would imply a new role for GPs. Physicians would thus be trained to become team leaders, spending more time coordinating the health and social care teams and seeing many fewer patients, mostly those with serious conditions *(54)*.

Chronic disease management and integrated care

As the emergence of new provider profiles and flexible practice models suggests, multidisciplinary cooperation between and beyond levels of care is needed, with the primary care team functioning as a coordination hub (Fig. 3.2).

Moreover, the organizational changes reflect and follow epidemiological trends. The increased prevalence of chronic diseases and multiple illnesses has persuaded several health systems that already have strong primary care settings to experiment with care models related to certain conditions such as diabetes, cardiovascular diseases and cancer. This in turn empowers primary care as a hub for coordination. The countries involved include Denmark, France, Ireland, Italy and the United Kingdom *(11)*. A commonly cited example is the disease management programmes introduced in Germany in 2002 for diabetes types 1 and 2, asthma and chronic obstructive pulmonary disease, ischaemic heart disease and breast cancer. By

Fig. 3.2. Primary care as a hub of coordination

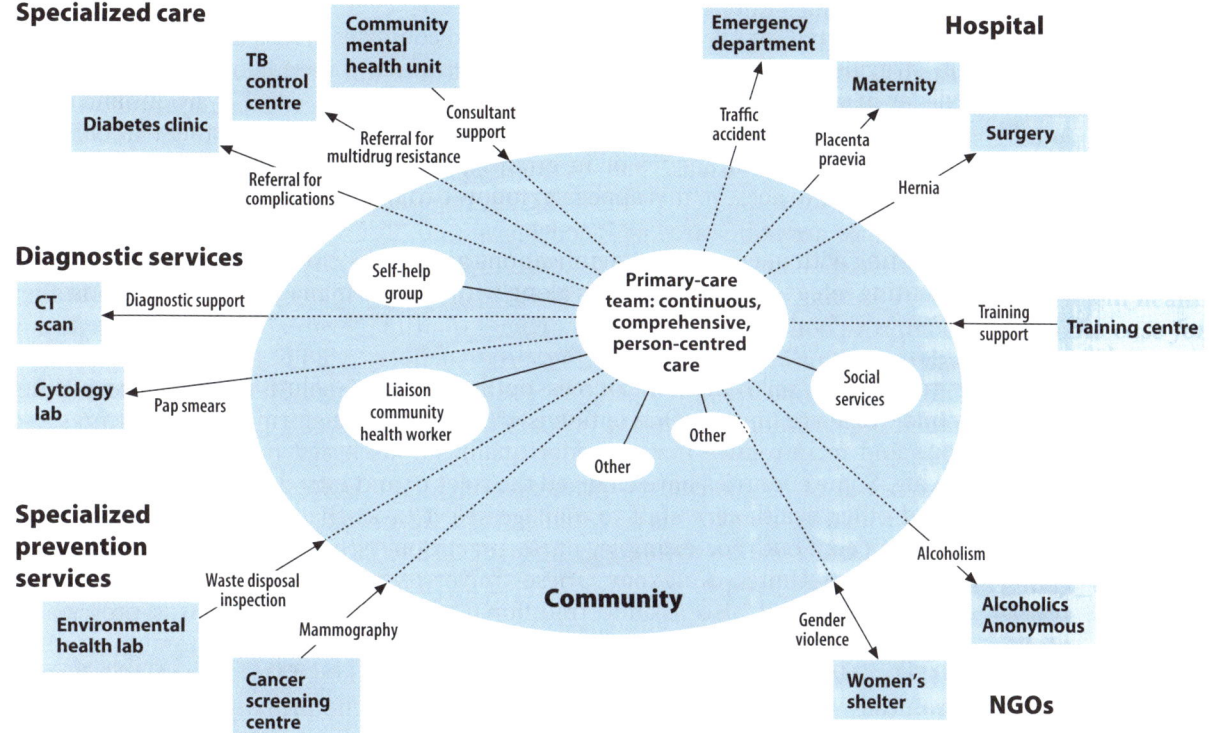

Source: The world health report 2008. Primary health care – Now more than ever (38).

2008, more than 4.7 million patients were enrolled in these programmes, many with GPs who had received specialized training in these conditions (55). In 2000, Zwisler, Schou & Sørensen (56) reported the launch of a clinical trial in Denmark for people with ischaemic heart disease, with the option for patients to receive integrated rehabilitative care in an ambulatory setting. Multidisciplinary and specifically trained staff teams were set up with a core team comprising a cardiologist, a nurse, a physical therapist, a dietitian and a secretary, and a peripheral team including a social worker and a psychiatrist. After the trial was evaluated in 2003, recommendations for the follow-up phase included adding a psychologist and a priest to the peripheral team (56).

Other countries have experimented with more comprehensive integrated care models or provider networks that focus on chronic conditions in a broader sense. An example with considerable impact on how primary care is perceived and developed is the concept of transmural care in the Netherlands from the early 1990s. The aim was to improve the quality of care for patients who could not return to a fully independent life by managing the interface between acute hospital care and primary care with a link to social care (57).

Implications for the future

Several important issues require attention before people-centred primary care can be fully renewed in the European Region. First, the investment in human resources required for primary care, including education and appropriate training, needs to be understood more clearly. Changing traditional roles and, for instance, increasing the tasks undertaken by nurses requires rethinking payment schemes or even designing alternative schemes around team-based remuneration.

Second, strategies need to be developed to manage the shift towards new multidisciplinary teams and networks, including involving the social sector.

Third, research is required into what works and what does not work. For example, findings on the effectiveness of new provider qualifications and practice settings are limited. Pilot studies suggest that nurses with wider roles seem to improve chronic care. Similarly, although some small-scale studies of disease management and integrated care programmes suggest that patients benefit from the new process of care, population-based evaluations and cost–effectiveness studies are still scarce or inconclusive *(57)*. Countries in transition towards a primary care orientation need to be able to monitor whether the distinctive features of people-centred care are gaining prominence in the practice of their primary care system before they can start to improve both the process and outcomes of primary care. Without this, assessing whether system reforms are actually changing service delivery will not be possible. The WHO Regional Office for Europe has developed a tool to support Member States in monitoring and evaluating their organizational models in primary care *(51)*.

Indeed, the renewal of people-centred primary care in the European Region needs to be complemented with a more vigorous research agenda. Revealingly, a Cochrane review could only find one valid study on how to integrate primary care services in low- and middle-income countries from the user's perspective *(38,58)*.

Sustaining performance through health financing policy

Reforms of the financing of health care have varied across the European Region according to countries' institutional, cultural, economic and political settings *(59)*. Most countries have upheld the broad values outlined in the Ljubljana Charter on Reforming Health Care *(2)*; some recent reforms have sought to improve equity, reduce financial barriers and ensure universal coverage. Reform has also focused on efforts to sustain the attainment of these objectives in the context of rising costs through a variety of means, including increasing the priority given to health in the allocation of public resources, diversifying and blending sources, and changing the flow of funds and pooling arrangements and exploring methods of purchasing care to improve efficiency. (Here, purchasing means the transfer of pooled resources from an agency – such as private or public insurance funds, local or national government agencies or other public organizations – to providers.)

A previous section has already examined universal coverage and the distribution of financial protection. This section focuses more specifically on the methods of financing health care and reforms used by countries in their efforts to sustain their performance on these objectives.

Reallocating public funds to health despite tighter fiscal constraints

Most governments in the Region have increased their commitment to funding health despite growing fiscal constraints over the past decade, although countries vary. Public spending on health as a share of GDP grew in most countries (Fig. 3.3). Given that most European countries also imposed tighter fiscal limits during this period (that is, tending to reduce total government spending as a share of GDP), this reflects decisions by most countries to increase the priority given to health in overall public spending. The data summarized in

Fig. 3.3. Public spending on health as a percentage of GDP, WHO European Region, 1997 and 2006

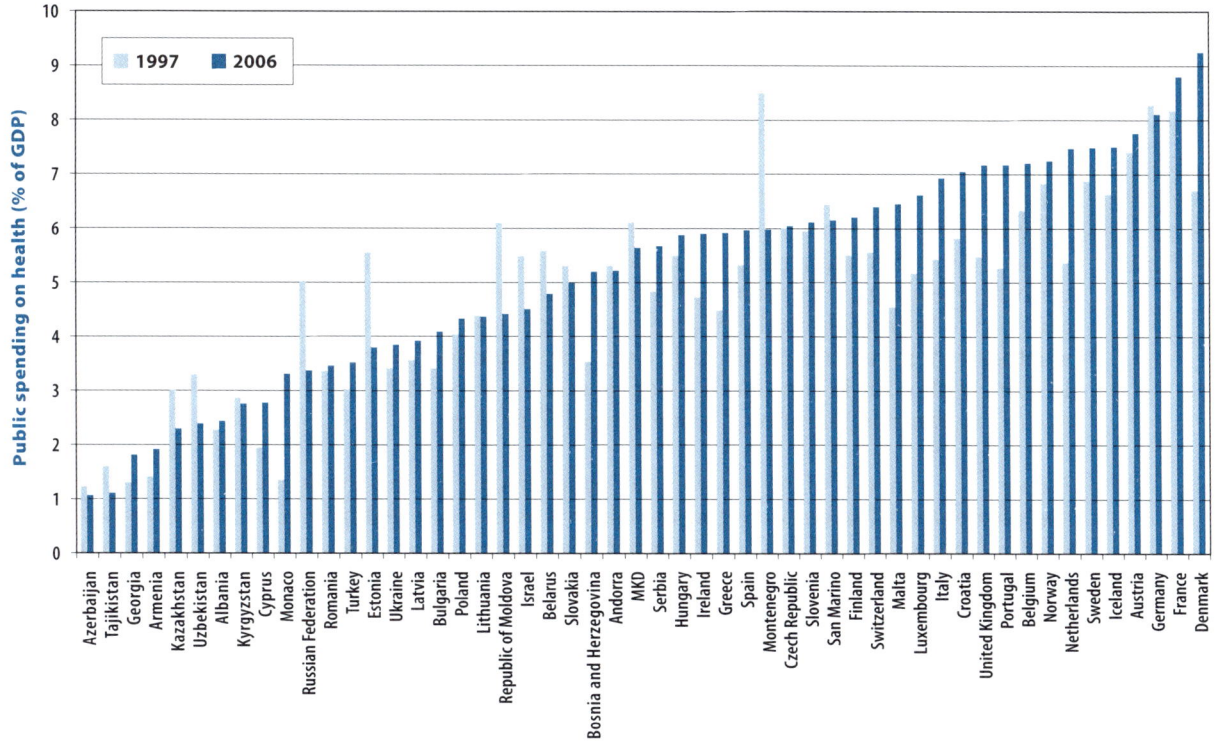

Note. MKD is the International Organization for Standardization (ISO) abbreviation for the former Yugoslav Republic of Macedonia. No data were available for Turkmenistan.
Source: European Health for All database (9).

Fig. 3.4 confirm this. Hence, one approach countries have used to sustain their performance is simply to increase the relative priority given to health in their decisions on allocating public resources.

The figures reveal important variation within the Region, however. In particular, although 24 of the 27 EU countries increased the share of health in total public spending during this period, 8 of 11 CIS countries (no data were available for Turkmenistan) experienced a decrease. The other countries present a mixed picture. Hence, while the overall pattern suggests a strong commitment to sustaining health system goals through increased spending, this was particularly true of EU countries. The pattern in many CIS countries leaves cause for concern about why their priorities are shifting away from health, especially since it already received a relatively low share of the budgets in most of these countries.

Beyond expenditure, the Member States in the WHO European Region broadly agree that they need to monitor and modify funding and pooling arrangements to ensure that they can maintain or increase their commitment to solidarity across different social and generational groups, even as they struggle to maintain or achieve financial balance and sustainability during the next decades. Some lessons therefore arise from the experience of health financing reforms in recent years. In particular, the health financing system has become fragmented in some countries and methods of purchasing services are often not aligned with efficiency and quality objectives; countries use various policy responses to tackle these problems.

Fig. 3.4. Percentage of total government spending devoted to health, WHO European Region, 1997 and 2006

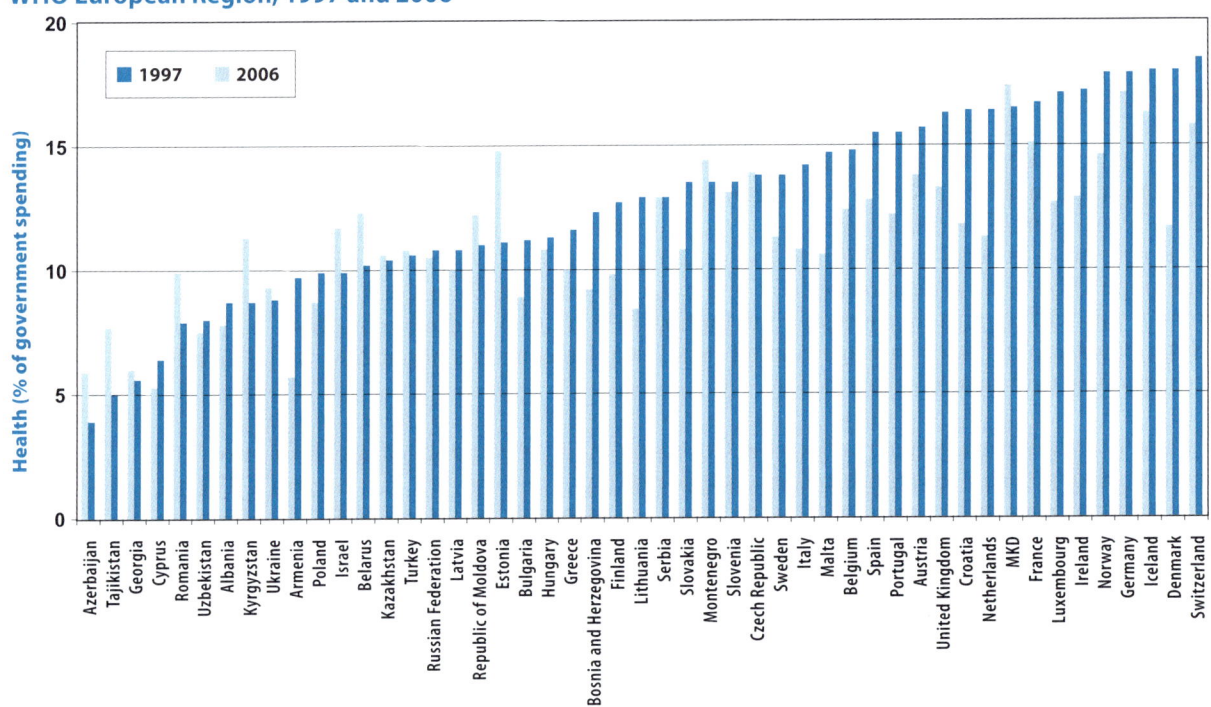

Note. MKD is the International Organization for Standardization (ISO) abbreviation for the former Yugoslav Republic of Macedonia. No data were available for Andorra, Monaco, San Marino and Turkmenistan.
Source: European Health for All database (9).

Diversification of sources and new combinations of revenue collection and pooling arrangements

In response to a combination of rising cost pressures and limitations on the scope for raising general and especially payroll tax rates, increasing numbers of countries have diversified their sources of public funding while ensuring or improving the coherence of their pooling arrangements. Policy-makers in the Czech Republic, France, Germany, the Netherlands and Switzerland have faced considerable pressure to expand the revenue base to incorporate broader sources of taxation.

Many countries in the eastern part of the European Region face similar challenges as they manage the recent shift from general tax revenue and universal population-based entitlement to dedicated (usually payroll) tax funding and contribution-based entitlement. There are important differences in motivation and historical experience between the CIS countries, the countries that emerged from the former Yugoslavia and the other central European and Baltic countries. Most of the third group introduced social health insurance arrangements that marked, at least in form, a return to the systems in place in the pre-Communist era. The difficulty insurance funds face in collecting contributions has led to shifting the collection responsibility to the central government tax agencies in Estonia, Hungary and Romania. Except for Bosnia and Herzegovina, the countries emerging from the former Yugoslavia switched to centralized single insurance funds in the early 1990s. Only five of the CIS countries, however, have introduced some form of compulsory health insurance: Georgia, Kazakhstan, Kyrgyzstan, the Republic of Moldova and the Russian Federation, although Georgia and Kazakhstan discontinued it (60).

The recent reforms in Germany reflect a response to the challenge facing many countries relying predominantly on payroll taxes for compulsory health insurance: their ability to sustain near-universal coverage and high levels of financial protection in the future without harmful effects on the labour market. Until 2009, about 90% of sickness fund revenue in Germany came from payroll contributions, which have risen significantly in recent years. At the current level of benefits, and maintaining the relative share of payroll and general revenues, average contribution rates would have to rise to 22–25% by 2025 and 26–30% by 2030 to keep the system in financial balance while maintaining the current level of benefits *(61)*. In response, the Government of Germany began in 2009 to moderate the growth of contribution rates by injecting more general revenue into the system *(62)*. In the Czech Republic, nearly 30% of the population will be over retirement age by 2030 versus 20% in 2003. If no changes are made, this will require the current contribution rate (13.5%) to double by about 2030 *(63)*. Such potential increases in wage-related taxation raise concerns about how they will affect employment and economic growth.

In a very different economic context, the Government of the Republic of Moldova introduced a compulsory health insurance reform, supported by a new payroll tax, in 2004. The aim was to transform the fragmented pooling structure inherited from the USSR, create a strong purchasing agency to inject new incentives into the system and increase the level of public funding for health care. Given the reality that a large share of the labour force is in the informal sector, however, it was recognized that the payroll tax alone would be insufficient to fund the desired level of benefits for the population. Part of the reform therefore included channelling general budget revenue to the new Health Insurance Fund to provide coverage for defined non-contributing population groups. The result was an unusual combination of funding sources for compulsory health insurance: about two thirds of the money managed by the Fund came from transfers from general revenue and only about one third from the payroll tax *(64)*.

Mitigating the effects of fragmentation in countries with multiple competing insurers: balancing insurance competition with solidarity

Some countries in the Region use compulsory health insurance, managed through competing insurers: Belgium, the Czech Republic, Germany, Israel, the Netherlands, the Russian Federation, Slovakia, Switzerland and, most recently, Georgia. By explicitly fragmenting available prepaid funds for health insurance, such competition potentially threatens solidarity and the extent of risk protection that can be offered from a given level of funding. Nearly all the countries that have done this have introduced measures to mitigate these potential effects. In the Czech Republic, for example, managing competition between insurers has limited their incentives to select or discriminate in enrolling individuals. A risk-equalization mechanism introduced initially in 1994 was greatly improved under a 2003 law and implemented over the next three years. This has had some success, effectively creating a virtual national pool by subjecting all prepaid funds to risk adjustment instead of the partial risk adjustment done previously. An important aim of this reform was to improve the efficiency of the health system by changing the focus of insurers' efforts from competing on pooling (by investing in efforts to attract people with the highest probability of a positive margin between revenue and expenditure) to competing on improving the purchasing of health services. Whereas an insurer previously profited by selecting rich, young or healthy clients, the new approach reduces the potential benefit of such selection. Because the reformed system better matches each insurer's income and its policy-holders' risk structure, insurers have stronger incentives to compete based on improved cost management and the overall quality of their services. Although improved purchasing practices have not yet materialized, a sufficient level of risk compensation is necessary to minimize strategic pooling behaviour by insurers *(60)*.

Incomplete reforms in health financing may create greater fragmentation in how funds flow to facilities; this in turn may create conflicting incentives and counteract the integrated delivery of care. In the Russian Federation, introducing mandatory health insurance has led to the creation of larger risk pools that increase the potential for enhanced solidarity. The allocation of these funds down the system via competing insurers, however, often accompanies rather than replaces the direct transfer of local government budgets to health facilities, which continues in many territories. The reform is therefore incomplete, and substantial fragmentation remains *(60)*.

Achieving the solidarity-based health system goals of sharing financial risks when the starting-point is a system of competing insurers, such as in both the Czech Republic and the Russian Federation, requires measures to increase the scope of risk pooling (which enhances the potential for greater solidarity within the health system) and to compensate insurers for the different risk profiles of members (to make risk selection unprofitable). The intent should be to divert the competitive energy of insurers towards administrative efficiency and the purchasing of health services, although considerable work is needed to define the areas in which competition delivers real benefits.

Promoting solidarity by centralizing financing

Although decentralization can be useful in achieving certain functions and objectives in health systems, a decentralized structure of pooling and allocating funds limits the scope for redistributing resources. Norway has moved to recentralize its system in recent years, allocating resources to 4 regional health authorities instead of 19 counties. The redistributional aspects of the reforms in Norway have faced substantial political challenges and, as a result, the reforms have not been fully achieved, but efficiency and productivity have improved somewhat *(65)*.

Kyrgyzstan (starting in 2001) and the Republic of Moldova (in 2004) replaced the decentralized budgetary system inherited from the USSR with a centralized system of pooling. Kyrgyzstan implemented this gradually over five years, while the Republic of Moldova did it in one year. In both cases, the main source of funds was general budget revenue, and the pooling reforms either combined this with payroll tax revenue or used it in an explicitly complementary manner in the new national health insurance fund. The centralization of pooling was combined with a shift to output- and capitation-based allocation to providers and greater managerial autonomy for providers. The reforms in each country led to a more equal distribution of government health spending across regions, a reduction in the burden of out-of-pocket spending and greater efficiency in provider operations, although substantial progress can still be made on all fronts *(66)*.

In Kyrgyzstan, after the rayon (district) pools were progressively consolidated to oblast (provincial) pools during the period 2001–2005, pooling was centralized to the national level in 2006. The impact of this was immediate, as shown in Fig. 3.5, which depicts government health spending per head by oblast in 2005 and in 2006 relative to Bishkek (the capital). The funding gap between Bishkek and other oblasts declined in all cases except one. In Naryn oblast, one of the poorest and geographically most challenging due to its mountainous terrain, per capita expenditure exceeded that of Bishkek. A single set of financing standards formed the basis for the allocation of funds across regions, and they were adjusted through new coefficients to account for the differences in the geographical and demographic characteristics of each region in an attempt to reflect differences in relative need and the cost of delivering services.

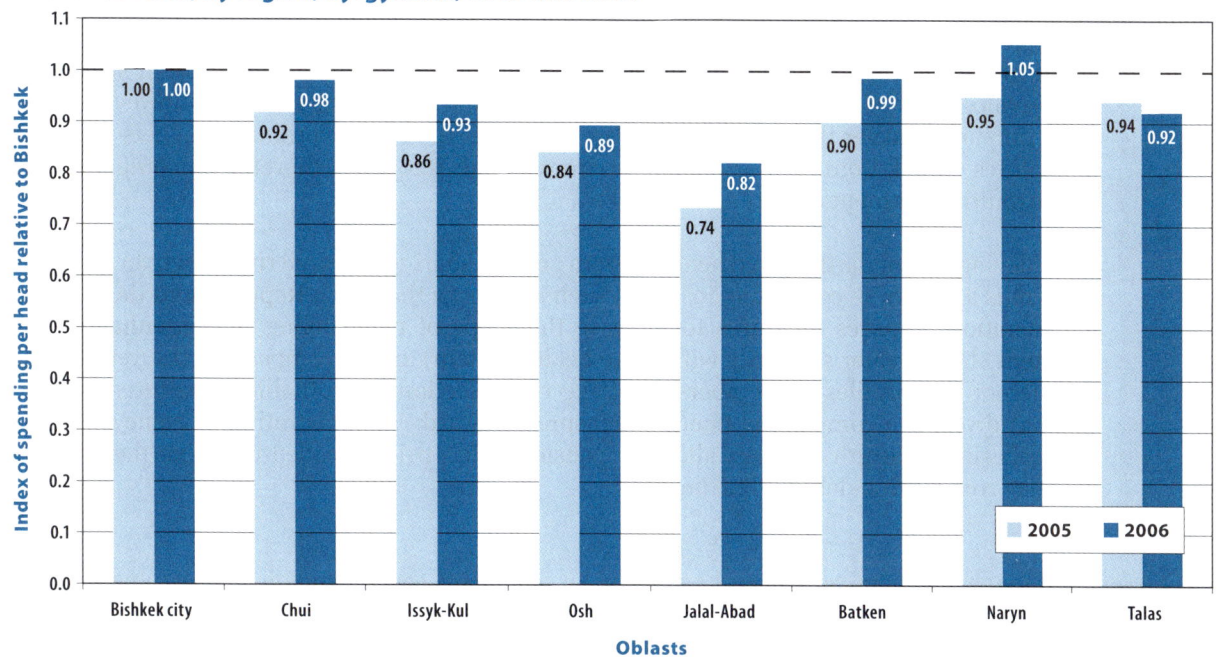

Fig. 3.5. Relative spending per head on the state benefit package (Mandatory Health Insurance Fund) by region, Kyrgyzstan, 2005 and 2006

Source: Financial management reports on execution of the state guaranteed benefit package and 2007 Ministry of Health performance indicator report (67).

Similarly, in the Republic of Moldova, the centralization of pooling from the rayon level in 2003 to the national level in 2004 was associated with improved equality in the distribution of public spending on health. Fig. 3.6 demonstrates that the variation in spending across rayons was greatly reduced in 2004 compared with 2003. The data for 2003 reflect local budget spending per head for each rayon, whereas for 2004 the data show spending per head by rayon by the Mandatory Health Insurance Fund.

Strategic purchasing of health care: resources allocated to providers linked with performance information or population needs

During the past decade, how to strengthen the purchasing of health care services to improve performance has attracted increasing attention. Many countries began to introduce some form of strategic purchasing model from the early 1990s. Purchasing strategically implies using methods that link the allocation of resources to information on, for example, the performance of providers or the needs of the population they serve. In contrast, passive purchasing typically takes the form of input-based or historical budgeting or untargeted fee-for-service reimbursement.

Health systems based on a vertically integrated model in which the national or regional government funds and delivers services have made many reforms to split the purchasing and providing functions and give purchasers a lever to improve provider performance. Following the internal market reform in the NHS in the United Kingdom – introduced in 1991 and then consolidated into regionally defined purchasers as primary care trusts in 2000 –, Italy, Portugal and some regions in Spain and Sweden also introduced purchaser–provider splits.

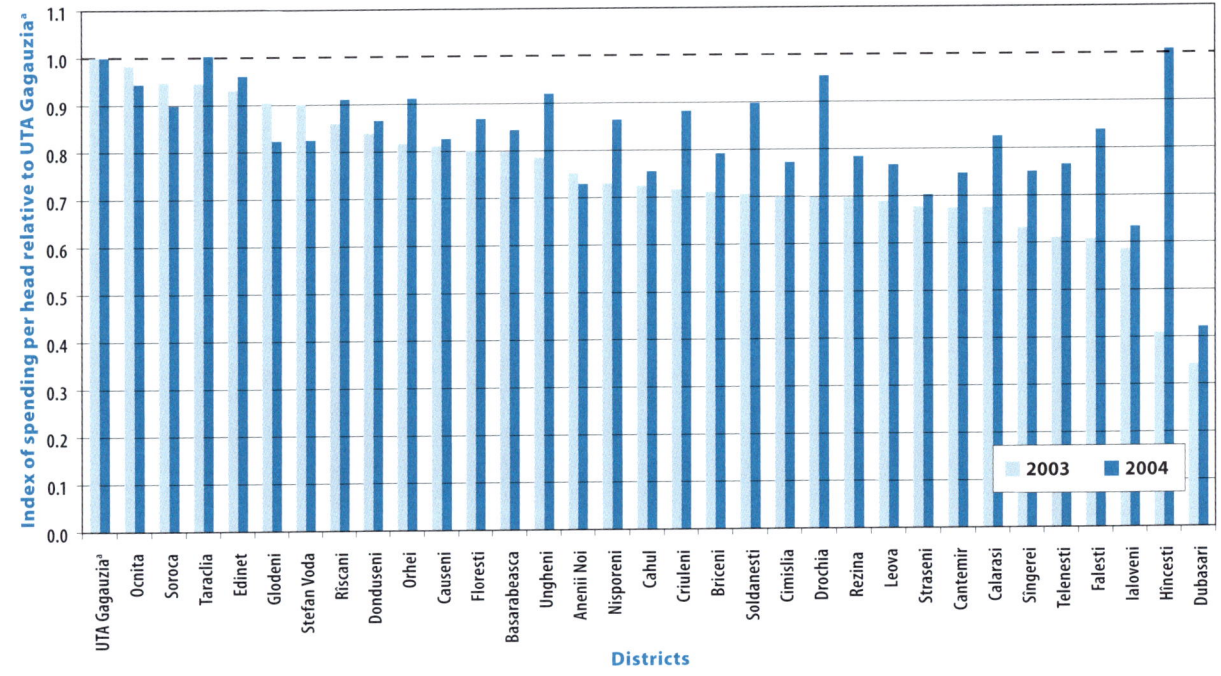

Fig. 3.6. Health spending per head in districts of the Republic of Moldova, 2003 and 2004

a Autonomous Territorial Unit of Gagauzia.
Source: Shishkin, Kacevicius, Ciocanu (64).

Many mechanisms are available, beginning with health needs assessment and the use of contracts, which may include quality monitoring and performance-based payment systems. In these contexts, methods of adjusting risk are used to ensure that the resources flowing to the purchasers match health care needs, which can enhance equity of access and allocative efficiency.

In some countries with a historical split between purchasing and providing functions and insurance funds making contracts with providers, policy-makers have sought to create or extend competition between funds managing compulsory social insurance revenue (including non-profit-making and profit-making insurers), partly to create incentives for strengthened purchasing to achieve efficiency and quality gains. Other reasons for introducing or expanding patient choice of insurer have been to improve responsiveness to consumers and to reduce variation in contributions. As noted above, this strategy faces challenges, especially the scope for risk selection, and the many constraints that limit competition among funds. Many of the measures taken to limit the effects of risk selection – such as nationally defined benefit packages, fee schedules and contribution rates – also limit the scope for insurers to innovate with new purchasing methods. Nevertheless, efforts have recently been made to facilitate competition by permitting selective contracting by insurers to leverage efficiency and quality improvements by providers. One positive development has been in Germany, where some aspects of strategic purchasing were integrated into the risk adjustment formula. In particular, the formula gives a financial incentive to insurers to enrol people with disabilities into disease management programmes (68).

Paying hospitals

An increasing number of countries have experimented with mechanisms to improve the efficiency and transparency of hospital services. Most European health systems pay hospitals through global budgets, although case-based payments (often called diagnosis-related groups) are increasingly being introduced to define the budgets or as a form of payment. Although hard budgets have the potential to contain costs, case-based payments bring incentives to increase both activity and transparency in typically opaque hospital accounting systems. The specific goals of introducing case-based payments in hospital care vary across countries, with some aiming to increase activity and reduce waiting times and others seeking to control costs and improve transparency in financing. All, however, broadly aim to create incentives for greater provider efficiency. Hospital case-based payment systems vary in design. For instance, the broader diagnosis–treatment combination in the Netherlands includes payment for both specialist physicians and hospitals in one package. Such an approach inevitably risks premature discharge along with increasing readmission rates, so careful monitoring is required *(69)*.

Overall, such case-based payments have been demonstrated to increase hospital activity, generate information on hospital costs and case mix, and encourage cost control per diagnosis. Although the incentives associated with case-based payments give rise to such advantages, they also have a disadvantage that can potentially undermine the gains: they encourage hospitals to select less costly cases within a category (cream skimming) and shift more expensive cases to other hospitals, overreport the complexity of cases (upcoding) and skimp on the quality (or more accurately, the quantity) of care provided per case *(70)*.

Paying physicians

Across the European Region, the main approaches for paying providers are salary, capitation and fees for services. In the public sector, most primary and outpatient care physicians are paid by salary or capitation or a combination. In primary care, capitation is the predominant form of payment in many countries, such as Croatia, England, Estonia, Hungary, Italy, Kazakhstan, Kyrgyzstan, Lithuania, the Netherlands, Poland, Romania and Slovakia. Fee-for-service payments prevail in Austria, Belgium, France, Germany (within an overall budget cap), Luxembourg and Switzerland. This method of payment is also the norm for privately delivered primary and outpatient care. For hospital physicians, however, salary payment is the most common method, except in Belgium and Switzerland. Fee-for-service systems have an incentive to increase activity, while salary and capitation methods may control costs but provide incentives to decrease activity and shift patients' costs onto other providers. Several studies have found evidence for the effects of payment method on physician behaviour *(71,72)*, and countries are increasingly experimenting with mixed payment schemes, which include elements of the different methods to maximize positive incentives and moderate negative ones *(69)*.

Some countries, especially in central and eastern Europe, have moved away from paying salaries to primary care providers towards paying fees for services or capitation. Other countries, such as those in western Europe, have extended targeted fee-for-service payments in addition to capitation, to increase preventive care and reward good performance. Purchasing mechanisms may be able to offset the effects of perverse incentives by carefully linking funds to compliance with quality indicators. Provider contracts in a few countries are being tied to quality indicators, which may include meeting accreditation standards, following quality assurance procedures or achieving quality and outcome targets. Similarly, some countries are moving towards performance-based payment systems for professionals with explicit financial incentives to reward certain behaviour and outcomes. The recent contract and payment reform for GPs in the United Kingdom rewards those achieving certain quality targets, but also has problems, similar to all types of performance-related pay. Most GPs already met the targets *(73)*, so that the budget was exceeded, leading to subsequent failure to increase fees with inflation and resulting low morale.

Although financial incentives are necessary, they are not sufficient to improve quality in service delivery, and work needs to be closely coordinated with initiatives in service delivery and stewardship.

Conclusion

Despite large and growing differences in the context within which health systems are developing across the European Region, all countries need to address the challenge posed by fragmentation in financial arrangements and need to move to align provider incentives with the objectives of health financing policy. These needs are heightened at times of economic recession, when fiscal constraints are likely to be very tight, thus constraining the capacity of governments to continue the past decade's trend towards increasing public spending on health. One clear message from countries' reform experience in recent years is that a focus on policy objectives, not on implementing particular mechanisms, should drive health financing policy. Basing policy choices on distinctions between broad health financing models such as Bismarck and Beveridge is not useful, as these have lost their relevance. What matters are the details: what is the source of funds, how they are collected, how funds are pooled, how services are purchased and how a population's entitlements and obligations are specified. Financing policy should aim to sustain good health system performance, orienting the system in accordance with the underlying values of equity, solidarity and participation while managing resources in a fiscally responsible manner (74).

Exercising stewardship for healthy public policies

As noted in Part 2, overall health status in the WHO European Region has improved during the past 15 years. Nevertheless, this improvement coexists with serious concerns, such as the high prevalence of noncommunicable diseases in most countries, inequality in access to health services and health outcomes between and within countries, a mismatch between health status, human resources and the health needs of the population and rising expenditure on health care. In some countries, these concerns have persisted despite decades of efforts to reform the health system. More recently, the global economic downturn – which comes at a time when governments are already struggling with major energy and environmental problems – threatens to exacerbate existing social and health inequalities and inequities. The current climate is triggering significant changes in social norms, lifestyles and health-related behaviour and is likely to have numerous and long-lasting effects on health systems.

In this context, pressure is growing on governments to do something tangible and, specifically, to improve the performance, efficiency and sustainability of health systems. With the mass media and public advocating more transparency and accountability, the stewardship function of health ministries and governments has received increased attention (see the section below on assessing health system performance for accountability). Health ministries in particular are being urged to exercise their diverse stewardship roles to ensure that governments implement healthy public policies to obtain better health outcomes, with envisaged consequent positive effects on the economy. Overall, ascertaining the relative influence of factors affecting the performance of the health system and determining the best ways to exercise effective stewardship seem to be important prerequisites for improving health outcomes.

Stewardship and health systems

Health system stewardship is one of health systems' four functions outlined in *The world health report 2000 (75)* as a way of conceptualizing and understanding health system governance. In contrast to managing or operating the system directly, government guides it. Government sets goals and objectives and the rules under which they are to be attained. This involves formulating strategic policy directions, ensuring good regulation and appropriate tools for implementing it, and fostering the necessary intelligence on the health system's performance to ensure accountability and transparency *(76)*. Thus, stewardship can also bring together the other three functions to generate the desired health system structure and overall performance.

The configuration of health system stewardship varies depending on the economic, political and social context and on the core values of countries' cultures. For example, the role of the private sector in delivering health services and the degree of decentralization to decision-making authorities at the subnational level vary depending on a country's circumstances, culture and history. Nevertheless, the Member States of the European Region have endorsed some specific roles of health system stewardship *(77)*:

- defining the vision for health and the strategy to achieve it;
- applying intelligence when defining the vision and evaluating outcomes;
- governing the health system in a way that is values based, ethical and conducive to the attainment of its goals;
- mobilizing the legal and regulatory powers of the health system to attain its goals;
- ensuring that the health system is designed so that it can adapt to changing needs; and
- exerting influence on other sectors than health and advocating better health.

This shows that the role of a health system steward is not limited to overseeing the health sector. Stewardship includes providing leadership and advocacy to influence and coordinate action with other branches of government (such as finance, trade, transport and agriculture) at the central and regional or local levels (for decentralized systems), the private sector and other stakeholders. This is required to ensure that all areas of policy appropriately consider health and that attention is paid to its social determinants *(78)*. This is crucial, since even high-income countries have dramatic differences in health that are closely linked with degrees of social disadvantage. Improving both the level and distribution of health status requires increasingly coordinated government action based on the principles of justice, participation and collaboration *(79)*. In addition, other government sectors and actors in society often manage measures that modify the risk factors for major diseases and the determinants of health. Broader societal health determinants – especially education, employment and the environment – influence the distribution of risk factors among population groups, thereby resulting in inequality in health (Fig. 3.7). Overall, health system stewardship has to be exercised to enhance healthy public policy, which "is characterized by an explicit concern for health and equity in all areas of policy and by an accountability for health impact" according to the Adelaide Recommendations on Healthy Public Policy *(81)*.

Health system stewards have to make the case for other sectors' taking health into consideration when making their own policies, and exert influence through coordination with partners by:

Fig. 3.7. Stewardship of factors influencing health

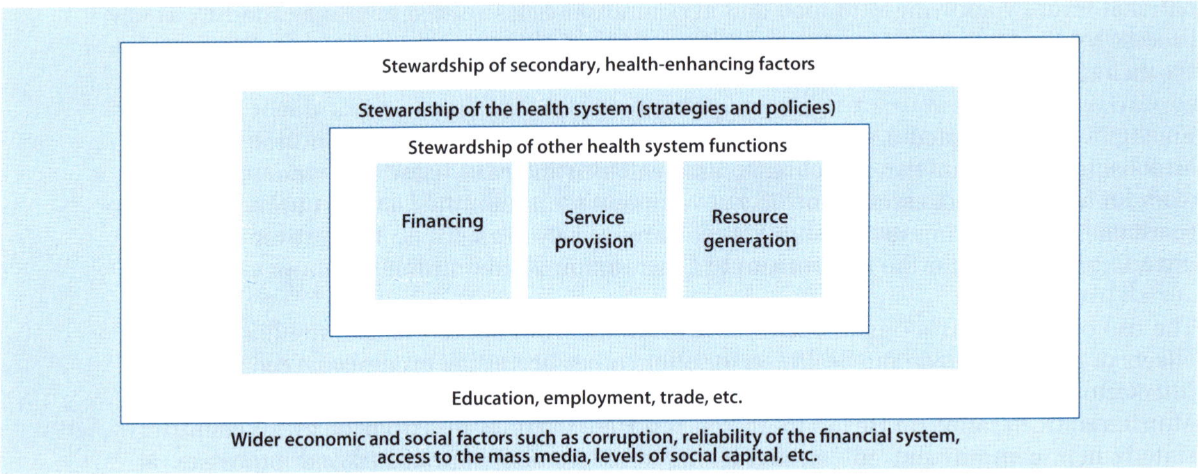

Stewardship of secondary, health-enhancing factors

Stewardship of the health system (strategies and policies)

Stewardship of other health system functions

Financing | Service provision | Resource generation

Education, employment, trade, etc.

Wider economic and social factors such as corruption, reliability of the financial system, access to the mass media, levels of social capital, etc.

Source: adapted from Davies *(80)*.

- collaborating and building coalitions across sectors in government and with actors outside government to attain the health system's goals;
- promoting initiatives to improve health or address its social determinants; and
- advocating the incorporation of health in all policies.

Stewards can thus play diverse roles in promoting healthy public policies. They can:

- lead the health agenda across government;
- support other ministries, for example, in developing their capacity to assess how their policies affect health;
- partner other ministries in developing and implementing policies affecting health, such as the food industry or environmental policies; or
- indicate the negative effects of certain policies through health impact assessments and therefore act as defenders if necessary.

Examples of stewardship for healthy public policies in practice

In Sweden, the health sector started multidisciplinary research on the determinants of health and facilitated the active participation of all political parties, the public and other stakeholders in the process of formulating public health goals. This led to the approval of the public health policy of 2003 *(82)*, one of the first formalized country health strategies based on the determinants of health. The 11 objectives and their specific, measurable targets are monitored and evaluated on behalf of a steering committee of ministers from different sectors chaired by the Minister for Elderly Care and Public Health.

In the United Kingdom, the national policy that explicitly addresses equity in health has identified intersectoral action as a key strategy. The establishment of health action zones in 1999 was designed to organize area-based and intersectoral action around the social determinants of health. In addition, health equity auditing was introduced to ensure that local community plans for health and development give priority to those with greatest need.

In Slovenia, the Ministry of Health started to implement health impact assessment at the national level by applying it to food and agriculture policies related to joining the EU. The process resulted in better cooperation between the agriculture and health sectors, leading to the inclusion of a food security pillar in the national action plan on food and nutrition.

Finally, Norway adopted a phased approach to reducing social inequality in health by first establishing a unit in the Directorate for Health to increase knowledge and strengthen work on health impact assessment. The government then submitted a report to the Storting (parliament) presenting its strategy for reducing social inequality in health over 10 years, including guidelines for the government and state administration *(83,84)*.

The use of health impact assessment in Finland and Slovenia to evaluate the likely health effects of policies outside the health sector offers other promising examples of coordination, intersectoral action and advocacy for better health, as reflected in the 2007 European Union Ministerial Declaration on Health in All Policies. Here the ministers from the 27 EU countries stated their commitment to "strengthening multisectoral approaches and processes at European, national, regional and local levels by which public health impacts can be effectively taken into account in all policies" *(85)*.

The examples above reflect the two key ways in which governments can improve their stewardship of the system: incorporating health considerations into all areas of policy (health in all policies) and monitoring and measuring health system performance (see the section below on assessing health system performance for accountability). The WHO European Member States explicitly endorsed both of these in the Tallinn Charter: Health Systems for Health and Wealth *(12)*.

Health in all policies: instruments and challenges

Health in all policies is a strategy to strengthen the link between health and other policies. This is a key approach for strengthening the stewardship function for public health to improve the health system's performance, and has been widely endorsed by policy-makers in recent years. It addresses the effects on health across all policies such as those on agriculture, education, the environment, government spending, housing and transport *(86)*. Key elements of this strategy are health impact assessment (see below), intersectoral mechanisms and intersectoral health targets. In this way, the core of health in all policies is improving the health of the population by examining the determinants of health, which can be influenced to improve health but are mainly otherwise beyond the remit of the health ministry *(87)*. Reaching out to engage in dialogue and collaborating with other ministries and sectors is therefore a key stewardship task.

The European Region, especially the EU, has a strong legal basis for health in all policies. The strategy was included in *The Health for All policy framework for the WHO European Region (76)*; EU Member States endorsed a European Council conclusion on health in all policies under the Finnish Presidency in 2006 *(88)*, and health in all policies is a principle of the health strategy adopted by the EU in 2007 *(89)*. Finally, EU Member States, along with WHO and the European Commission, endorsed the European Union Ministerial Declaration on Health in All Policies *(85)*. In addition, the 1992 Treaty establishing the European Community essentially provides a mandate for the EU institutions actively to support health in all policies *(90)*. The Treaty of Lisbon *(91)* envisages the "protection of human health" as an element in defining and implementing other policies.

Some instruments have been applied to implement health in all policies *(87)*. For example, legal mandates for assessing the health implications of policies and legal responsibility to follow and report population health trends and policies affecting them are important instruments in institutionalizing health in other policies. Other examples include:

- parliamentary reporting on public health and public health policy at the national and local levels;
- developing permanent intersectoral committees to prepare, implement and follow up health in all policies; or
- other intersectoral mechanisms that include formal consultation in the form of, for example, requests for formal statements on policy proposals and more informal mechanisms and contacts.

Health impact assessment helps to inform decision-makers on the health effects of pending decisions and their alternatives *(92)*. It is used not only to assess health implications but also to help make them visible and be considered seriously in policy-making processes. The scope of health impact assessment varies from a small desk-based assessment of the directions of likely health effects of policy options to an assessment aiming at accurately estimating the magnitude of the effects. Investment in health impact assessment should be proportional to the importance of the policy decision. This tool has been used in different countries and at different political administrative levels. It can be applied to policies, programmes and projects and, in addition to the examples already provided, has been quite frequently used in Finland, the Netherlands and the United Kingdom *(93)*. Lithuania is one of the first countries to legally mandate health impact assessment *(94)*.

The influence of health impact assessment on decisions may vary, but ample evidence indicates that it can be substantial *(95)*. In addition, economic evaluation conducted in England and Wales has concluded that the benefits of health impact assessment exceed the costs *(96)*. The remaining challenge, however, is to demonstrate to the stakeholders of other sectors the advantage of using health impact assessment systematically and to find implementation strategies suitable to the particular context.

Other mechanisms facilitate health in all policies, although they all depend on the context and have not been subject to systematic or comparative analysis. They include intersectoral committees, interservice groups, public health expert panels, consensus conferences, formal consultations in drafting legislation and public referenda *(97)*. Finland's Ministry of Social Affairs and Health has used bilateral policy dialogues and health policy reporting between ministries to strengthen intersectoral cooperation on the determinants of health *(83)*.

Further, intersectoral health targets can be used to strengthen stewardship. Targets have the capacity to support dialogue, inform the allocation of resources and influence the management and behaviour of organizations and individuals. They are an important mechanism for determining achievement levels for measuring performance. Health targets are a common mechanism for stewardship in formulating health policy throughout the Region *(98–102)*. The most recent and comprehensive mapping exercise showed that most countries are using health targets in formulating comprehensive health policies *(75)*.

Health targets are a demanding tool, however, as defining and monitoring them require sophisticated technical skills, political will and an adequate infrastructure. Many countries have made use of targets, such as England, Germany and Hungary. In general, experience shows that health targets produce few effects unless they are embedded in adequate accountability frameworks and supported by suitable health intelligence *(103,104)*.

Conclusion

In recent years, therefore, governments have changed the tools they use to regulate the delivery of services and the extent to which political, managerial and fiscal functions are decentralized or recentralized from the central to the regional levels *(105)* to achieve broad health system goals. There are, however, some challenges in implementing health in all policies *(87)*:

1. success in implementation is limited by the extent to which health policies or intersectoral action of selected sectors on their own can improve the determinants of health;
2. the costs of the strategies are important decision-making points, and any health policy measures that negatively influence the cost structure of another public policy area will encounter difficulty;
3. the promotion of local health agendas and measures will have limited effects if the determinants of other policies are set at the national, regional and global levels; and
4. the health effects of specific policy changes are not necessarily direct and immediate but may only become evident much later.

Tackling these challenges requires building the capacity for intersectoral action and basing decisions on an increasing evidence base and reliable information and data.

One of the six WHO global priorities in stewardship *(106)* is to support Member States in building coalitions across government ministries, with the private sector and with communities to act on key determinants of health and to ensure that the health needs of the most vulnerable people are properly addressed. Achieving this objective requires not only episodic action but also the building of robust social institutions capable of exerting continued influence on society. Health system stewards must therefore strike a balance between the medium-term outcomes necessary to respect the pace of political life and the long-term actions required to promote better health through healthy public policies.

Assessing health system performance for accountability

Improving the performance of countries' health systems is a priority issue across the European Region, especially in the current economic climate in which obtaining the greatest value from existing resources is paramount. In this regard, health system performance assessment is a recognized approach among the countries in the WHO European Region *(107)*. It has been given renewed recognition and impetus by the Tallinn Charter *(12)*, through which Member States committed themselves to transparency and being accountable for health system performance to achieve measurable results.

Accountability for better health outcomes and health system stewardship

Assessing a health system's performance involves measuring and analysing how well it is meeting its ultimate goals, such as better health status and better financial protection for the population, and increased responsiveness or efficiency for the health system *(75,106)* and how its performance against intermediary objectives – such as access, coverage, quality and safety of health services *(106)* – contributes to reaching these goals.

A fully developed approach to assessing health system performance has the following attributes.

- It is regular, systematic and transparent. Reporting mechanisms are defined beforehand and cover the whole assessment. It is not bound in time by a reform agenda or national health plan end-point, although it might be revised at regular intervals better to reflect emerging priorities and to revise targets with the aim of achieving them.
- It is comprehensive and balanced in scope, covers the whole health system and is not limited to specific programmes, objectives or levels of care. The performance of the system as a whole is more than the sum of the performance of each of its constituents.
- It is analytical and uses complementary sources of information to assess performance. Performance indicators are supported in their interpretation by policy analysis, complementary information (qualitative assessments) and reference points: trends over time, local, regional or international comparisons or comparisons to standards, targets or benchmarks.
- In meeting these criteria, health system performance assessment needs to be transparent and promote the accountability of the health system steward. These two elements are mutually reinforcing, and this section focuses on examining how countries can use health system performance assessment to drive performance and ensure accountability.

Accountability has two main characteristics: rendering an account (providing information) and then holding accountable (imposing sanctions or rewards for the accountable party) *(108)*. Health system performance assessment corresponds to a performance accountability approach grounded in management science, which aims to demonstrate and account for performance based on agreed targets *(109)* and, as such, differs from accountability for compliance with procedures and rules (also known as hierarchical control). It holds stakeholders to account for both the performance of their national, regional and local health systems and for their action to improve performance. Fig. 3.8 describes some of the accountability relationships in health systems.

A commitment to accountability is not only an answer to external audiences but also a constructive tool for organizational development, enhancement of management practices, self-evaluation and strategic planning *(110)*. More specifically, building coherence between strategy, performance management and accountability by measuring performance can lead to improved performance and increased value for health systems *(111–114)*.

In addition, the release of publicly available report cards has enhanced accountability for health system performance to the public by documenting the relative performance of national health systems, often with related international rankings *(5)*. Such scorecards have raised awareness and interest in health systems' performance at all levels. Moreover, by creating a focused platform for bringing public and mass-media attention to differences between health

Fig. 3.8. Map of some important accountability relationships in the health system

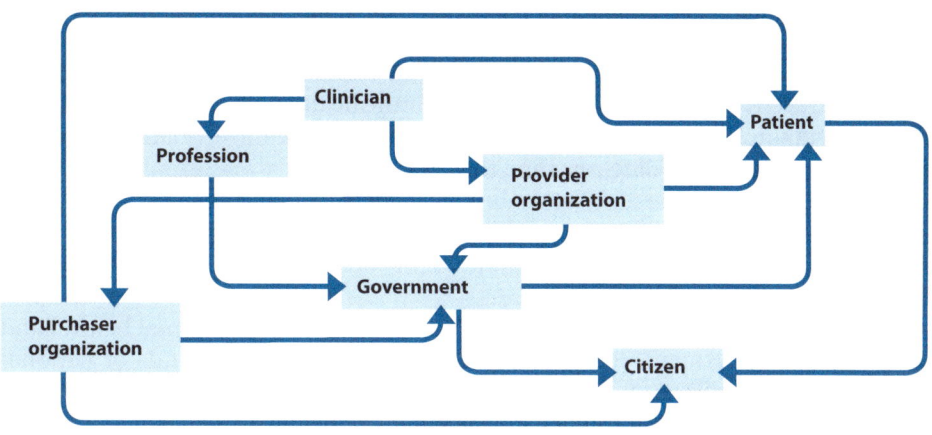

Source: Smith, Mossialos, Papanicolas (108).

systems, international comparisons have become a powerful tool for alerting national policy-makers to deficiencies and prompting remedial action. Such comparisons may also force health system stewards to explain publicly the reasons for variation and their own system's potentially lower scores in given areas. Although many methodological challenges related to comparable data and aggregation of indicators in league tables remain (108,115), the responses to such reports as *The world health report 2000* (75) or the OECD *Health at a glance 2007* (116) indicate the power of such comparisons. Although mass-media and consumer reports have so far focused primarily on the quality of health care providers, through scoring, they are now stepping into the wider sphere of international health system comparisons with, for instance, the development of the Euro health consumer index (117).

Assessing health system performance can also improve performance more directly. Embedding strategic performance information into decision-making processes supports policy-makers in assessing and readjusting strategies, plans, policies and related targets to move towards achieving health system goals. Health system performance assessment, linked to accountability and strategy, thus supports stewardship by ensuring that: health systems are strategically oriented towards improving health outcomes for the population, policy decisions are informed by appropriate intelligence related to health problems and determinants of health, all government policies contribute to better health and healthy public policies are promoted across all areas of government. This is consistent with the core responsibilities of health system stewards: ensuring that a strategic policy direction is formulated, ensuring good regulation and appropriate tools for implementing it and fostering the intelligence on health system performance needed to ensure accountability and transparency (107).

Assessing health system performance in European countries

Most countries in the WHO European Region have incorporated elements of health system performance assessment into their oversight arrangements. Very few, however, have developed systems that have formalized and integrated all of its attributes with the potential substantially to improve performance.

Table 3.4 presents an overview of the implementation of health system performance assessment in selected European countries. Consistent with the approach presented above, it reviews the characteristics of health system performance assessment and identifies strengths and weaknesses in implementation. For example, a "–" score under "Regular, systematic and transparent" means that the assessment is not released regularly or that the results are not shared broadly and transparently with health system stakeholders and the public at large. Conversely, a "+" score on the "Link to health system performance management" column means that performance information is clearly linked to strategy and that processes are in place to ensure that it is used systematically at different stages of the decision-making process, for policy development, resource allocation or accountability decisions. A "–/+" score indicates that the situation is still unclear.

Table 3.4. Overview of health system performance characteristics in select countries in the WHO European Region

Country	Performance assessment			Accountability and performance management	
	Regular, systematic and transparent	Comprehensive and balanced in scope	Depth of analysis	Link to accountability	Link to health system performance management
Armenia	–/+	–	+	–	–
England (United Kingdom)	+	+	+	+	+
Estonia	+	+	+	+	–
Georgia	–	+	+	–	–
Kyrgyzstan	+	+	+	+	+
Netherlands	+	+	+	+	+
Portugal	+	+	–/+	+	–
Sweden	+	–	+	+	+

Based on this table, the next section discusses five countries in which specific attributes of health system performance assessment have been implemented and how these translate into practice.

The Netherlands: regular, systematic and transparent assessment of health system performance

In the Netherlands, the Ministry of Health, Welfare and Sport commissioned the National Institute for Public Health and the Environment (RIVM) to develop and release performance assessment reports for the health care system in the Netherlands in 2007 and 2008. The reports are published annually on the RIVM web site (118).

The framework for assessing health system performance focuses on the technical quality of health care while keeping a broader perspective on health and its other determinants. It measures performance through 110 indicators. The selected system goals and indicator domains are in accordance with the policy of the Ministry of Health, Welfare and Sport.

England: comprehensive assessment of health system performance

Since 1999, England has developed three different systems of performance assessment for the NHS. The NHS performance assessment framework (119) is based on six areas of performance: health improvement, fair access, effective delivery of appropriate health care, efficiency, patient care experience, and health outcomes of NHS care. The annual star rating system, which ran from 2001 to 2005, gave different types of organization a rating from zero (failing) to three stars (high performing) based on assessment against a set of key targets and a balanced scorecard of three domains (which varied by type of organization). Failing key targets put an organization at risk of being zero-rated, while attaining three stars required good performance on key targets and the balanced scorecard. Since 2006, organizations have been assessed through an annual health check, which has two components: financial management and quality care.

The framework is used: to assess the NHS' performance, covering quality and efficiency, to encourage benchmarking between similar NHS organizations and to underpin national and local performance and accountability arrangements.

Kyrgyzstan: health system performance assessment supported by in-depth analysis addressing performance drivers

In Kyrgyzstan, the Department of Strategic Planning and Reform Implementation of the Ministry of Health regularly assesses core health system performance. The Republic Centre for Health System Development and Information Technologies supports the Ministry. The Centre is an autonomous public entity responsible for supporting policy development and implementation by generating knowledge, in-depth analysis of performance and training.

Health system performance and the impact of reforms have been monitored and published regularly since 2004 *(120)*. The 2008 report, assessing the impact of the implementation of the health system reform programme, showed that, halfway through the programme, key performance indicators demonstrate strong and sustained progress towards meeting targets on financial protection, access, efficiency and transparency, and mixed results in terms of health and quality of care indicators *(121)*.

Portugal: linking health system performance assessment and accountability structures and processes

In Portugal, the National Health Plan 2004–2010 *(122)* targets performance improvement objectives for the health system and monitors progress on targets related to the plan. The set of performance indicators is available on the Internet and monitored and released regularly *(123)*.

The National Health Plan has many characteristics of a framework for health system performance assessment through its scope and regular reporting mechanisms. To ensure the implementation of the plan, structures (such as the Office of the High Commissioner for Health) and processes (coordination mechanisms through an interministerial committee) were established to clarify roles and responsibilities, coordinate implementation and ensure accountability across the government and health system for achieving health system targets.

Sweden: linking performance assessment and management of health system performance

In Sweden, the National Board of Health and Welfare *(124)* monitors and evaluates health services to determine whether the services delivered are aligned with the goals set out by the national government. If the scope of the assessment is related to health services, the link to the national goals is important from a health system perspective.

With the Swedish Association of Local Authorities and Regions, the Board published a report on health care quality and efficiency in 21 county councils and health care regions in Sweden *(125)* that serves two purposes. The first is to inform the public and to stimulate the debate on health care quality and efficiency. Second, the results are used to support local and regional efforts to improve health care services in terms of clinical quality, health outcomes, patient experience and efficient resource use.

International trends, key challenges and the way forward

As the discussion and Table 3.4 have highlighted, the implementation of health system performance assessment varies widely across the WHO European Region. Data and quantitative indicators are produced and to some extent made public in all countries, but analysis is very often fragmented and not linked to regular and systematic accountability and performance management processes. Rather than building additional parallel systems, developing full frameworks for health system performance assessment in many countries would mean bringing isolated initiatives together, complementing them and making sense of the data already available to assess performance from a health system standpoint and inform strategic priorities.

The impetus generated by the Tallinn Charter *(12)* has created high awareness of the essential role of health system performance assessment in successful stewardship of the health system. This commitment was further reinforced in the context of the economic recession during the first Tallinn Charter follow-up meeting in February 2009, when European Member States agreed on plans to take the Tallinn Charter forward *(126)*. In addition, they requested support and facilitation at the international level to develop a common framework for health system performance assessment, to select minimum and tailored sets of performance indicators and to develop processes for cross-country learning and benchmarking *(126)*. Some of the challenges and ways forward in implementing full performance assessments across the Region are described below.

Many issues around information systems and data quality or the selection of indicators are used to explain why health system performance assessment is still underdeveloped. The lack of standardization in methods and data often results in inconsistency, which might prevent performance information from being used for comparison over time, across organizations, across health care settings or across regions. Nevertheless, even if limitations still exist, major advances have been achieved in recent years with the support of international organizations such as WHO, OECD and the European Commission. A consensus is increasingly being built on data standardization and a focus on a limited number of health system performance indicators *(108,127)*. Advances at the international level are likely to benefit the national level, with more coherence in information systems to adapt to international reporting requirements and build on international best practices.

The fragmentation of performance measurement and monitoring systems often creates major bottlenecks, reflecting a lack of coordination and communication within different levels of government and the health system, especially as each stakeholder monitors processes and outcomes on specific programmes. The challenge lies in aligning performance assessment and accountability based on strategy, by cascading performance indicators at the macro, meso and micro levels while recognizing and adapting to the different levels of responsibility. The intention is to reach greater clarity in the roles and responsibilities of health system actors to achieve health outcomes, which should translate into clearer performance expectations and better performance management approaches driving improvement. A better alignment of information systems, indicator selection and accountability structures and processes (both nationally and internationally) would probably benefit many countries in the European Region.

Effective communication and wide dissemination are required to create platforms to introduce important changes in health systems. From this perspective, information on performance should be interpreted in ways that are simple and clear to policy-makers *(128)* and can be communicated effectively to the public. Further, health system performance assessment has to be built into integrated performance management systems, through which important indicators are used systematically in decision-making processes across government. These processes relate to strategy and policy development, target setting, performance measurement, resource allocation and improving accountability and performance.

Member States in the Region vary widely in terms of the availability and quality of data, accountability structures and processes, citizens' participation, transparency, and the maturity of their culture of performance measurement and continuous quality improvement. If accountability relationships are to function properly, no system of performance information should be viewed in isolation from the broader design within which the measurement is embedded *(108)*. National ownership and fostering of a culture of measurement, transparency and continuous performance improvement are crucial to improve health system performance based on research evidence and performance information. This culture grows as data are used, information systems improve and policy-makers are equipped to translate performance information into evidence-informed decision-making.

The WHO Regional Office for Europe supports health ministries and governments in using better performance information to steer complex reforms in environments of growing financial constraints and rising expectations. Future priorities for action, as indicated by Member States, will be:

- developing a common framework for assessing health system performance;
- based on the experience of other international organizations, selecting a core and a tailored set of performance indicators to enable both international comparisons and in-depth assessment of health system performance at the national level; and
- developing mechanisms for cross-country learning and benchmarking *(126)*.

References

1. Saltman RB, Figueras J. Analysing the evidence on European health reforms. *Health Affairs*, 1998, 17:85–108.
2. *Ljubljana Charter on Reforming Health Care*. Copenhagen, WHO Regional Office for Europe, 1996 (http://www.euro.who.int/AboutWHO/Policy/20010927_5, accessed 27 May 2009).
3. Dowling B, Glendinning C, eds. *The new primary care: modern, dependable, successful?* Maidenhead, Open University Press/McGraw-Hill Education, 2003.
4. Starfield B. *Primary care: balancing health needs, services, and technology*. New York, Oxford University Press, 1998.
5. Saltman RB, Rico A, Boerma WGW, eds. *Primary care in the driver's seat? Organizational reform in European primary care*. Maidenhead, Open University Press/McGraw-Hill Education, 2006 (http://www.euro.who.int/observatory/Publications/20060117_1, accessed 27 May 2009).

6. *Putting commissioning into practice*. London, Audit Commission, 2007.
7. McKee M, Healy J. *Hospitals in a changing Europe*. Maidenhead, Open University Press/McGraw-Hill Education, 2002.
8. Castoro C et al. *Day surgery: making it happen*. Copenhagen, WHO Regional Office for Europe on behalf of the European Observatory on Health Systems and Policies, 2007 (Policy Brief No. 12; http://www.euro.who.int/observatory/Publications/20020527_16, accessed 27 May 2009).
9. European Health for All database [online database]. Copenhagen, WHO Regional Office for Europe, 2009 (http://www.euro.who.int/hfadb, accessed 27 May 2009).
10. Nolte E, McKee M, eds. *Caring for people with chronic conditions: a health system perspective*. Maidenhead, Open University Press/McGraw-Hill Education, 2008.
11. Singh D. *How can chronic disease management programmes operate across care settings and providers?* Copenhagen, WHO Regional Office for Europe, 2008 (http://www.euro.who.int/document/hsm/6_hsc08_ePB_9.pdf, accessed 27 May 2009).
12. *The Tallinn Charter: Health Systems for Health and Wealth*. Copenhagen, WHO Regional Office for Europe, 2008 (http://www.euro.who.int/document/e91438.pdf, accessed 27 May 2009).
13. Busse R et al. Being responsive to citizens' expectations? The role of health services in responsiveness and satisfaction. In: Figueras J et al., eds. *Health systems, health and wealth: assessing the case for investing in health systems*. Copenhagen, WHO Regional Office for Europe, 2008 (http://www.euro.who.int/document/hsm/3_hsc08_eBD3.pdf, accessed 28 June 2009).
14. World Health Survey [web site]. Geneva, World Health Organization, 2009 (http://www.who.int/healthinfo/survey/en/index.html, accessed 27 May 2009).
15. Hurst J, Siciliani L. *Tackling excessive waiting times for elective surgery: a comparison of policies in twelve OECD countries*. Paris, Organisation for Economic Co-operation and Development, 2003 (OECD Health Working Papers, No. 6).
16. Coulter A, Parsons S, Askham J. *Where are the patients in decision-making about their own care?* Copenhagen, WHO Regional Office for Europe, 2008 (http://www.euro.who.int/document/hsm/3_hsc08_ePB_6.pdf, accessed 27 May 2009).
17. Legido-Quigley H et al. *Assuring the quality of health care in the European Union. A case for action*. Copenhagen, WHO Regional Office for Europe on behalf of the European Observatory on Health Systems and Policies, 2008 (http://www.euro.who.int/InformationSources/Publications/Catalogue/20080606_1, accessed 27 May 2009).
18. Merkur S et al. (2008). *Do lifelong learning and revalidation ensure that physicians are fit to practise?* Copenhagen, WHO Regional Office for Europe, 2008 (http://www.euro.who.int/document/hsm/9_hsc08_ePB_12.pdf, accessed 27 May 2009).
19. McDaid D et al. *How can European health systems support investment in and the implementation of population health strategies?* Copenhagen, WHO Regional Office for Europe, 2008 (http://www.euro.who.int/document/hsm/1_hsc08_ePB_2.pdf, accessed 27 May 2009).
20. Pelletier-Fleury N et al. Preventive service delivery: a new insight into French general practice. *Health Policy*, 2007, 83:268–276.
21. MacArthur I, Shevkun E. Restructuring public health services. In: McKee M, Healy J, Falkingham J, eds. *Health care in central Asia*. Maidenhead, Open University Press/McGraw-Hill Education, 2002.
22. Bobak M et al. Modernizing public health. In: Figueras J et al., eds. *Health systems in transition: learning from experience*. Copenhagen, WHO Regional Office for Europe, 2004 (http://www.euro.who.int/observatory/Publications/20040720_2, accessed 27 May 2009).

23. Kulzhanov M, Rechel B. *Kazakhstan: health system review*. Copenhagen, WHO Regional Office for Europe on behalf of the European Observatory on Health Systems and Policies, 2007 (http://www.euro.who.int/observatory/Hits/TopPage, accessed 27 May 2009).
24. Ahmedov M et al. *Uzbekistan: health system review*. Copenhagen, WHO Regional Office for Europe on behalf of the European Observatory on Health Systems and Policies, 2007 (http://www.euro.who.int/observatory/Hits/TopPage, accessed 27 May 2009).
25. Dubois C-A, McKee M, Nolte E, eds. *Human resources for health in Europe*. Copenhagen, WHO Regional Office for Europe on behalf of the European Observatory on Health Systems and Policies, 2006 (http://www.euro.who.int/observatory/Publications/20060112_1, accessed 27 May 2009).
26. Buchan J. *How can the migration of health service professionals be managed so as to reduce any negative effects on supply?* Copenhagen, WHO Regional Office for Europe, 2008 (http://www.euro.who.int/document/hsm/7_hsc08_ePB_10.pdf, accessed 27 May 2009).
27. Simoens S, Hurst J. *The supply of physician services in OECD countries*. Paris, Organisation for Economic Co-operation and Development, 2006.
28. Polluste K et al. Public health reforms in Estonia: impact on the health of the population. *British Medical Journal*, 2005, 331:210–213.
29. Sogoric S et al. Countries selecting public health priorities – A "bottom-up" approach (Croatian experience). *Collegium Antropologicum*, 2005, 29:111–119.
30. Gulis G et al. Transition and public health in the Slovak Republic. *British Medical Journal*, 2005, 331: 213–215.
31. Buchan J. Migration of health workers in Europe: policy problem or policy solution? In: Dubois C-A, McKee M, Nolte E, eds. *Human resources for health in Europe*. Copenhagen, WHO Regional Office for Europe on behalf of the European Observatory on Health Systems and Policies, 2006 (http://www.euro.who.int/observatory/Publications/20020522_2, accessed 27 May 2009).
32. Mrazek M, Mossialos E. Regulating pharmaceutical prices in the European Union. In: Mossialos E, Mrazek M, Walley T, eds. *Regulating pharmaceuticals in Europe: striving for efficiency, equity and quality*. Copenhagen, WHO Regional Office for Europe on behalf of the European Observatory on Health Systems and Policies, 2004 (http://www.euro.who.int/observatory/Publications/20020522_2, accessed 27 May 2009).
33. Velasco-Garrido M, Busse R. *Health technology assessment: an introduction to objectives, role of evidence and structure in Europe*. Copenhagen, WHO Regional Office for Europe on behalf of the European Observatory on Health Systems and Policies, 2005 (Policy Brief No. 8; http://www.euro.who.int/observatory/Publications/20020527_16, accessed 27 May 2009).
34. Sorenson C et al. *How can the impact of health technology assessments be enhanced?* Copenhagen, WHO Regional Office for Europe, 2008 (http://www.euro.who.int/document/hsm/2_hsc08_ePB_5.pdf, accessed 27 May 2009).
35. Zentner A et al. Methods for the comparative evaluation of pharmaceuticals. *GMS Health Technology Assessment*, 2005, 1:Doc09.
36. Sorenson C et al. *Ensuring value for money in health care: the role of health technology assessment in the European Union*. Copenhagen, WHO Regional Office for Europe on behalf of the European Observatory on Health Systems and Policies, 2008 (http://www.euro.who.int/observatory/Publications/20020522_2, accessed 27 May 2009).
37. *Primary health care: report of the International Conference on Primary Health Care, Alma-Ata, USSR, September 6–12, 1978*. Geneva, World Health Organization, 1978.

38. *The world health report 2008. Primary health care – Now more than ever.* Geneva, World Health Organization, 2008 (http://www.who.int/whr/2008/en/index.html, accessed 27 May 2009).
39. Kelley E, Hurst J. *Health care quality indicators project. Conceptual framework paper.* Paris, Organisation for Economic Co-operation and Development, 2006 (OECD Health Working Papers, No. 23; http://www.oecd.org/dataoecd/1/36/36262363.pdf, accessed 27 May 2009).
40. Starfield B et al. Continuity and coordination in primary care: their achievement and utility. *Medical Care*, 1976, 14:625–636.
41. Saultz JW. Defining and measuring interpersonal continuity of care. *Annals of Family Medicine*, 2003, 1:134–143 (http://www.annfammed.org/cgi/content/full/1/3/134, accessed 27 May 2009).
42. Boerma WGW. Coordination and integration in European primary care. In: Saltman RB, Rico A, Boerma WGW, eds. *Primary care in the driver's seat? Organizational reform in European primary care.* Maidenhead, Open University Press/McGraw-Hill Education, 2006 (http://www.euro.who.int/Document/E87932_chapt1.pdf, accessed 27 May 2009).
43. Boerma WGW. *Profiles of general practice in Europe. An international study of variation in the tasks of general practitioners.* Utrecht, NIVEL, 2003 (http://www.nivel.nl/pdf/profiles-of-general-practice-in-europe.pdf, accessed 27 May 2009).
44. Boecken J. *Gesundheitsmonitor Deutschland 2006.* Gütersloh, Bertelsmann Stiftung, 2006.
45. Atun R. *Evaluating reforms undertaken in PHC services in the framework of the Manas Program (1996–2005).* Bishkek, Manas Health Policy Analysis Project, 2006.
46. Lee TH et al. The future of primary care. *New England Journal of Medicine*, 2008, 359:2085–2086.
47. Ibraimova C, Isaeva T, Smith B. *Report of a time utilization study of family group practice physicians in Kyrgyzstan.* Bishkek, USAID ZdravPlus Project, 2009.
48. Leppo K. The rise, stagnation and revitalization of PHC in Finland, 1970–2010. *International Conference Dedicated to the 30th Anniversary of the Alma-Ata Declaration on Primary Health Care, Almaty, Kazakhstan, 15–16 October 2008.*
49. Fujisawa R, Lafortune G. *The remuneration of general practitioners and specialists in 14 OECD countries: what are the factors influencing variations across countries?* Paris, Organisation for Economic Co-operation and Development, 2008 (OECD Health Working Papers, no. 41).
50. Boerma WGW et al. *Primary care quality management in Slovenia.* Copenhagen, WHO Regional Office for Europe, 2008 (http://www.euro.who.int/Slovenia/Publications/20080307_1, accessed 27 May 2009).
51. Kringos DS et al. *Evaluation of the organizational model of primary care in Turkey.* Copenhagen, WHO Regional Office for Europe, 2008 (http://www.euro.who.int/document/e92219.pdf, accessed 27 May 2009).
52. Busse R, Schlette S. *Focus on prevention, health and aging, new health profession.* Gütersloh, Bertelsmann Stiftung, 2007 (Health Policy Developments, 7/8).
53. Dubois CA, Singh D, Jiwani I. The human resource challenge in chronic care. In: Nolte E, McKee M, eds. *Caring for people with chronic conditions: a health system perspective.* Maidenhead, Open University Press/McGraw-Hill Education, 2008.
54. Casado D. *Integrating health and social care.* Gütersloh, Health Policy Monitor, 2003 (http://www.hpm.org/survey/es/b2/4, accessed 3 July 2009).
55. Van Lente EJ et al. Auswirkungen der Disease-Management-Programme auf die Versorgung chronisch kranker Patienten in Deutschland – eine Zwischenbilanz. *Gesundheits- und Sozialpolitik*, 2008, 62(3):10–18.

56. Zwisler A-DO, Schou L, Sørensen LV, eds. *Cardiac rehabilitation: rationale, methods and experience from Bispebjerg Hospital.* Copenhagen, Cardiac Rehabilitation Unit, Department of Cardiology, Bispebjerg Hospital, 2004 (http://www.cardiacrehabilitation.dk/rehab_uk, accessed 27 May 2009).
57. Nolte E, McKee M. Integration and chronic care: a review. In: Nolte E, McKee M, eds. *Caring for people with chronic conditions: a health system perspective.* Maidenhead, Open University Press/McGraw-Hill Education, 2008.
58. Briggs CJ, Garner P. Strategies for integrating primary health services in middle- and low-income countries at the point of delivery. *Cochrane Database of Systematic Reviews,* 2006, (2):CD003318.
59. Mossialos E et al., eds. *Funding health care: options for Europe.* Maidenhead, Open University Press/McGraw-Hill Education, 2002 (http://www.euro.who.int/observatory/Publications/20020524_21, accessed 27 May 2009).
60. Kutzin J et al. Reforms in the pooling of funds. In: Kutzin, J, Cashin C, Jakab M, eds. *Implementing health financing reform: lessons for and from countries in transition.* Copenhagen, WHO Regional Office for Europe on behalf of the European Observatory on Health Policies and Systems (in press).
61. Sauerland D. Financing health care in Germany. *6th European Conference on Health Economics, Budapest, Hungary, 6–9 July 2006.*
62. Cheng T-M, Reinhardt UE. Shepherding major health system reforms: a conversation with German Health Minister Ulla Schmidt. *Health Affairs,* 2008, 27:w204–w213.
63. Hroboň P. The Czech health system: its presence and future. *Hungarian Parliament Conference on Health Insurance Reform 2007–2009, Budapest, Hungary, 25–26 January 2007.*
64. Shishkin S, Kacevicius G, Ciocanu M. *Evaluation of Moldova's 2004 health financing reform.* Copenhagen, WHO Regional Office for Europe, 2008 (http://www.euro.who.int/financing/policy/20061103_1, accessed 27 May 2009).
65. Magnussen J. The recentralization of health care in Norway – Expectations and effects. *WHO European Ministerial Conference on Health Systems: Health Systems, Health and Wealth, Tallinn, Estonia, 25–27 June 2008.*
66. Kutzin J, Jakab M, Shishkin S. From scheme to system: social health insurance funds and the transformation of health financing in Kyrgyzstan and Moldova. *Advances in Health Economics* (in press).
67. *Financial management reports on execution of the state guaranteed benefit package and 2007 Ministry of Health performance indicator report.* Bishkek, Ministry of Health, Kyrgyzstan, 2007.
68. Busse R. Risk structure compensation in Germany's statutory health insurance. *European Journal of Public Health,* 2001, 11:174–177.
69. Saltman RB et al. Assessing health reform trends. In: Figueras J et al., eds. *Health systems, health and wealth: assessing the case for investing in health systems.* Copenhagen, WHO Regional Office for Europe, 2008 (http://www.euro.who.int/document/hsm/3_hsc08_eBD3.pdf, accessed 28 June 2009).
70. Busse R et al. Hospital case payment systems in Europe. Editorial. *Health Care Management Science,* 2006, 9:211–213.
71. Chaix-Couturier C et al. Effects of financial incentives on medical practice: results from a systematic review of the literature and methodological issues. *International Journal for Quality in Health Care,* 2000, 12:133–142.
72. Gosden T et al. Capitation, salary, fee-for-service and mixed system of payment: effects on the behaviour of primary care physicians. *Cochrane Database of Systematic Reviews,* 2000, (3):CD002215.
73. White C. GP contract settlement under threat. *British Medical Journal,* 2006, 332:10.

74. Kutzin J. *Health financing policy: a guide for decision-makers*. Copenhagen, WHO Regional Office for Europe, 2008 (http://www.euro.who.int/document/e91422.pdf, accessed 27 May 2009).
75. *The world health report 2000. Health systems: improving performance*. Geneva, World Health Organization, 2000 (http://www.who.int/whr/2000/en, accessed 27 May 2009).
76. *The Health for All policy framework for the WHO European Region: 2005 update*. Copenhagen, WHO Regional Office for Europe, 2005 (European Health for All Series, No. 7; http://www.euro.who.int/InformationSources/Publications/Catalogue/20051201_1, accessed 27 May 2009).
77. *Stewardship/governance of health systems in the WHO European Region*. Copenhagen, WHO Regional Office for Europe, 2008 (EUR/RC58/9 + EUR/RC58/Conf.Doc./4; http://www.euro.who.int/document/rc58/rc58_edoc09.pdf, accessed 27 May 2009).
78. Figueras J et al. Health systems, health, wealth and societal well-being: an introduction. In: Figueras J et al., eds. *Health systems, health and wealth: assessing the case for investing in health systems*. Copenhagen, WHO Regional Office for Europe, 2008 (http://www.euro.who.int/document/hsm/3_hsc08_eBD3.pdf, accessed 28 June 2009).
79. Commission on Social Determinants of Health. *Closing the gap in a generation: health equity through action on the social determinants of health*. Geneva, World Health Organization, 2008 (http://www.who.int/social_determinants/thecommission/finalreport/en/index.html, accessed 27 May 2009).
80. Davies P. Stewardship: what is it and how can we measure it? *Meeting on Health Economics in Developing and Transitional Countries: the Changing Role of the State, York, United Kingdom, 26 July 2001*.
81. *Adelaide Recommendations on Healthy Public Policy. Second International Conference on Health Promotion, Adelaide, South Australia, 5–9 April 1998*. Geneva, World Health Organization, 1998 (http://www.who.int/hpr/NPH/docs/adelaide_recommendations.pdf, accessed 27 May 2009).
82. Public health objectives [web site]. Stockholm, Government of Sweden, 2009 (http://www.regeringen.se/sb/d/2942, accessed 27 May 2009).
83. Stahl R et al., eds. *Health in all policies*. Helsinki, Ministry of Social Affairs and Health, 2006.
84. *National strategy to reduce social inequalities in health*. Oslo, Ministry of Health and Care Services, 2007 (Report No. 20 (2006–2007) to the Storting; http://ec.europa.eu/health/ph_determinants/socio_economics/documents/norway_rd01_en.pdf, accessed 27 May 2009).
85. *European Union Ministerial Declaration on Health in All Policies*. Rome, Ministry of Health, 2007.
86. Dahlgren G, Whitehead M. *Policies and strategies to promote equity in health*. Copenhagen, WHO Regional Office for Europe, 1992 (http://whqlibdoc.who.int/euro/-1993/EUR_ICP_RPD414(2).pdf, accessed 27 May 2009).
87. Wismar M et al. Introduction. In: Ståhl T et al., eds. *Health in all policies: prospects and potentials*. Helsinki, Ministry of Social Affairs and Health, 2006.
88. Council of the European Union. *Council conclusions on health in all policies (HiAP) (EPSCO)*. Brussels, European Commission, 2006.
89. *Together for health: a strategic approach for the EU 2008–2013*. Brussels, Commission of the European Communities, 2007 (white paper COM(2007) 630 final; http://ec.europa.eu/health/ph_overview/Documents/strategy_wp_en.pdf, accessed 27 May 2009).

90. *Treaty on European Union*. Brussels, European Commission, 1992 (http://europa.eu/abc/treaties/index_en.htm, accessed 27 May 2009).
91. *Treaty of Lisbon*. Brussels, European Commission, 2007 (http://europa.eu/abc/treaties/index_en.htm, accessed 27 May 2009).
92. Kemm J. What is HIA and why might it be useful? In: Wismar M et al., eds. *The effectiveness of health impact assessment: scope and limitations of supporting decision-making in Europe*. Copenhagen, WHO Regional Office for Europe, 2007 (http://www.euro.who.int/InformationSources/Publications/Catalogue/20071015_1, accessed 27 May 2009).
93. Blau J et al. The use of health impact assessment across Europe. In: Ståhl T et al., eds. *Health in all policies: prospects and potentials*. Helsinki, Ministry of Social Affairs and Health, 2006.
94. Striÿka M et al. A local-level HIA in the transport sector: following legal requirements in Lithuania. In: Wismar M et al., eds. *The effectiveness of health impact assessment: scope and limitations of supporting decision-making in Europe*. Copenhagen, WHO Regional Office for Europe, 2007 (http://www.euro.who.int/InformationSources/Publications/Catalogue/20071015_1, accessed 27 May 2009).
95. Wismar M et al., eds. *The effectiveness of health impact assessment: scope and limitations of supporting decision-making in Europe*. Copenhagen, WHO Regional Office for Europe, 2007 (http://www.euro.who.int/InformationSources/Publications/Catalogue/20071015_1, accessed 27 May 2009).
96. O'Reilly J et al. *Cost benefit analysis of health impact assessment*. London, Department of Health, 2006.
97. Ritsatakis A, Järvisalo J. Opportunities and challenges for including health components in the policy-making process. In: Ståhl T et al., eds. *Health in all policies: prospects and potentials*. Helsinki, Ministry of Social Affairs and Health, 2006.
98. van de Water HPA, van Herten LM. *Health policies on target? Review of health target and priority setting in 18 European countries*. Leiden, TNO, 1998.
99. Welteke R et al. Das NRW-Gesundheitszielkonzept im europäischen und internationalen Vergleich. In: Geene R, Luber E, eds. *Gesundheitsziele: Planung in der Gesundheitspolitik*. Frankfurt am Main, Mabuse-Verlag, 2000.
100. Busse R, Wismar M. Health target programmes and health care services – any link? A conceptual and comparative study. Part 1. *Health Policy*, 2002, 59:209–221.
101. Wismar M, Busse R. Outcome-related health targets – political strategies for better health outcomes – a conceptual and comparative study. Part 2. *Health Policy*, 2002, 59:223–241.
102. Claveranne J-P, Teil A. *Les modalités de définition des objectifs et stratégies de santé. Description et analyse de dispositifs des pays de l'Union Europeenne et d'Amerique du Nord. Tome I, analyses transversales*. Lyon, GRAPHOS-CNRS, 2003.
103. Wismar M et al. Health targets and (good) governance. *Euro Observer*, 2006, 8(1):1–8.
104. Wismar M et al. *Health targets in Europe: learning from experience*. Copenhagen, WHO Regional Office for Europe on behalf of the European Observatory on Health Systems and Policies, 2008 (http://www.euro.who.int/observatory/Publications/2007/20081105_1, accessed 27 May 2009).
105. Saltman RB et al., eds. *Decentralization in health care: strategies and outcomes*. Maidenhead, Open University Press/McGraw-Hill Education, 2007.
106. *Everybody's business. Strengthening health systems to improve health outcomes: WHO's framework for action*. Geneva, World Health Organization, 2007 (http://www.who.int/healthsystems/strategy/en/index.html, accessed 27 May 2009).

107. *Strengthened health systems save more lives: an insight into WHO's European health systems strategy*. Copenhagen, WHO Regional Office for Europe, 2005 (http://www.euro.who.int/financing, accessed 27 May 2009).
108. Smith PC, Mossialos E, Papanicolas I. *Performance measurement for health system performance improvement: experiences, challenges and prospects*. Copenhagen, WHO Regional Office for Europe on behalf of the European Observatory on Health Systems and Policies, 2008 (http://www.euro.who.int/document/hsm/2_hsc08_ebd2.pdf, accessed 27 May 2009).
109. Brinkerhoff D. *Accountability and health systems: overview, framework, and strategies*. Bethesda, MD, Partners for Health Reform Plus Project, Abt Associates Inc., 2003 (Technical Report No. 018).
110. Panel on Accountability and Governance in the Voluntary Sector. *Building on strength: improving governance and accountability in Canada's voluntary sector: final report*. Ottawa, Voluntary Sector Roundtable, 1999.
111. Berwick DM, James B, Coye MJ. Connections between quality measurement and improvement. *Medical Care*, 2003, 41(Suppl. 1):I30–I38.
112. Bevan G, Hood C. What's measured is what matters: targets and gaming in the English public health care system. *Public Administration*, 2006, 84:517–538.
113. Bevan G, Hood C. Have targets improved performance in the English NHS? *British Medical Journal*, 2006, 332:419–422.
114. Porter M, Teisberg E. *Redefining health care: creating value-based competition on results*. Cambridge, MA, Harvard Business School Press, 2006.
115. McKee M. *The world health report 2000. Advancing the debate*. Copenhagen, WHO Regional Office for Europe, 2001 (http://www.who.int/health-systems-performance/regional_consultations/euro_mckee_background.pdf, accessed 27 May 2009).
116. *Health at a glance 2007*. Paris, Organisation for Economic Co-operation and Development, 2009 (http://www.oecd.org/health/healthataglance, accessed 27 May 2009).
117. *The Euro health consumer index 2008*. Brussels, Health Consumer Powerhouse, 2008 (http://www.healthpowerhouse.com/index.php?option=com_content&view=article&id=55&itemid=54, accessed 27 May 2009).
118. *Dutch health care performance report 2008*. Bilthoven, National Institute for Public Health and the Environment, 2007 (http://www.rivm.nl/vtv/root/o33.html, accessed 27 May 2009).
119. *The NHS performance assessment framework*. London, Department of Health, 1999 (http://www.dh.gov.uk/en/Publicationsandstatistics/Publications/PublicationsPolicyAndGuidance/DH_4009190, accessed 27 May 2009).
120. Republic Center for Health System Development and Information Technologies [web site]. Bishkek, Kyrgyz Republic Center for Health System Development and Information Technologies, 2009 (http://eng.chsd.med.kg/News/ViewNews.aspx?SectionID=28, accessed 27 May 2009).
121. *Kyrgyzstan's Manas Taalimi mid-term review reveals effective donor collaboration, program integration and significant achievements in the health sector*. Bishkek, donors.kg, 2008 (http://www.donors.kg/en/news/?news=323, accessed 27 May 2009).
122. *Portuguese National Health Plan 2004–2010*. Lisbon, Ministry of Health of Portugal, 2004 (http://www.acs.min-saude.pt/en/national-health-plan, accessed 27 May 2009).
123. *Portuguese National Health Plan: indicators and targets*. Lisbon, Ministry of Health of Portugal, 2004 (http://www.acs.min-saude.pt/pns/en, accessed 27 May 2009).

124. National Board of Health and Welfare [web site]. Stockholm, National Board of Health and Welfare, 2009 (http://www.socialstyrelsen.se/en, accessed 27 May 2009).
125. *Quality and efficiency in Swedish health care: regional comparisons 2007.* Stockholm, Swedish Association of Local Authorities and Regions and National Board of Health and Welfare, 2009 (http://www.socialstyrelsen.se/en/showpub.htm?GUID={1482B3AF-ED64-4B31-983F-7788AC43D020}, accessed 27 May 2009).
126. *First Regional Follow-up Meeting on the Tallinn Charter: Health Systems for Health and Wealth, Copenhagen, Denmark, 5–6 February 2009.* Copenhagen, WHO Regional Office for Europe, 2009 (http://www.euro.who.int/healthsystems/20090128_1, accessed 27 May 2009).
127. *Strategy on European Community health indicators (ECHI).* Brussels, European Commission, 2004 (http://ec.europa.eu/health/ph_information/dissemination/echi/echi_en.htm, accessed 27 May 2009).
128. Lavis J. Research, public policy-making, and knowledge-translation processes: Canadian efforts to build bridges. *Journal of Continuing Education in the Health Professions*, 2006, 26:37–45.

Part 4.
Annex

Table 1. Population of the WHO European Region, 2007 (or latest available year) and 2020 (projected)

Member State	Total population (millions)		Average population density per km² (2007)	Total fertility rate		Population aged < 15 (% of total)		Population aged ≥ 65 (% of total)	
	2007	2020		2007	2020–2025	2007	2020	2007	2020
Albania	3.2	3.3	109.5	1.3	1.8	26.9	20.9	8.2	12.0
Andorra	0.1	–	177.5	1.2	–	–	–	–	–
Armenia	3.2	3.2	108.4	1.4	1.8	19.0	21.1	10.8	12.5
Austria	8.3	8.5	98.8	1.4	1.5	15.5	13.9	17.0	19.9
Azerbaijan	8.6	9.8	98.0	2.3	2.0	23.5	24.1	7.0	7.5
Belarus	9.7	9.1	46.9	1.4	1.4	14.8	15.0	14.6	14.9
Belgium	10.5	11.0	341.9	1.7	1.8	17.6	16.7	16.7	20.3
Bosnia and Herzegovina	3.9	3.7	76.5	1.2	1.3	24.3	13.4	6.3	17.3
Bulgaria	7.7	7.0	69.1	1.4	1.6	14.0	14.6	17.1	20.5
Croatia	4.6	4.3	78.5	1.4	1.6	15.7	14.6	17.0	20.4
Cyprus	0.9	1.0	83.3	1.4	1.6	18.0	16.8	12.3	15.8
Czech Republic	10.3	10.6	130.2	1.4	1.6	14.3	15.7	14.5	19.5
Denmark	5.5	5.6	125.0	1.9	1.8	18.8	16.6	14.9	20.1
Estonia	1.3	1.3	29.8	1.6	1.8	15.3	18.3	16.6	18.6
Finland	5.3	5.5	15.6	1.8	1.8	17.0	16.6	16.5	22.3
France	60.9	64.9	111.3	1.9	1.8	18.4	17.4	16.4	20.9
Georgia	4.4	4.0	63.1	1.5	1.7	20.4	17.5	14.2	16.1
Germany	82.7	80.4	230.9	1.4	1.4	14.1	12.3	19.3	23.0
Greece	11.2	11.3	84.5	1.4	1.5	14.3	13.8	18.6	20.7
Hungary	10.1	9.8	108.3	1.3	1.5	15.5	14.9	15.7	19.3
Iceland	0.3	0.4	3.0	2.1	1.9	21.0	19.4	11.5	14.6
Ireland	4.3	5.1	60.3	2.0	1.8	20.4	20.3	11.0	13.8
Israel	7.2	8.3	334.9	2.9	2.3	28.3	24.9	9.9	12.8
Italy	59.4	60.4	195.6	1.4	1.5	14.1	13.4	19.8	23.0
Kazakhstan	15.5	16.7	5.6	2.5	2.0	24.0	25.4	7.8	8.2
Kyrgyzstan	5.2	6.2	25.8	2.7	2.0	30.7	27.4	5.5	6.0
Latvia	2.3	2.1	35.4	1.4	1.6	13.9	16.1	17.2	18.3
Lithuania	3.4	3.1	52.1	1.4	1.5	15.6	14.9	15.7	17.9
Luxembourg	0.5	0.5	181.7	1.6	1.8	18.7	16.7	14.3	15.2
Malta	0.4	0.4	1 270.2	1.4	1.4	16.5	13.7	13.8	20.1
Monaco	0.04	–	16 842.1	1.8	–	–	–	–	–
Montenegro	0.6	0.6	45.2	–	1.8	20.3	17.8	12.6	15.2
Netherlands	16.4	17.1	393.6	1.7	1.8	18.0	16.1	14.6	19.7
Norway	4.8	5.2	14.4	1.9	1.8	19.5	17.6	14.7	18.0
Poland	38.5	37.5	122.0	1.3	1.4	16.0	14.5	13.4	18.3
Portugal	10.6	10.8	115.1	1.3	1.5	15.7	13.9	16.9	20.6
Republic of Moldova	3.6	3.4	105.9	1.3	1.6	17.9	18.2	10.3	13.9
Romania	21.5	20.4	90.5	1.3	1.4	15.3	14.6	14.9	17.4
Russian Federation	141.9	135.4	8.3	1.3	1.6	14.8	16.7	14.0	15.4
San Marino	0.03	–	518.3	1.2	–	15.9	–	15.6	–
Serbia	7.4	9.8	83.9	1.4	1.7	15.5	17.0	17.2	16.6
Slovakia	5.4	5.4	110.2	1.3	1.4	16.6	15.1	11.7	16.1
Slovenia	2.0	2.0	99.2	1.4	1.6	13.9	14.5	16.0	20.3
Spain	43.6	48.6	85.7	1.4	1.7	14.5	15.6	16.8	18.7
Sweden	9.1	9.7	20.2	1.9	1.8	17.1	17.3	17.3	21.0
Switzerland	7.3	7.9	181.3	1.4	1.6	15.9	14.6	16.1	20.2
Tajikistan	6.7	8.4	46.1	3.5	2.5	35.9	32.8	4.4	3.9
The former Yugoslav Republic of Macedonia	2.0	2.0	79.4	1.5	1.6	20.7	16.0	10.7	14.8
Turkey	70.6	83.9	93.7	2.2	1.9	26.4	23.1	7.1	7.5
Turkmenistan	5.0	5.8	10.0	2.6	2.0	39.2	26.4	3.8	5.1
Ukraine	45.5	42.9	77.2	1.3	1.6	14.3	16.0	16.3	16.9
United Kingdom	61.0	65.1	248.8	1.8	1.8	17.6	17.4	16.0	18.5
Uzbekistan	26.9	31.2	59.2	2.6	2.0	33.0	25.8	4.5	5.4

Sources: The data for 2007 (or the latest available year) come from the European Health for All database (Copenhagen, WHO Regional Office for Europe, 2009 (http://www.euro.who.int/hfadb, accessed 27 May 2009)). The 2020 data are medium variant projections from World population prospects: the 2008 revision population database (New York, United Nations, 2009 (http://esa.un.org/unpp/index.asp?panel=2, accessed 27 May 2009)).

Table 2. Basic socioeconomic indicators in the WHO European Region, 2007 or latest available year

Member State	Human Development Index	GDP (US$ per capita)	Real GDP (international dollars (PPP) per capita)	Total government expenditure (% of GDP)	Population aged ≥ 25 (% of total) with:			Population in the labour force (% of total)	Unemployment rate (%)
					primary education	secondary education	postsecondary education		
Albania	0.801	2 439	5 316	30.4	–	–	–	43.5	13.8
Andorra	0.921	–	–	19.2	–	–	–	–	–
Armenia	0.775	1 017	4 945	21.8	–	–	–	43.0	6.7
Austria	0.948	38 924	33 700	49.7	49.3	94.0	6.1	48.6	6.8
Azerbaijan	0.746	1 026	5 016	25.3	8.6	70.1	14	51.0	1.2
Belarus	0.804	2 330	7 918	47.9	32.5	45.8	12.5	49.3	1.0
Belgium	0.946	37 522	32 119	51.8	60.6	28.7	5.2	43.1	11.5
Bosnia and Herzegovina	0.803	2 183	7 032	37.0	27.2	65.5	7.3	52.9	31.1
Bulgaria	0.824	3 109	9 032	38.9	49.1	35.7	15	39.7	9.0
Croatia	0.850	7 724	13 042	43.4	53.8	39.5	6.4	43.8	11.1
Cyprus	0.903	18 668	22 699	44.0	–	–	–	50.1	4.5
Czech Republic	0.891	13 949	20 538	44.9	31.7	58.6	8.5	50.9	5.3
Denmark	0.949	50 765	33 973	53.3	–	41.6	19.6	52.1	3.4
Estonia	0.860	8 331	15 478	33.4	41.2	45.1	13.7	49.8	4.7
Finland	0.952	39 643	32 153	50.5	45.06	37.86	17.07	50.5	6.9
France	0.952	35 445	30 386	53.6	51.7	36.9	11.4	44.2	9.8
Georgia	0.754	1 151	3 365	28.2	–	–	–	50.6	13.8
Germany	0.935	35 241	29 461	46.9	–	18.0	4.3	50.0	10.3
Greece	0.926	23 991	23 381	37.5	62.6	28.7	8.7	47.2	8.8
Hungary	0.874	11 212	17 887	49.8	59.2	30.7	10.1	41.8	7.4
Iceland	0.968	54 657	36 510	42.4	–	–	–	60.0	2.9
Ireland	0.959	51 567	38 505	33.8	41.75	46.3	13.1	51.1	4.5
Israel	0.932	17 194	25 864	46.3	24.9	40.0	35.1	39.6	7.3
Italy	0.941	31 659	28 529	48.2	31.46	22.9	7.54	41.8	6.1
Kazakhstan	0.794	2 717	7 857	27.0	36.9	50.7	12.4	55.0	7.3
Kyrgyzstan	0.696	433	1 927	28.5	–	51.3	12.5	45.0	8.1
Latvia	0.855	5 868	13 646	35.6	40.3	46.3	13.4	48.2	4.9
Lithuania	0.862	6 480	14 494	33.5	30.4	57.0	12.6	48.0	4.3
Luxembourg	0.944	67 795	60 228	42.3	39.7	40.3	10.8	43.0	4.2
Malta	0.878	13 256	19 189	44.9	47.6	40.1	4.47	43.1	6.5
Monaco	0.925	–	–	21.3	21.8	41.1	23.58	–	2.5
Montenegro	–	–	–	29.9	–	–	–	–	30.3
Netherlands	0.953	40 860	32 684	45.2	14.0	64.0	22	53.0	4.2
Norway	0.968	72 016	41 420	42.1	0.2	81.3	18.7	54.9	2.5
Poland	0.870	8 969	13 847	43.3	44.3	47.8	7.9	45.4	13.8
Portugal	0.897	18 335	20 410	47.6	77.6	14.8	7.7	53.1	8.0
Republic of Moldova	0.708	615	2 100	37.0	29.8	58.9	11.3	52.4	1.9
Romania	0.813	3 374	9 060	31.2	29.8	63.2	6.9	47.0	7.3
Russian Federation	0.802	4 042	10 845	31.9	–	49.0	14.1	51.7	7.2
San Marino	0.916	–	–	44.6	68.9	28.7	2.4	66.2	1.6
Serbia	–	–	–	38.0	–	–	–	–	18.1
Slovakia	0.863	10 219	15 871	38.4	38.6	50.9	9.5	50.0	11.0
Slovenia	0.917	16 115	22 273	46.0	48.3	42.9	8.8	52.1	7.7
Spain	0.949	27 825	27 169	38.5	65.3	25.5	8.4	48.5	8.5
Sweden	0.956	43 267	32 525	55.3	32.4	43.0	23	51.9	5.4
Switzerland	0.955	51 970	35 633	36.4	24.0	57.0	19	56.4	3.8
Tajikistan	0.673	322	1 356	22.7	22.8	65.5	11.7	33.7	2.7
The former Yugoslav Republic of Macedonia	0.801	2 637	7 200	35.0	56.2	30.6	6.7	42.8	34.9
Turkey	0.806	9 305	13 669	24.2	77.8	21.9	10.8	46.2	10.3
Turkmenistan	0.713	1 294	3 838	21.6	–	–	–	46.7	–
Ukraine	0.788	1 366	6 848	43.6	–	40.5	6.5	47.7	6.8
United Kingdom	0.946	39 793	33 238	44.9	89.0	–	11	51.0	5.0
Uzbekistan	0.702	456	2 063	32.1	–	–	–	44.6	0.4

Table 3. Improving health outcomes in the WHO European Region

Member State	Life expectancy at birth (years), 2007[a]		Healthy life expectancy at birth (years), 2007		Probability of dying before age 5 years (per 1000 live births)		Maternal mortality ratio (per 100 000 live births)		Perinatal deaths (per 1000 births), 2007[a]
	Males	Females	Males	Females	National data reports, 2007[a]	WHO estimates, 2004	National data reports, 2007[a]	WHO/UNICEF/UNFPA/World Bank estimates, 2005	
Albania	73.7	78.9	64	64	12.4	18.5	15.1	92	11.5
Andorra	–	–	72	76	–	6.5	0.0	–	0.0
Armenia	70.0	75.9	59	63	13.4	32.0	15.0	76	15.3
Austria	77.6	83.2	70	74	4.4	5.0	3.9	4	3.1
Azerbaijan	71.3	76.3	59	60	14.5	89.5	34.9	82	8.9
Belarus	64.6	76.3	58	66	6.9	10.0	6.8	18	4.0
Belgium	74.6	81.1	70	74	5.9	4.5	5.3	8	7.4
Bosnia and Herzegovina	69.5	76.0	65	68	16.1	15.5	21.6	3	–
Bulgaria	69.1	76.3	63	69	14.5	15.0	10.0	11	11.0
Croatia	72.6	79.4	66	70	6.1	7.5	9.7	7	4.9
Cyprus	78.8	82.6	69	71	4.0	5.0	11.5	10	–
Czech Republic	73.8	80.3	68	72	4.0	4.5	2.6	4	3.6
Denmark	75.7	80.5	70	73	4.0	5.0	14.0	3	3.1
Estonia	67.3	78.2	61	71	7.3	8.0	0.0	25	4.3
Finland	76.1	83.2	70	75	3.5	4.0	1.7	7	3.3
France	77.5	84.6	71	76	4.4	4.5	7.4	8	6.9
Georgia	69.3	76.7	62	67	19.4	44.5	20.2	66	16.3
Germany	77.2	82.4	71	75	4.6	5.0	6.1	4	5.6
Greece	77.2	82.0	71	74	4.3	5.0	1.8	3	5.3
Hungary	68.8	77.2	62	69	7.5	8.0	8.2	6	4.9
Iceland	79.7	83.5	73	75	3.4	2.5	0.0	4	1.9
Ireland	77.5	82.2	71	74	4.3	6.0	1.4	1	5.1
Israel	78.2	82.1	72	74	5.5	6.0	7.3	4	4.8
Italy	78.6	84.3	73	76	4.3	4.5	2.0	3	4.6
Kazakhstan	60.8	72.3	53	60	18.6	72.5	47.5	140	14.1
Kyrgyzstan	63.5	71.7	55	59	35.5	67.5	60.9	150	21.8
Latvia	65.8	76.5	59	68	10.3	11.0	25.8	10	6.5
Lithuania	64.9	77.3	58	68	7.2	9.5	6.2	11	5.2
Luxembourg	77.0	82.2	71	75	3.2	5.5	18.6	12	3.6
Malta	77.7	82.3	71	74	6.7	6.0	0.0	8	4.1
Monaco	–	–	71	76	–	4.0	0.0	–	12.2
Montenegro	71.4	76.9	65	66	11.0	–	–	–	6.8
Netherlands	78.2	82.7	72	74	4.8	5.5	5.0	6	5.7
Norway	78.3	83.0	72	74	3.9	4.0	8.5	7	3.6
Poland	71.0	79.8	64	70	7.1	7.5	2.9	8	5.0
Portugal	74.9	81.6	69	73	5.2	5.5	8.2	11	4.2
Republic of Moldova	65.2	72.7	58	63	14.0	28.0	18.4	22	10.3
Romania	69.7	76.9	63	68	14.2	20.0	15.4	24	10.0
Russian Federation	60.5	73.3	55	65	13.0	16.0	23.8	28	9.0
San Marino	78.9	83.2	74	76	0.5	3.5	0.0	–	0.0
Serbia	70.9	76.5	64	66	8.1	–	12.7	–	6.9
Slovakia	70.3	78.2	64	70	8.6	8.5	5.6	6	5.3
Slovenia	74.8	82.1	69	74	3.8	4.5	15.1	6	3.9
Spain	77.1	83.8	71	76	4.7	4.5	3.9	4	4.7
Sweden	78.9	83.2	72	75	3.5	3.5	4.7	3	4.3
Switzerland	79.4	84.4	73	76	5.1	5.0	8.2	5	7.6
Tajikistan	71.2	76.3	58	57	16.6	117.5	43.4	170	15.1
The former Yugoslav Republic of Macedonia	71.1	76.1	65	66	13.0	14.0	0.0	10	15.3
Turkey	71.1	75.6	64	67	26.6	32.0	21.2	44	8.1
Turkmenistan	62.5	69.8	53	57	53.2	102.5	15.6	130	9.5
Ukraine	62.3	73.8	55	64	12.3	18.0	15.2	18	9.0
United Kingdom	77.7	81.9	71	73	5.8	5.5	7.3	8	8.2
Uzbekistan	68.2	73.0	58	60	20.8	68.5	25.0	24	7.5

[a] Data from 2007 or the latest available year.

Table 4. Factors influencing health – environment, lifestyle and behaviour – in the WHO European Region, 2007 or latest available year

Member State	Population (% of total) with:		Deaths due to work-related accidents (per 100 000)	Regular daily smokers in the population aged ≥ 15 (% of total)	Pure alcohol consumption (litres per capita)	Road traffic accidents involving alcohol (per 100 000)	People killed or injured in road traffic accidents (per 100 000)	First admissions to drug treatment centres (per 100 000)
	homes connected to water supply system	access to hygienic means of sewage disposal						
Albania	68	89	–	39.0	1.7	0.5	35.5	–
Andorra	–	100	1.5	36.0	–	7.5	205.3	–
Armenia	85	84	0.5	27.0	1.1	2.3	54.5	3.0
Austria	100	100	2.4	23.2	10.5	34.7	655.9	30.6
Azerbaijan	47	55	1.5	17.7	3.1	1.0	43.1	6.2
Belarus	61	–	2.2	27.5	4.8	7.7	93.7	13.1
Belgium	100	100	1.0	22.0	8.9	41.0	616.5	–
Bosnia and Herzegovina	82	93	0.6	37.6	8.3	–	176.9	–
Bulgaria	99	100	1.7	32.7	5.0	5.4	143.3	–
Croatia	94	93	1.7	27.4	10.3	88.0	503.6	39.0
Cyprus	100	100	1.8	23.9	9.0	2.4	316.4	–
Czech Republic	87	75	1.8	25.4	13.7	27.3	327.3	37.4
Denmark	100	100	0.9	24.0	9.8	20.1	146.5	24.7
Estonia	87	82	1.6	29.9	13.4	42.2	237.5	89.7
Finland	97	100	0.9	20.6	8.2	19.3	178.5	–
France	99	96	1.0	25.4	10.0	–	185.9	51.3
Georgia	58	83	1.5	27.8	1.3	2.8	107.7	6.3
Germany	100	93	1.1	33.9	10.7	29.4	531.9	–
Greece	84	96	1.0	37.6	7.7	13.1	197.5	17.3
Hungary	91	56	1.2	30.4	11.6	28.8	347.1	40.3
Iceland	100	100	2.0	19.5	5.5	7.9	348.8	76.6
Ireland	97	96	1.5	24.0	10.6	–	203.8	57.1
Israel	100	100	1.1	23.2	1.7	4.8	542.2	25.2
Italy	99	100	1.4	22.4	7.6	5.1	553.9	59.3
Kazakhstan	61	72	2.2	23.1	2.2	8.2	146.1	206.9
Kyrgyzstan	48	60	0.4	20.0	2.4	6.1	96.0	8.2
Latvia	–	–	2.6	30.4	8.4	32.3	262.6	14.7
Lithuania	–	–	2.9	26.5	8.6	28.8	270.8	9.4
Luxembourg	100	100	2.1	25.0	14.6	31.3	248.8	–
Malta	100	100	1.7	23.4	5.4	0.3	297.6	96.6
Monaco	100	100	10.7	–	–	53.3	833.3	–
Montenegro	–	–	0.2	–	–	–	–	–
Netherlands	98	100	0.4	29.1	7.8	12.8	209.5	30.1
Norway	100	100	0.8	22.0	4.8	–	247.4	–
Poland	95	80	1.3	29.0	6.7	15.1	174.6	–
Portugal	82	100	2.9	20.9	9.4	21.5	506.0	44.8
Republic of Moldova	41	68	1.5	27.1	10.2	7.8	100.8	10.3
Romania	49	51	1.9	21.4	7.4	1.4	39.4	–
Russian Federation	81	87	2.0	35.8	8.9	71.6	198.8	11.9
San Marino	100	100	–	22.7	–	–	–	–
Serbia	–	–	–	26.2	–	–	–	–
Slovakia	83	100	1.6	28.0	9.5	20.9	205.8	16.4
Slovenia	98	98	2.1	18.9	8.8	88.3	728.2	13.7
Spain	99	97	1.6	26.4	10.0	10.6	316.3	51.5
Sweden	100	100	0.8	15.9	5.6	11.7	300.9	–
Switzerland	100	100	0.6	22.0	9.4	34.4	365.1	–
Tajikistan	40	53	0.4	–	0.3	0.3	36.4	8.6
The former Yugoslav Republic of Macedonia	–	–	0.2	36.0	1.9	10.0	212.3	3.5
Turkey	93	88	2.3	27.4	1.2	26.8	273.9	2.2
Turkmenistan	52	62	3.5	14.0	0.7	1.8	46.9	64.6
Ukraine	78	99	2.1	36.0	5.2	6.3	128.2	26.2
United Kingdom	100	96	0.3	25.0	9.3	18.8	449.9	16.8
Uzbekistan	53	57	–	12.5	1.0	–	57.6	10.7

Table 5. Health system financing, immunization and Stop TB Strategy in the WHO European Region

Member State	Total health expenditure, WHO estimates, 2005		General government health expenditure, 2005, as:		Children immunized (%), 2007[a]		People receiving social or disability benefits (per 100 000), 2007[a]	TB under DOTS (%)	
	As % of GDP	Per capita (international dollars (PPP))	% of total health expenditure	% of total government expenditure	With DTP3	Against measles		Cases detected, 2006[a]	Treatment success, 2005[a]
Albania	6.5	353	40.3	8.6	98	97	–	37	77
Andorra	6.3	2 697	70.5	23.1	96	94	1 596	125	80
Armenia	5.4	270	32.9	8.2	88	92	4 920	59	72
Austria	10.2	3 485	75.7	15.6	85	77	–	46	75
Azerbaijan	3.9	193	24.8	3.8	95	97	3 392	50	59
Belarus	6.6	515	75.8	10.5	95	99	5 263	40	73
Belgium	9.6	3 071	71.4	13.2	99	92	2 561	55	66
Bosnia and Herzegovina	8.8	779	58.7	14	91	96	0	62	97
Bulgaria	7.7	734	60.6	12.1	95	96	–	94	86
Croatia	7.4	1 001	81.3	13.9	96	96	8 642	0	–
Cyprus	6.1	1 550	43.2	6	97	87	–	42	63
Czech Republic	7.1	1 447	88.6	14.1	98	97	5 593	57	72
Denmark	9.4	3 169	83.6	14.8	75	89	3 518	62	83
Estonia	5.0	846	76.9	11.5	95	96	8 390	66	72
Finland	7.5	2 299	77.8	11.6	99	98	5 353	0	–
France	11.2	3 406	79.9	16.6	96	93	458	0	–
Georgia	8.6	318	19.5	5.9	98	97	945	109	73
Germany	10.7	3 250	76.9	17.5	90	95	8 363	54	71
Greece	10.1	2 949	42.8	11.5	88	88	1 238	0	–
Hungary	7.8	1 329	70.8	11.1	100	100	7 023	49	45
Iceland	9.4	3 354	82.5	18.3	97	95	4 347	71	100
Ireland	8.2	3 125	79.5	19.2	92	87	295	0	–
Israel	7.8	2 143	66.5	11.2	96	97	3 593	31	78
Italy	8.9	2 494	76.6	14.1	96	87	2 681	71	74
Kazakhstan	3.9	306	64.2	9.3	93	100	2 635	69	71
Kyrgyzstan	6.0	113	39.5	8.4	94	99	2 149	63	85
Latvia	6.4	860	60.5	10.8	98	97	6 466	85	74
Lithuania	5.9	862	67.3	11.9	95	97	6 223	109	70
Luxembourg	7.7	5 521	90.7	16.5	99	96	–	4	–
Malta	8.4	1 733	77.4	14.6	74	79	2 751	36	100
Monaco	4.6	5 447	74.9	16.3	99	99	–	–	–
Montenegro	8	106	75.5	20.3	92	90	1 682	–	–
Netherlands	9.2	3 187	64.9	13.2	96	96	5 829	36	84
Norway	9.1	4 331	83.5	18	93	92	6 205	39	91
Poland	6.2	844	69.3	9.9	99	98	8 114	67	77
Portugal	10.2	2 034	72.3	15.5	97	95	3 443	88	89
Republic of Moldova	7.5	170	55.5	11.3	97	96	3 646	69	62
Romania	5.5	507	70.3	12.4	97	97	94	79	82
Russian Federation	5.2	561	62	10.1	98	99	3 978	44	58
San Marino	7.3	3 191	85.7	14	92	92	–	0	0
Serbia	8.0	395	71.9	15.1	94	95	–	–	–
Slovakia	7.1	1 130	74.4	13.8	99	99	3 644	43	92
Slovenia	8.5	1 959	72.4	13.4	97	96	–	71	84
Spain	8.2	2 242	71.4	15.3	96	97	–	0	–
Sweden	9.2	3 012	81.7	13.6	99	96	6 031	58	64
Switzerland	11.4	4 088	59.3	18.6	95	86	3 425	0	–
Tajikistan	5.0	67	22.8	5	86	85	2 032	33	86
The former Yugoslav Republic of Macedonia	7.8	569	70.4	15.8	95	96	15 882	66	84
Turkey	5.7	618	71.4	13.9	96	96	447	80	91
Turkmenistan	4.8	308	66.7	14.9	98	99	–	58	81
Ukraine	7.0	488	52.8	8.4	98	98	5 318	65	–
United Kingdom	8.2	2 598	87.1	16	92	86	–	0	–
Uzbekistan	5.0	171	47.7	7.4	97	100	921	48	81

[a] Or latest available year.

Note. WHO computed the figures to ensure comparability; they are not necessarily the official statistics of Member States, which may use alternative rigorous methods.

Table 6. Human resources for health in the WHO European Region, 2007 or latest available year

Member State	Number per 100 000					Number graduated per 100 000			
	Physicians	GPs	Nurses	Dentists	Pharmacists	Physicians	Nurses	Dentists	Pharmacists
Albania	115.0	50.9	404.3	32.9	39.2	6.2	9.2	2.3	1.2
Andorra	303.0	47.5	326.1	57.2	88.8	2.4	18.3	1.2	1.2
Armenia	343.7	58.1	413.0	36.1	5.1	8.9	34.7	2.2	1.0
Austria	374.9	153.0	634.6	54.0	59.5	19.4	34.4	1.2	2.4
Azerbaijan	377.4	17.6	725.4	29.4	18.8	14.3	8.8	1.8	4.1
Belarus	484.1	40.2	1 197.6	49.3	30.9	13.2	20.7	2.2	1.7
Belgium	422.8	177.3	1 341.3	83.5	116.0	8.4	55.3	1.1	3.7
Bosnia and Herzegovina	141.8	20.4	437.2	16.1	7.9	2.9	66.3	2.6	2.1
Bulgaria	364.4	65.0	421.0	84.0	12.5	14.6	15.9	2.0	1.2
Croatia	259.0	65.0	523.6	71.7	57.2	9.6	–	3.5	3.2
Cyprus	252.9	–	436.0	92.8	20.8	0.0	–	–	–
Czech Republic	356.6	71.4	842.7	67.3	56.0	7.7	47.2	1.3	2.6
Denmark	319.8	77.5	961.3	79.2	69.1	21.7	41.2	4.2	2.3
Estonia	328.5	63.5	655.2	87.5	64.7	7.9	44.1	2.9	4.7
Finland	331.0	95.0	855.3	85.3	155.1	7.0	49.8	1.0	7.0
France	341.6	166.6	793.2	68.0	115.7	6.0	35.5	1.3	3.9
Georgia	454.6	23.3	363.4	27.8	5.7	37.9	37.7	1.7	2.8
Germany	348.4	99.0	781.2	76.3	59.9	8.5	–	1.9	2.1
Greece	534.6	125.5	326.8	127.2	69.2	13.3	7.4	2.7	1.3
Hungary	278.0	64.9	903.9	42.2	54.5	10.0	36.6	1.9	2.4
Iceland	368.0	77.9	943.3	94.0	102.5	13.1	39.1	1.3	3.9
Ireland	302.9	71.7	1 549.8	58.5	96.9	16.7	41.6	1.5	3.3
Israel	352.6	70.5	579.0	108.8	74.0	4.3	22.4	0.9	2.5
Italy	365.4	91.6	700.7	62.8	74.7	11.5	17.7	2.7	4.1
Kazakhstan	370.6	24.2	692.3	36.9	81.7	28.4	45.1	1.4	3.4
Kyrgyzstan	238.0	35.4	543.2	19.6	1.7	17.3	64.4	2.2	0.9
Latvia	304.9	54.9	548.0	68.2	–	4.9	24.3	1.5	4.0
Lithuania	406.7	77.5	734.8	71.0	81.3	7.8	30.1	3.4	2.9
Luxembourg	290.0	92.5	1 023.1	78.5	85.0	–	12.8	0.0	–
Malta	331.7	82.7	583.5	42.8	154.0	14.7	7.8	2.0	8.3
Monaco	664.3	32.1	1 621.4	121.4	217.9	–	85.7	0.0	–
Montenegro	196.9	32.1	507.8	39.6	16.8	–	–	–	–
Netherlands	393.2	52.9	1 505.0	49.5	17.5	12.3	36.1	1.7	0.8
Norway	380.4	74.9	1 546.8	86.1	67.9	10.4	77.5	2.2	1.9
Poland	203.2	–	468.8	32.0	58.9	6.1	39.1	2.1	2.2
Portugal	342.6	56.1	481.4	58.3	97.8	7.0	23.9	3.1	4.9
Republic of Moldova	312.2	56.7	754.9	43.8	83.7	9.0	11.6	2.1	0.4
Romania	192.1	68.7	397.4	20.2	4.2	11.9	15.9	3.7	2.8
Russian Federation	431.0	27.3	806.2	32.0	8.1	10.7	27.2	1.8	1.9
San Marino	251.7	–	507.7	36.4	52.1	–	–	0.0	–
Serbia	271.1	68.9	557.4	33.3	25.9	15.9	–	5.2	5.0
Slovakia	313.3	43.3	631.6	45.3	49.0	9.9	85.6	0.9	3.1
Slovenia	237.3	48.8	764.8	59.9	47.0	6.4	21.5	2.1	6.1
Spain	375.7	76.8	743.7	56.2	92.0	8.7	20.2	2.5	5.2
Sweden	357.9	60.4	1 083.4	83.1	72.7	10.0	49.8	2.3	5.1
Switzerland	385.0	52.4	832.8	51.4	57.0	7.9	49.9	1.6	1.6
Tajikistan	201.3	20.8	446.6	15.2	10.3	8.0	20.5	0.7	0.6
The former Yugoslav Republic of Macedonia	254.2	96.2	369.8	57.6	44.5	8.4	9.3	5.7	5.1
Turkey	151.0	47.4	200.9	24.8	34.7	6.9	8.6	1.4	1.4
Turkmenistan	243.8	63.6	431.4	14.1	19.5	5.6	6.2	0.2	0.3
Ukraine	308.4	32.0	783.4	41.1	47.8	14.6	23.9	3.7	5.7
United Kingdom	212.6	67.3	498.6	43.9	58.6	6.4	48.8	1.3	1.3
Uzbekistan	266.6	20.1	1 012.0	17.7	3.4	12.9	160.3	1.0	12.3

Table 7. Health service delivery in the WHO European Region, 2007 or latest available year

Member State	Hospitals per 100 000	Non-inpatient health care establishments per 100 000	Beds per 100 000				Private in-patient hospital beds as % of all beds	Admissions per 100	
			Hospital	Acute care hospital	Psychiatric hospital	Nursing and elderly homes		Inpatient care	Acute care hospital
Albania	1.5	73.8	291.5	255.6	23.1	7.8	–	8.7	–
Andorra	2.4	113.2	261.6	194.7	14.6	170.4	25.6	–	9.3
Armenia	4.2	32.8	406.8	349.7	45.4	31.3	–	8.9	8.5
Austria	3.3	–	776.3	638.9	62.9	–	27.7	27.9	26.6
Azerbaijan	8.7	41.2	793.3	725.9	48.3	18.8	0.7	6.2	6.0
Belarus	7.2	69.0	1 122.9	–	69.9	178.6	0.1	28.5	–
Belgium	2.0	–	525.1	470.2	148.8	1 199.7	62.3	16.4	16.2
Bosnia and Herzegovina	1.0	30.3	303.6	327.5	37.2	–	–	8.2	7.2
Bulgaria	4.4	21.9	636.4	755.4	58.2	–	6.4	22.8	14.8
Croatia	1.7	70.7	534.6	352.4	93.9	–	0.4	16.5	14.6
Cyprus	12.3	–	371.5	350.8	26.7	–	50.1	7.9	7.8
Czech Republic	3.3	233.9	810.5	595.5	107.0	70.0	28.7	21.5	20.2
Denmark	1.1	–	349.5	310.7	60.4	230.6	2.0	15.2	17.8
Estonia	4.3	62.2	557.0	380.2	56.2	549.9	9.8	18.9	16.8
Finland	6.5	4.3	682.5	233.6	84.1	–	3.6	24.6	18.9
France	4.7	–	716.8	361.8	92.6	110.7	35.2	18.8	16.3
Georgia	6.0	14.4	331.9	291.5	28.1	6.8	–	6.5	6.3
Germany	4.1	–	829.1	572.9	108.4	917.8	27.1	22.6	19.8
Greece	2.8	15.3	481.7	394.4	87.3	30.7	28.1	18.4	14.5
Hungary	1.8	4.1	712.6	413.4	30.4	85.5	3.0	20.9	18.5
Iceland	6.8	40.6	750.8	368.2	117.9	812.0	8.9	17.2	16.5
Ireland	4.1	–	533.9	274.2	85.1	511.3	–	14.2	14.0
Israel	5.3	–	583.2	203.1	48.1	321.6	32.9	18.2	17.2
Italy	2.2	30.8	393.9	336.3	13.0	332.8	23.4	14.6	14.0
Kazakhstan	6.8	52.8	772.1	527.7	62.8	129.2	6.0	17.4	16.4
Kyrgyzstan	2.8	15.2	506.0	387.4	43.3	54.0	1.6	15.1	14.5
Latvia	4.1	116.8	757.1	523.3	137.0	–	6.3	23.4	20.4
Lithuania	4.9	28.8	814.0	509.3	102.3	437.3	0.3	23.8	21.2
Luxembourg	8.4	–	633.4	508.9	63.3	951.4	–	19.4	18.4
Malta	2.2	–	780.3	269.4	169.4	537.8	5.1	–	10.8
Monaco	7.1	0.0	1 957.1	1 553.6	210.7	1 217.9	–	53.9	–
Montenegro	1.8	31.3	397.8	308.4	49.7	–	–	10.9	9.9
Netherlands	1.2	–	480.8	340.2	137.1	1 040.5	–	10.6	10.5
Norway	1.5	–	391.2	284.2	57.0	865.1	1.3	18.8	16.9
Poland	2.1	26.3	516.2	410.8	64.8	–	4.7	17.8	–
Portugal	1.9	21.9	345.4	298.5	61.8	–	24.0	11.4	11.2
Republic of Moldova	2.3	19.7	612.0	493.2	54.9	79.7	0.7	17.2	16.3
Romania	1.9	54.5	654.3	505.2	77.3	–	0.6	24.3	–
Russian Federation	4.5	9.0	965.9	931.3	112.3	15.2	–	23.7	22.9
San Marino	–	–	716.0	–	–	–	–	–	–
Serbia	1.4	2.3	540.3	–	–	–	–	14.2	9.4
Slovakia	2.7	163.3	678.8	601.6	82.4	–	5.1	18.9	18.4
Slovenia	1.4	3.2	466.2	376.7	67.8	–	1.1	17.9	17.2
Spain	1.7	–	337.0	271.0	46.6	32.7	34.3	11.9	11.7
Sweden	0.9	11.2	522.0	282.3	48.8	27.0	19.0	15.6	15.2
Switzerland	4.5	–	553.9	364.8	105.8	1 167.1	–	17.0	16.4
Tajikistan	6.8	49.8	612.0	546.9	24.7	14.6	0.2	11.2	11.1
The former Yugoslav Republic of Macedonia	2.7	81.4	462.7	326.4	58.5	29.4	1.0	9.4	9.2
Turkey	1.9	22.8	263.8	253.5	9.6	26.5	9.3	12.4	12.2
Turkmenistan	2.3	35.7	406.5	303.9	32.9	8.1	0.2	13.9	12.8
Ukraine	5.6	14.6	873.0	711.9	93.9	100.7	–	21.9	20.8
United Kingdom	2.7	–	389.7	241.6	82.9	429.3	4.3	15.3	21.4
Uzbekistan	3.3	20.7	483.2	399.8	28.9	34.8	3.3	16.3	15.6

Definitions of the indicators included in the tables

Introductory note

Most definitions are those used by the European Health for All database (HFA-DB), which is the main source of the statistical data in the tables. Other sources of definitions are indicated as appropriate.

Terms are listed in the order in which they are presented in each table.

Table 1

Total mid-year population
Estimate of resident (de jure) population on 1 July of given calendar year, usually calculated as an average of end-year estimates. The central statistical office is the source in most countries. This data item is used as the denominator to calculate most other indicators. Although de facto population would be preferable, the de jure population is used because it is more commonly available, particularly in age-disaggregated form. In some countries, however, particularly in those affected by armed conflict in the 1990s, the difference between official population estimates and the population actually residing in the country (de facto population) may be too large. In such cases special efforts should be made to provide estimates for de facto population to be used as a denominator.
Source: European Health for All database (HFA-DB) [online database]. Copenhagen, WHO Regional Office for Europe, 2009 (http://www.euro.who.int/hfadb, accessed 27 May 2009).

Average population density per km^2
Simple ratio of the mid-year population to the country area.
Source: European Health for All database (HFA-DB) [online database]. Copenhagen, WHO Regional Office for Europe, 2009 (http://www.euro.who.int/hfadb, accessed 27 May 2009).

Total fertility rate
Average number of children that would be born per woman if all women lived to the end of their childbearing years and bore children according to a given set of age-specific fertility rates. It is computed by summing the age-specific fertility rates for all ages and multiplying by the interval into which the ages are grouped. Data are usually provided by country statistical offices. Reports of the World Bank, the United Nations Development Programme (UNDP) and country statistical yearbooks are used as data sources for the HFA-DB.
Source: European Health for All database (HFA-DB) [online database]. Copenhagen, WHO Regional Office for Europe, 2009 (http://www.euro.who.int/hfadb, accessed 27 May 2009).

Population aged < 15 (% of total)
Estimate of the resident (de jure) population aged 0–14 years on 1 July of given calendar year. Usually it is calculated as an average of end-year estimates. The central statistical office is the source in most countries.
Source: European Health for All database (HFA-DB) [online database]. Copenhagen, WHO Regional Office for Europe, 2009 (http://www.euro.who.int/hfadb, accessed 27 May 2009).

Population aged ≥ 65 (% of total)
Estimate of resident (de jure) population aged 65 years and above on 1 July of given calendar year, usually calculated as an average of end-year estimates. The central statistical office is the source in most countries.
Source: European Health for All database (HFA-DB) [online database]. Copenhagen, WHO Regional Office for Europe, 2009 (http://www.euro.who.int/hfadb, accessed 27 May 2009).

Table 2

Human Development Index
Composite index measuring average achievement in three basic dimensions of human development: a long and healthy life, knowledge and a decent standard of living. UNDP reports are used as a data source for the HFA-DB. For details on how the Index is calculated, see the latest UNDP human development report.
Sources: European Health for All database (HFA-DB) [online database]. Copenhagen, WHO Regional Office for Europe, 2009 (http://www.euro.who.int/hfadb, accessed 27 May 2009) and UNDP.

GDP [gross domestic product] in US$ per capita
Total output of goods and services for final use produced by an economy, by both residents and non-residents, regardless of the allocation to domestic and foreign claims. The WHO Regional Office for Europe uses World Bank reports as a common data source, and the Organisation for Economic Co-operation and Development (OECD) health database as the primary data source for OECD member states.
Source: European Health for All database (HFA-DB) [online database]. Copenhagen, WHO Regional Office for Europe, 2009 (http://www.euro.who.int/hfadb, accessed 27 May 2009).

Real GDP in international dollars (PPP) per capita
GDP expressed in purchasing power parity (PPP) is adjusted to the relative domestic purchasing power of the national currency as compared to the US dollar, rather than using the official exchange rate. Multipliers (PPPs) are estimated periodically, using the cost of the standard basket of goods. The WHO Regional Office for Europe uses OECD and UNDP as common data sources.
Source: European Health for All database (HFA-DB) [online database]. Copenhagen, WHO Regional Office for Europe, 2009 (http://www.euro.who.int/hfadb, accessed 27 May 2009).

Total government expenditure as % of GDP
Total government expenditure corresponds to the consolidated outlays of all levels of government (central/federal, provincial/regional/state/district and municipal/local governments) social security institutions and extrabudgetary funds, including capital outlays.
Source: European Health for All database (HFA-DB) [online database]. Copenhagen, WHO Regional Office for Europe, 2009 (http://www.euro.who.int/hfadb, accessed 27 May 2009).

Population with primary education (% of total)
Proportion of the population aged 25 years or more with the highest level of education attained corresponding to primary, incomplete primary or no formal schooling. The main data source is the Institute for Statistics of the United Nations Educational, Scientific and Cultural Organization (UNESCO). Some countries provided data directly to the WHO Regional Office for Europe.

Source: European Health for All database (HFA-DB) [online database]. Copenhagen, WHO Regional Office for Europe, 2009 (http://www.euro.who.int/hfadb, accessed 27 May 2009).

Population with secondary education (% of total)
Proportion of the population aged 25 years or more with the highest level of education attained corresponding to secondary education (lower or higher level). The main data source is the UNESCO Institute for Statistics. Some countries provided data directly to the WHO Regional Office for Europe.
Source: European Health for All database (HFA-DB) [online database]. Copenhagen, WHO Regional Office for Europe, 2009 (http://www.euro.who.int/hfadb, accessed 27 May 2009).

Population with postsecondary education (% of total)
Proportion of the population aged 25 years or more with the highest level of education attained corresponding to postsecondary education. The main data source is the UNESCO Institute for Statistics. Some countries provided data directly to the WHO Regional Office for Europe.
Source: European Health for All database (HFA-DB) [online database]. Copenhagen, WHO Regional Office for Europe, 2009 (http://www.euro.who.int/hfadb, accessed 27 May 2009).

Population in the labour force (% of total)
Economically active population as a percentage of the total population. The data source for HFA-DB is the International Labour Organization (ILO) yearbook of labour statistics.
Source: European Health for All database (HFA-DB) [online database]. Copenhagen, WHO Regional Office for Europe, 2009 (http://www.euro.who.int/hfadb, accessed 27 May 2009).

Unemployment rate (%)
Ratio of the unemployed people to the total labour force. The ILO definition is applied, in which the unemployed comprise all people above a specified age who were without work, currently available for work or seeking work during the reference period. The WHO Regional Office for Europe uses the ILO yearbook of labour statistics as a common source of data.
Sources: European Health for All database (HFA-DB) [online database]. Copenhagen, WHO Regional Office for Europe, 2009 (http://www.euro.who.int/hfadb, accessed 27 May 2009) and *Yearbook of labour statistics 2008* (Geneva, International Labour Organization, 2008).

Table 3

Life expectancy at birth (years)
Average number of years that a newborn baby is expected to live if current mortality rates continue to apply, calculated by the WHO Regional Office for Europe for all countries that report detailed mortality data to WHO, using Wiesler's method. Mortality data are disaggregated by age: 0, 1–4, 5–9, 10–14, etc., 80–84, ≥ 85 years. Unfortunately, some countries cannot ensure complete registration of all deaths and births. As a result, life expectancy calculated using incomplete mortality data is higher than it actually is, and intercountry comparisons should be made with caution. In some cases, underregistration of deaths may reach 20%. Particularly high levels of mortality underregistration are observed in countries that were affected by armed conflict during the 1990s. In one such country (Georgia), the lack of sufficiently accurate population estimates used as denominator aggravates this problem.

Source: European Health for All database (HFA-DB) [online database]. Copenhagen, WHO Regional Office for Europe, 2009 (http://www.euro.who.int/hfadb, accessed 27 May 2009).

Healthy life expectancy at birth (years)

Equivalent number of years in full health that a newborn child can expect to live based on the current mortality rates and prevalence distribution of health states in the population. Healthy life expectancy at birth is based on life expectancy but includes an adjustment for time spent in poor health. The source of the data is the January 2009 draft of *World health statistics 2009*.

Source: *World health statistics 2009*. Geneva, World Health Organization, 2009 (http://www.who.int/whosis/whostat/2009/en/index.html, accessed 4 June 2009).

Probability of dying before age 5 years (per 1000 live births), national data reports

Number of deaths per 1000 live births until 5 years of age. The figures are taken from the appropriate cells of the relevant life tables and as such are by-products of the life expectancy calculations, i.e. (1 − L5 probability to survive by 5) x 1000. Unfortunately, some countries cannot ensure complete registration of all deaths and births. Thus, under-5 mortality rates calculated using incomplete mortality data are lower than they actually are and intercountry comparisons should be made with caution. Particularly high levels of mortality underregistration are observed in the countries of central Asia and the Caucasus, some countries of the former Yugoslavia and Albania.

Source: European Health for All database (HFA-DB) [online database]. Copenhagen, WHO Regional Office for Europe, 2009 (http://www.euro.who.int/hfadb, accessed 27 May 2009).

Probability of dying before age 5 years (per 1000 live births), WHO estimates

WHO headquarters makes these estimates, using special techniques, and publishes them in the annual world health reports. Data from various sources, including surveys, have been used when routine vital statistics were unavailable or incomplete. The estimates were also partially harmonized with survey-based estimates used by the United Nations Children's Fund (UNICEF) and other organizations. These estimates may differ significantly from the official national figures for some countries, where the registration of deaths and births is incomplete.

Source: European Health for All database (HFA-DB) [online database]. Copenhagen, WHO Regional Office for Europe, 2009 (http://www.euro.who.int/hfadb, accessed 27 May 2009).

Maternal mortality ratio (per 100 000 live births), national data reports

A maternal death is death of a woman while pregnant or within 42 days of termination of pregnancy, irrespective of the duration and the site of the pregnancy, from any cause related to or aggravated by the pregnancy or its management, but not from accidental or incidental causes (International Statistical Classification of Diseases and Related Health Problems, tenth revision (ICD-10) code: O00-O99). Two sources of information on maternal mortality are used to calculate this indicator:

- routine mortality data by cause regularly reported to WHO (in most cases from central statistical offices); and
- hospital data reported to health ministries.

Normally, the numbers of maternal deaths from both sources should be identical. This is the case in most western countries, but differences arise in some countries, mainly in the eastern part of the WHO European Region, owing to national practices of death certification and

coding. In such cases, hospital data are likely to be accurate. Since the January 2001 version of HFA-DB, the maternal mortality rate has been calculated using both data sources (when both figures are reported) and HFA-DB uses the larger figure. Nevertheless, experts argue that, even in countries with good vital registration systems, maternal mortality is actually about 50% higher than the official figures. WHO, UNICEF and the United Nations Population Fund (UNFPA) have therefore developed adjusted estimates for selected years.
Source: European Health for All database (HFA-DB) [online database]. Copenhagen, WHO Regional Office for Europe, 2009 (http://www.euro.who.int/hfadb, accessed 27 May 2009).

Maternal mortality ratio (per 100 000 live births), WHO/UNICEF/UNFPA/World Bank estimates
WHO and UNICEF, with the participation of UNFPA and the World Bank, have developed an approach to estimating maternal mortality that seeks to generate estimates for countries with no data and to correct available data for underreporting and misclassification. These estimates may differ significantly from the national statistics reported by the countries to WHO. The source of the estimates is the WHO, UNICEF, UNFPA and World Bank publication on maternal mortality.
Source: *Maternal mortality in 2005. Estimates developed by WHO, UNICEF, UNFPA and the World Bank*. Geneva, World Health Organization, 2007 (http://www.who.int/making_pregnancy_safer/documents/9789241596213/en, access 27 May 2009).

Perinatal deaths (per 1000 births)
Number of weight-specific (≥ 1000 g) fetal deaths and early neonatal deaths per 1000 births (live births and stillbirths). If weight-specific data are not available, any available data provided according to national criteria are used as a proxy.
Source: European Health for All database (HFA-DB) [online database]. Copenhagen, WHO Regional Office for Europe, 2009 (http://www.euro.who.int/hfadb, accessed 27 May 2009).

Table 4

Population with homes connected to a water supply system (% of total)
Percentage based on data from various sources. Definitions and estimation methods used may differ significantly between countries and time periods. For more detail, see HFA-DB.
Source: European Health for All database (HFA-DB) [online database]. Copenhagen, WHO Regional Office for Europe, 2009 (http://www.euro.who.int/hfadb, accessed 27 May 2009).

Population with access to hygienic means of sewage disposal (% of total)
Percentage with access to a sewage system, septic tank or other hygienic means of sewage disposal based on data from various sources. Definitions and estimation methods used may differ significantly between countries and time periods. For more detail, see HFA-DB.
Source: European Health for All database (HFA-DB) [online database]. Copenhagen, WHO Regional Office for Europe, 2009 (http://www.euro.who.int/hfadb, accessed 27 May 2009).

Deaths due to work-related accidents (per 100 000)
Number of deaths per 100 000 population due to work-related accidents: those occurring at or in the course of work which may result in death, personal injury or disease. The data source is the ILO yearbook of labour statistics. All industries are included, but commuting accidents (on the way to or from work) are excluded. National definitions and registration practices are understood to vary significantly.

Source: European Health for All database (HFA-DB) [online database]. Copenhagen, WHO Regional Office for Europe, 2009 (http://www.euro.who.int/hfadb, accessed 27 May 2009).

Regular daily smokers in the population aged ≥ 15 (% of total)
Percentage of the population aged 15 years and above that regularly smokes each day, measured using a standard questionnaire during a health interview of a representative sample of this population. Many countries regularly carry out health interview surveys. The WHO Regional Office for Europe collects most of the data in HFA-DB from multiple sources. When only male and female values are available, the total is calculated as the average of the male and the female rates. More details on the sources may be available from the WHO Regional Office for Europe (http://data.euro.who.int/tobacco).
Source: European Health for All database (HFA-DB) [online database]. Copenhagen, WHO Regional Office for Europe, 2009 (http://www.euro.who.int/hfadb, accessed 27 May 2009).

Pure alcohol consumption (litres per capita)
Estimated amount of pure ethanol in spirits, wine, beer and other alcoholic drinks consumed per head in a country during a calendar year. It is calculated from official statistics on local production, sales, imports and exports, taking account of stocks and home production whenever possible. Pure alcohol is estimated at 4.5% in beer and 14% in wine. The WHO Regional Office for Europe calculates estimates on the basis of data collected mainly from three sources:

- publications on world drink trends formerly issued by Produktschap woor Gedistilleerde Dranken (Schiedam, Netherlands);
- the Food and Agriculture Organization of the United Nations (FAO); and
- WHO national counterparts.

Additional data are available in the specialized alcohol database maintained by the Regional Office (http://data.euro.who.int/alcohol/) and in the Global Information System on Alcohol and Health (http://apps.who.int/globalatlas/default.asp) maintained by WHO headquarters.
Source: European Health for All database (HFA-DB) [online database]. Copenhagen, WHO Regional Office for Europe, 2009 (http://www.euro.who.int/hfadb, accessed 27 May 2009).

Road traffic accidents involving alcohol (per 100 000)
Number of road traffic accidents involving one or more people under the influence of alcohol per 100 000 population. This includes accidents involving personal injury, but not those with only material damage. A road traffic accident is defined according to the Inland Transport Committee of the United Nations Economic Commission for Europe (UNECE). From 2002 onward, the data source is UNECE statistics on road traffic accidents in Europe.
Source: European Health for All database (HFA-DB) [online database]. Copenhagen, WHO Regional Office for Europe, 2009 (http://www.euro.who.int/hfadb, accessed 27 May 2009).

People killed or injured in road traffic accidents (per 100 000)
Number of people killed or injured in road traffic accidents per 100 000 population. See also the definition above. From 2002 onwards the data source is UNECE statistics on road traffic accidents in Europe.
Source: European Health for All database (HFA-DB) [online database]. Copenhagen, WHO Regional Office for Europe, 2009 (http://www.euro.who.int/hfadb, accessed 27 May 2009).

First admissions to drug treatment centres (per 100 000)
Number of people per 100 000 population who were admitted for the first time for treatment of conditions related to drug abuse during the calendar year.
Source: European Health for All database (HFA-DB) [online database]. Copenhagen, WHO Regional Office for Europe, 2009 (http://www.euro.who.int/hfadb, accessed 27 May 2009).

Table 5

Total health expenditure as % of GDP, WHO estimates
Sum of general government and of private expenditure on health. WHO produced the estimates for this indicator, basing them as much as possible on the national health accounts classification (see 2006 world health report (http://www.who.int/whr/2006/en) for details). The sources include both nationally reported data and estimates from international organizations – such as the International Monetary Fund (IMF), the World Bank, the United Nations and OECD – so they may differ from official national statistics reported by countries.
Source: European Health for All database (HFA-DB) [online database]. Copenhagen, WHO Regional Office for Europe, 2009 (http://www.euro.who.int/hfadb, accessed 27 May 2009).

Total health expenditure per capita (in international dollars (PPP)), WHO estimates
Sum of general government and of private expenditure on health, as expressed in international dollars (US$ PPP – see definition in discussion of GDP above). WHO produced the estimates for this indicator, basing them as much as possible on the national health accounts classification (see 2006 world health report (http://www.who.int/whr/2006/en) for details). The sources include both nationally reported data and estimates from international organizations – such as IMF, the World Bank, the United Nations and OECD – so they may differ from official national statistics reported by countries.
Source: European Health for All database (HFA-DB) [online database]. Copenhagen, WHO Regional Office for Europe, 2009 (http://www.euro.who.int/hfadb, accessed 27 May 2009).

General government health expenditure as % of total health expenditure
General government expenditure on health is the sum of outlays for health maintenance, restoration or enhancement paid for in cash or supplied in kind by government entities, such as the health ministry, other ministries, parastatal organizations or social security agencies (without double counting government transfers to social security and extrabudgetary funds). It includes transfer payments to households to offset medical care costs and extrabudgetary funds to finance health services and goods. The revenue base of these entities may comprise multiple sources, including external funds. Total expenditure on health includes funds mobilized by the system; it is the sum of general government expenditure on health and private expenditure on health.

WHO produced the estimates for this indicator, basing them as much as possible on the national health accounts classification (see 2006 world health report (http://www.who.int/whr/2006/en) for details). The sources include both nationally reported data and estimates from international organizations – such as IMF, the World Bank, the United Nations and OECD – so they may differ from official national statistics reported by countries.
Source: European Health for All database (HFA-DB) [online database]. Copenhagen, WHO Regional Office for Europe, 2009 (http://www.euro.who.int/hfadb, accessed 27 May 2009).

General government health expenditure as % of total government expenditure
General government expenditure is the consolidated outlays of all levels of government (central/federal, provincial/regional/state/district, municipal/local governments), social security institutions and extrabudgetary funds, including capital outlays. It is provided by the central bank/finance ministry to IMF or by the United Nations Statistics Department. General government expenditure on health is the sum of outlays for health maintenance, restoration or enhancement paid for in cash or supplied in kind by government entities, such as the health ministry, other ministries, parastatal organizations or social security agencies (without double counting government transfers to social security and extrabudgetary funds). It includes transfer payments to households to offset medical care costs and extrabudgetary funds to finance health services and goods. The revenue base of these entities may comprise multiple sources, including external funds.

WHO produced the estimates for this indicator, basing them as much as possible on the national health accounts classification (see 2006 world health report (http://www.who.int/whr/2006/en) for details). The sources include both nationally reported data and estimates from international organizations – such as IMF, the World Bank, the United Nations and OECD – so they may differ from official national statistics reported by countries.
Source: European Health for All database (HFA-DB) [online database]. Copenhagen, WHO Regional Office for Europe, 2009 (http://www.euro.who.int/hfadb, accessed 27 May 2009).

Children immunized with DTP3 (%)
Percentage of infants reaching their first birthday in a given calendar year who have been fully vaccinated against diphtheria with three doses of DPT (diphtheria–pertussis–tetanus) or DT (diphtheria–tetanus) vaccine. Data are reported annually to and are available from the WHO Regional Office for Europe.
Source: European Health for All database (HFA-DB) [online database]. Copenhagen, WHO Regional Office for Europe, 2009 (http://www.euro.who.int/hfadb, accessed 27 May 2009).

Children immunized against measles (%)
Percentage of children reaching their second birthday who have been fully vaccinated against measles (one dose). Data are reported annually to and are available from the WHO Regional Office for Europe.
Source: European Health for All database (HFA-DB) [online database]. Copenhagen, WHO Regional Office for Europe, 2009 (http://www.euro.who.int/hfadb, accessed 27 May 2009).

People receiving social or disability benefits (per 100 000)
This indicator is self-explanatory.
Source: European Health for All database (HFA-DB) [online database]. Copenhagen, WHO Regional Office for Europe, 2009 (http://www.euro.who.int/hfadb, accessed 27 May 2009).

TB under DOTS, cases detected (%)
Tuberculosis (TB) case detection means that TB is diagnosed in a patient and is reported within the national surveillance system, and then to WHO. The case detection rate under the DOTS strategy for TB control is calculated as the number of cases notified within areas covered by a DOTS programme divided by the estimated number of cases in the whole country, expressed as a percentage.

WHO estimates of TB incidence, prevalence and deaths are based on a consultative and analytical process; they are revised annually to reflect new information gathered through surveillance and from special studies, such as surveys of the prevalence of infection and

disease. For details of estimation methods, see the WHO headquarters web site (http://www.who.int/tb/publications/global_report/2006/methods/en/index.html).
Source: European Health for All database (HFA-DB) [online database]. Copenhagen, WHO Regional Office for Europe, 2009 (http://www.euro.who.int/hfadb, accessed 27 May 2009).

TB under DOTS, treatment success (%)
Treatment success in DOTS programmes is the percentage of new smear-positive patients that are cured (negative on sputum smear examination), plus the percentage that complete a course of treatment, without bacteriological confirmation of cure.

WHO estimates of TB incidence, prevalence and deaths are based on a consultative and analytical process; they are revised annually to reflect new information gathered through surveillance and from special studies, such as surveys of the prevalence of infection and disease. For details of estimation methods, see the WHO headquarters web site (http://www.who.int/tb/publications/global_report/2006/methods/en/index.html).
Source: European Health for All database (HFA-DB) [online database]. Copenhagen, WHO Regional Office for Europe, 2009 (http://www.euro.who.int/hfadb, accessed 27 May 2009).

Table 6

Physicians per 100 000
Number of physicians per 100 000 population.

In 2006, the following definition was harmonized with the Statistical Office of the European Communities (EUROSTAT) and OECD. Physicians (medical doctors) – as defined by the International Standard Classification of Occupations (ISCO) 88 (code 2221) – apply preventive and curative measures; improve or develop concepts, theories and operational methods; and conduct research in the area of medicine and health care. Practising physicians provide services directly to patients. Their tasks include: conducting medical examinations and making diagnoses; prescribing medication and giving treatment for diagnosed illnesses, disorders or injuries; giving specialized medical or surgical treatment for particular types of illnesses, disorders or injuries; and giving advice on and applying preventive medicine methods and treatments. The number of physicians at the end of the calendar year includes:

- people who have completed studies in medicine at university level (with an adequate diploma) and who are licensed to practice;
- interns and resident physicians (with an adequate diploma and providing services under supervision of other medical doctors during a postgraduate internship in a health care facility);
- salaried and self-employed physicians delivering services irrespective of the place of service provision; and
- foreign physicians licensed to practice and actively practising in the country.

The group excludes: students who have not yet graduated; dentists and stomatologists/dental surgeons; physicians working in administration, research and other posts that exclude direct contact with the patients; unemployed and retired physicians; and those working outside the country.
Source: European Health for All database (HFA-DB) [online database]. Copenhagen, WHO Regional Office for Europe, 2009 (http://www.euro.who.int/hfadb, accessed 27 May 2009).

General practitioners per 100 000
Number of general practitioners (GPs) per 100 000 population.

GPs, including assistant GPs, include only physicians (preferably as physical persons) working in outpatient establishments in specialties such as general practice and family, internal and general medicine. GPs do not limit their practice to certain disease categories, and assume the responsibility for providing or referring for the provision of continuing and comprehensive medical care. In most eastern European countries the general practitioner roughly corresponds to the "district therapeutist".
Source: European Health for All database (HFA-DB) [online database]. Copenhagen, WHO Regional Office for Europe, 2009 (http://www.euro.who.int/hfadb, accessed 27 May 2009).

Nurses per 100 000
Number of nurses per 100 000 population.

A nurse is a person who has completed a programme of basic nursing education and is qualified and authorized in her or his country to practise nursing in all settings for the promotion of health, prevention of illness, care of the sick and rehabilitation. Basic nursing education is a formally recognized programme of study (normally at least two years, including university level) that provides a broad and sound foundation for the practice of nursing and for postbasic education that develops specific competency.

As some countries have difficulties in separating statistics on midwives from the total number of nursing personnel, it is recommended that midwives be included in the broader category of nurses, but, whenever possible, statistics also be provided separately for midwives. In addition, including feldshers (physician's assistants – a category of health personnel working in some eastern European countries) under the broad category of nurses is proposed.

The number of nurses at the end of the calendar year includes only active nurses: those working in hospitals, primary health care, nursing homes, etc. The number of nurses includes: qualified nurses, first- and second-level nurses, feldshers, midwives and nurse specialists. It excludes: nursing auxiliaries and other personnel without formal education in nursing.
Source: European Health for All database (HFA-DB) [online database]. Copenhagen, WHO Regional Office for Europe, 2009 (http://www.euro.who.int/hfadb, accessed 27 May 2009).

Dentists per 100 000
Number of dentists per 100 000 population.

In 2006, the following definition was harmonized with EUROSTAT and OECD. Dentists – as defined by ISCO 88 (code 2222) – apply medical knowledge in the field of dentistry; improve or develop concepts, theories and operational methods; and conduct research. Dentistry is the provision of comprehensive care regarding the teeth and oral cavity, including prevention, diagnosis and treatment of aberrations and diseases. Practising dentists provide services directly to patients. Their tasks include: making diagnoses, advising on and giving necessary dental treatment and giving surgical, medical and other forms of treatment for particular types of dental and oral diseases and disorders. The number of dentists at the end of the calendar year includes:
- people who have completed studies in dentistry/stomatology at university level (granted an adequate diploma) and who are licensed to practise;

- interns (with an adequate diploma and providing services under supervision of other dentists or dental specialists during their postgraduate internship in a health care facility);
- salaried and self-employed dentists delivering services irrespective of the place of service provision; and
- foreign dentists licensed to practice and actively practising in the country.

It excludes: students who have not yet graduated; dentists working in administration, research and other posts that exclude direct contact with the patients; unemployed and retired dentists, and those working outside the country.
Source: European Health for All database (HFA-DB) [online database]. Copenhagen, WHO Regional Office for Europe, 2009 (http://www.euro.who.int/hfadb, accessed 27 May 2009).

Pharmacists per 100 000
Number of pharmacists per 100 000 population.

In 2006, the following definition was harmonized with EUROSTAT and OECD. Pharmacists as defined by ISCO 88 (code 2224) apply pharmaceutical concepts and theories by preparing and dispensing or selling medicaments and drugs. Practising pharmacists prepare, dispense or sell medicaments and drugs directly to patients (clients) and provide advice. Their tasks include:

- preparing and directing the preparation of medicaments according to prescriptions of medical and dental practitioners, or establishing formulae;
- checking prescriptions to ensure that recommended dosages are not exceeded and that instructions are understood by patients or other people administering medicaments, and advising on possible drug incompatibility; and
- dispensing medicaments and drugs in hospitals or selling them in pharmacies.

The number of pharmacists at the end of the calendar year includes: people who have completed studies in pharmacology at university level (granted an adequate diploma) and who are licensed to practice pharmacology; salaried and self-employed pharmacists delivering services irrespective of the place of service provision; and foreign pharmacists licensed to practise pharmacology and actively practising in the country. It excludes: students who have not yet graduated; pharmacists working in administration, research and other posts that exclude direct contact with the patients (clients); unemployed and retired pharmacists; and pharmacists working outside the country.
Source: European Health for All database (HFA-DB) [online database]. Copenhagen, WHO Regional Office for Europe, 2009 (http://www.euro.who.int/hfadb, accessed 27 May 2009).

Physicians graduated per 100 000
Number of students per 100 000 population graduated from university medical faculties or similar medical institutions in a given year. Only people eligible to practise as a physician are included. Dentists, pharmacists and graduates of public health faculties are excluded.
Source: European Health for All database (HFA-DB) [online database]. Copenhagen, WHO Regional Office for Europe, 2009 (http://www.euro.who.int/hfadb, accessed 27 May 2009).

Nurses graduated per 100 000
See above definitions.

Dentists graduated per 100 000
See above definitions.

Pharmacists graduated per 100 000
See above definitions.

Table 7

Hospitals per 100 000
Number of hospitals per 100 000 population. A hospital is a residential establishment equipped with inpatient facilities for twenty-four-hour medical and nursing care, and diagnosis, treatment and rehabilitation of the sick and injured, usually for both medical and surgical conditions, and staffed with professionally trained medical practitioners, including at least one physician. The hospital may but does not need to also provide services on an outpatient basis. The term hospitals includes general, specialized, acute care and long-stay hospitals, but not balneological institutes, health resorts, sanatoria, nursing homes for the physically and mentally disabled, homes for the elderly (that is, establishments providing principally custodial care), day centres and day hospitals.

Variations in interpreting the meaning of a nursing home are a major source of differences between countries in the content of data on hospitals. Whenever possible, a distinction is recommended to be made between institutions providing principally nursing care (nursing hospitals) and those providing principally custodial care (nursing homes). The former should be counted as hospitals, while the latter should not.
Source: European Health for All database (HFA-DB) [online database]. Copenhagen, WHO Regional Office for Europe, 2009 (http://www.euro.who.int/hfadb, accessed 27 May 2009).

Non-inpatient health care establishments per 100 000
Number of non-inpatient health care establishments per 100 000 population, including all health care establishments providing outpatient care – such as outpatient departments of hospitals, polyclinics, ambulatories, medical centres, medical aid posts, etc. – that are staffed with at least one health professional (physician or nurse). Establishments providing only dental care should be excluded.
Source: European Health for All database (HFA-DB) [online database]. Copenhagen, WHO Regional Office for Europe, 2009 (http://www.euro.who.int/hfadb, accessed 27 May 2009).

Hospital beds per 100 000
Number of hospital beds per 100 000 population. In 2006, the following definition was harmonized with EUROSTAT and OECD. Total hospital beds are all hospital beds that are regularly maintained and staffed and immediately available for the care of admitted patients. This includes: beds in all hospitals (including general hospitals (HP.1.1 in the System of Health Accounts (SHA) classification), mental health and substance abuse hospitals (HP.1.2), and other specialty hospitals (HP.1.3)), and both occupied and unoccupied beds. The term excludes: surgical tables, recovery trolleys, emergency stretchers, beds for same-day care, cots for healthy infants, beds in wards that were closed for any reason, provisional and temporary beds and beds in nursing and residential care facilities (HP.2).
Source: European Health for All database (HFA-DB) [online database]. Copenhagen, WHO Regional Office for Europe, 2009 (http://www.euro.who.int/hfadb, accessed 27 May 2009).

Acute care hospital beds per 100 000
Number of acute care hospital beds per 100 000 population. In 2006, the following definition was harmonized with EUROSTAT and OECD. Curative care (acute care) beds in hospitals (HP.1) are hospital beds that are available for curative care (HC.1 in the SHA classification, excluding psychiatry). This group includes beds accommodating patients where the principal clinical intent is to do one or more of the following: manage labour (obstetric), cure non-mental illness or provide definitive treatment of injury, perform surgery, relieve symptoms of non-mental illness or injury (excluding palliative care), reduce severity of non-mental illness or injury, protect against exacerbation and/or complication of non-mental illness and/or injury that could threaten life or normal functions, and perform diagnostic or therapeutic procedures. It excludes beds allocated for other functions of care (such as psychiatric care, rehabilitation, long-term care and palliative care), in mental health and substance abuse hospitals (HP.1.2), for rehabilitation (HC.2) and for palliative care.
Source: European Health for All database (HFA-DB) [online database]. Copenhagen, WHO Regional Office for Europe, 2009 (http://www.euro.who.int/hfadb, accessed 27 May 2009).

Psychiatric hospital beds per 100 000
Number of psychiatric hospital beds per 100 000 population. In 2006, the following definition was harmonized with EUROSTAT and OECD. Psychiatric care beds in hospitals (HP.1) are hospital beds accommodating patients with mental health problems (part of HC.1 in the SHA classification). This group includes: all beds in mental health and substance abuse hospitals (HP.1.2), and those in the psychiatric departments of general hospitals (HP.1.1) and specialty (other than mental health and substance abuse) hospitals (HP.1.3). It excludes beds allocated to non-mental curative care (part of HC.1) or long-term nursing care in hospitals (HC.3), and those for rehabilitation (HC.2) and palliative care.
Source: European Health for All database (HFA-DB) [online database]. Copenhagen, WHO Regional Office for Europe, 2009 (http://www.euro.who.int/hfadb, accessed 27 May 2009).

Nursing and elderly home beds per 100 000
Number of beds per 100 000 population in nursing homes for the physically and mentally disabled who need assistance in daily living activities on a continuing basis and in homes for the elderly: that is, establishments providing principally custodial care. While nursing and elderly homes are different types of establishment in many countries, to a large extent they provide similar services.
Source: European Health for All database (HFA-DB) [online database]. Copenhagen, WHO Regional Office for Europe, 2009 (http://www.euro.who.int/hfadb, accessed 27 May 2009).

Private inpatient hospital beds as % of all beds
Percentage of inpatient beds not owned by central or local government or social security establishments, including non-profit-making and profit-making private beds.
Source: European Health for All database (HFA-DB) [online database]. Copenhagen, WHO Regional Office for Europe, 2009 (http://www.euro.who.int/hfadb, accessed 27 May 2009).

Inpatient care admissions per 100
Number of admissions per 100 population. Admission is the hospitalization of a patient in an inpatient facility normally involving a stay of at least 24 hours. In the case of death or discharge to another health establishment, the actual stay may be shorter than 24 hours. These cases are registered as one-day hospitalizations. Discharge is the conclusion of a period of inpatient care, whether a patient returned to his or her home, was transferred to another

inpatient facility or died. The number of admissions/discharges excludes: a transfer from one department to another at the same hospital, day-cases of day patients, weekend leave (when a patient is released temporarily and the hospital bed is still reserved) and cases where hospital personnel provide treatment at patients' homes. Newborn babies are not included.
Source: European Health for All database (HFA-DB) [online database]. Copenhagen, WHO Regional Office for Europe, 2009 (http://www.euro.who.int/hfadb, accessed 27 May 2009).

Acute care hospital admissions per 100
The same as above, except that only short-stay hospitals are taken into account.
Source: European Health for All database (HFA-DB) [online database]. Copenhagen, WHO Regional Office for Europe, 2009 (http://www.euro.who.int/hfadb, accessed 27 May 2009).